The mathematical theory
of infectious diseases
and its applications

Books on cognate subjects

The advanced theory of statistics (3 vol.)
         SIR MAURICE KENDALL & ALAN STUART

Multivariate analysis   SIR MAURICE KENDALL

Time-Series   SIR MAURICE KENDALL

The analysis of multiple time-series*   M. H. QUENOUILLE

The estimation of animal abundance and related parameters
             G. A. F. SEBER

The linear hypothesis: a general theory*   G. A. F. SEBER

Stochastic point processes and their applications*   S. K. SRINIVASAN

The analysis of categorical data*   R. L. PLACKETT

Inequalities on distribution functions*   H. J. GODWIN

Statistical method in biological assay   D. J. FINNEY

The logit transformation: with special reference to its
   uses in bioassay*   W. D. ASHTON

An introduction to symbolic programming*   P. WEGNER

* A volume in "Griffin's Statistical Monographs and Courses"

Complete statistical catalogue available from Charles Griffin &
Co. Ltd

The Mathematical Theory of Infectious Diseases
and its Applications

Norman T. J. Bailey, M.A., D.Sc.

Unit of Health Statistical Methodology, World Health Organization,
Geneva. Formerly Professor of Biomathematics, Cornell University
Graduate School of Medical Sciences, and Member of
the Sloan-Kettering Institute for Cancer Research

Second edition

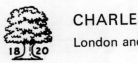

CHARLES GRIFFIN & COMPANY LTD

London and High Wycombe

CHARLES GRIFFIN & COMPANY LIMITED
Registered Office:
5A Crendon Street, High Wycombe, Bucks HP13 6LE

First published   1957
    (entitled *The mathematical theory of epidemics*)
Second edition   1975
ISBN: 0 85264 231 8

Set by E W C Wilkins Ltd, London & Northampton
Printed in Great Britain by Compton Printing Ltd, Aylesbury

... je souhaite seulement que dans une question qui regarde de si près le bien de l'humanité, on ne décide rien qu'avec toute la connoissance de cause qu'un peu d'analyse & de calcul peut fournir.

Daniel Bernoulli, 1760

Preface to the Second Edition

On the 30th April 1760 the Swiss mathematician Daniel Bernoulli (who was also a qualified physician) presented a paper to the Académie Royale des Sciences in Paris, in which, for the first time apparently, a mathematical model was used to study the population dynamics of an infectious disease. Bernoulli was specifically concerned with investigating the mortality caused by smallpox and with assessing the risks and advantages associated with preventive inoculation (or variolation), a controversial technique which, before the discovery of vaccination, was attracting increasing attention. In his mathematical discussion Bernoulli formulated and solved the relevant differential equations, and evaluated the results in terms of their bearing on the value of the control measure involved. Thus the theoretical work not only grew out of a real health problem, but the conclusions were all directly related to practical action.

This approach seems to me to be as valid now as it was in Bernoulli's day. Since that time over two centuries have elapsed, and we may well ask why progress has apparently been so slow, though an acceleration in new developments has been very evident in recent years. One explanation is that it was psychologically necessary to await the establishment of an unmistakable physical basis for the cause of infectious disease. This occurred in the second half of the 19th century, and undoubtedly laid the foundations for a thoroughgoing mathematical study of population phenomena. Preliminary investigations began to be elaborated in the opening years of the present century, when the whole climate of opinion about the understanding and possible control of medical and biological processes was undergoing a radical transformation. By the time the first edition of this book appeared in 1957 the total number of primarily mathematical references to the population theory of infectious disease was still only around 100. This figure had increased to approximately 200 by 1967, and to-day stands at about 500, the current rate of increase being faster than exponential.

The need for a revised edition of the original book is thus obvious, especially as there still seems to be no other broad survey of the relevant literature. In reflecting on the field covered, it appeared that the earlier title, *The Mathematical Theory of Epidemics,* was unduly restrictive. Even in the 1957 edition there were discussions of endemic phenomena, as well as of purely epidemic outbreaks. Moreover, the number of illustrative applications then available was very small, but this has greatly increased. Further, we now have the possibility of discussing a much wider range of mathematical techniques, as well as being able to investigate many additional important epidemiological factors.

Accordingly, it seems desirable to indicate the increase in scope in the title, for which *The Mathematical Theory of Infectious Diseases and its Applications* seems more suitable. The subject-matter includes epidemics, recurrent epidemics, endemics, spatial factors, carrier models, host-vector and parasitic disease models, multistate models, interference phenomena, immunization programs, and public health control. At the same time there have been many advances in mathematical treatments and techniques. Important developments have occurred in the handling of both deterministic and stochastic formulations. And the great strides made in recent years in computer technology have opened up quite new opportunities for parameter estimation and simulation studies.

Given the wealth of material now available, the task of presentation entails some obvious difficulties. First of all, a drastic selection of subject-matter is inevitable. And this in turn raises questions of how to choose contributions of the highest priority. Personal bias seems inescapable, but at least the rationale adopted should be expressed explicitly. I believe that the ultimate justification for the development of infectious disease theory lies in its ability to facilitate practical applications, and I have made special efforts to emphasize the latter. The book is accordingly now divided into three parts. The first part deals with matters of general orientation. The second part covers general theory, in so far as this tends to provide insight into the mechanisms underlying actual phenomena and to provide a technical basis for the investigation and control of specific diseases. Practical applications are reviewed in the third part, which includes a broad range of topics aimed at facilitating epidemiological understanding and public health control.

I am convinced that purely academic investigations are largely a waste of time, but that more applied mathematical work on infectious diseases could, if pursued with vigour and imagination, greatly help to alleviate and prevent at least some of the human suffering which exists at the present time on an astronomical scale.

I should like to express my indebtedness to the Publishers for persuading me to undertake the labour of preparing this second edition, which I should otherwise not have attempted. It is also a pleasure to acknowledge the support I have received from my friend and colleague, Dr Klaus Dietz, with whom I have had constant discussions over a number of years. Dr Dietz also read and commented on Chapter 17, though the responsibility for the final presentation is entirely mine. I should, in addition, like to thank all those authors who over a long period of time have been kind enough to send me pre-publication drafts of their papers, as well as subsequent reprints. It should be noted that several tables and figures included in the first edition, and there acknowledged, have also been incorporated in the present edition. For the inclusion of new material I must thank the Regents of the University of California for permission to reprint the diagrams in Fig. 9.1–9.4, which originally appeared in Vol. 4 of the

Fifth Berkeley Symposium on Mathematical Statistics and Probability, published by the University of California Press. Finally, I should like to take this opportunity of thanking Mrs Ruth Scott-Smith for her assistance with the preparation of the typescript.

NORMAN T. J. BAILEY

Geneva
May 1975

From Preface to the First Edition

It is just about fifty years ago that the mathematical theory of epidemics, in the modern sense of the phrase, was first started by the work of William Hamer and Ronald Ross. Considerable progress has since been made, and this has been accelerated in recent years by the availability of new mathematical methods of handling random processes. A great number of interesting and valuable results are widely scattered in the literature, but there appears to be no single text-book giving a systematic treatment of the whole field. The present volume attempts to meet this need. Some selection of the existing material has been inevitable, but the bibliography has been made as complete as possible so far as predominantly mathematical references are concerned.

This book is primarily intended for those who wish to learn more about the use of mathematical and statistical methods in understanding the mechanisms underlying the spread of infectious diseases. It is, however, by no means addressed exclusively to professional mathematicians and statisticians, although some sections rely fairly heavily on rather specialized techniques. The theories discussed should be of general interest to all those who are involved in any form of biometrical investigation. Moreover, many of the results obtained may well have considerable relevance to the work of general practitioners, epidemiologists and Medical Officers of Health, who are all concerned more with the practical implications of the theory than with its mode of derivation. Those who do not want to follow the mathematical arguments in detail should be able to learn enough for their purpose from the general discussions of the basic models used and of the consequences that flow from them.

The mathematical theory of epidemics appears at present to be developing fairly rapidly. If it is to continue in the future as a useful branch of applied mathematics then there must be adequate co-operation between mathematician and epidemiologist. The theory is only likely to have valuable applications in so far as it is developed in the context of a proper understanding of the epidemiological realities. Many of the models used in this book are of necessity over-simplified: nevertheless, useful results are already available. Future refinements should enable much further progress to be made.

I have greatly enjoyed writing this book on a subject which has fascinated me ever since Dr A. M. McFarlan first drew my attention to it at Cambridge in 1948. It is a pleasure therefore to acknowledge my indebtedness to Dr McFarlan for stimulating my interest and for many useful subsequent discussions. I have also derived great benefit from continued contacts with Dr R. E. Hope Simpson, of the Cirencester Public Health Laboratory, who has not only introduced me to many practical aspects of field epidemiology but has also very kindly allowed me to make use of much of his own excellent but unpublished data.

I am indebted to the editors of *Biometrika* and of the *Journal of the Royal Statistical Society,* Series B, for allowing me to draw freely on my own papers in these journals. In particular, the Biometrika Trustees have kindly permitted the reprinting of Fig. 4.1, 4.2, 5.1, 5.2 and 5.3, which originally appeared in two papers of mine in *Biometrika*; and, with the agreement of Dr P. Whittle, the use of Fig. 5.4, which is a redrawn version of a diagram he exhibited in the same journal.* I should also like to thank the University of California Press for permission to make considerable use of two excellent papers by Professor Bartlett and Mr D. G. Kendall in Vol. 4 of the *Third Berkeley Symposium on Mathematical Statistics and Probability.* The Appendix Tables were computed on EDSAC and are published here for the first time by permission of the Director of the University Mathematical Laboratory, Cambridge.

NORMAN T. J. BAILEY

Oxford,
August 1957

---

* These diagrams appear in the second edition with the numbers 5.1, 5.2, 6.1, 6.2, 6.3 and 6.4, respectively.

Contents

xiii

Part 1

Orientation

1

General introduction

The fearful toll of human life and happiness exacted through the ages by wide-spread disease and pestilence affords a spectacle that is both fascinating and repellent. A recital of the astronomical number of casualties suffered in this way by the human race is almost stupefying in its effect, and makes the consequences of all past wars seem almost trivial in comparison. Thus in Europe in the 14th century there were some 25 million deaths out of a population of perhaps 100 million from the Black Death alone. The death-rate in many places was even higher, whole towns and villages being virtually annihilated. In 1520 the Aztecs lost about half their population of $3\frac{1}{2}$ million from smallpox; the downfall of their empire in 1521 was due more to smallpox than to Cortes. It has been estimated that Russia suffered about 25 million cases of typhus in the years from 1918 to 1921 with a death-rate of approximately 10 percent. In the world pandemic of influenza in 1919 the total number of deaths is thought to have been in the region of 20 million over twelve months. Examples such as these could be multiplied *ad nauseam*.

Although the great scourges of history may now seem to be no more than unpleasant memories, there are no grounds for complaisant optimism. It is true that many previously widespread diseases are gradually disappearing from the modern world. Tuberculosis, for example, has steadily declined in prevalence, though the world total of active cases is still about 15 million. Smallpox, on the other hand, seems very close to virtual extinction. Nevertheless, there are many diseases, especially those of a parasitic nature, whose global prevalence continues to exist on a staggering scale.

Thus, over the centuries, malaria has been eradicated from many areas of the world where it was previously endemic, by the simple procedure of draining swamps and marshes. But there are still nearly 350 million people living in areas of the world where malaria is endemic, and where no organized anti-malaria programmes have yet been instituted. The probability is that very high proportions of these populations are seriously affected. Again, schistosomiasis is estimated to affect approximately 200 million people. The figure for

3

filariasis is in the neighbourhood of 250 millions, while the prevalence of hookworm disease is put at around 450 million. In spite of much progress in treating trachoma, the total number of people involved is of the order of 400–500 million.

This list is by no means complete. There are several other diseases, for each of which the victims may be counted in tens of millions, such as leprosy or onchocerciasis. One consequence of this is that, in the worst hit areas of the world, mainly in developing countries, a large number of people suffer from multiple infections by different serious diseases. The total load of human misery and suffering from communicable disease in the world today is incalculable, and presents a formidable challenge to public health authorities, epidemiologists, parasitologists, entomologists, biomathematicians, and any other experts whose skills may have some bearing on the problems involved.

There is in the modern world an additional risk which threatens developing and developed countries alike. It is therefore worth emphasizing what is no doubt already realized by certain government departments. Progress in understanding the nature of epidemic processes will not only assist the prevention of infectious disease, but will also increase the power and scope of the deliberately organized outbreaks contemplated by specialists in bacteriological warfare. As long as there remain in existence biological warfare laboratories whose purpose is to evolve new, unfamiliar and highly virulent organisms, against which mankind is by definition virtually unprotected, then there will continue to be serious danger not only from the deliberate use of the material for its intended wartime purpose but also from the accidental release of organisms through a failure of peacetime security. Although decisions to prosecute such researches must rest primarily with the community as a whole, or at least with its elected representatives, it is the duty of responsible scientists working in special fields to point out to the general public the risks, which are immense in this case, inherent in their activities.

Modern medicine can now do much to alleviate or cure many infectious diseases once they have been contracted, but by far the most spectacular results have been in the field of prevention. The elimination of poverty and hunger, and the provision of adequate social and public health measures such as quarantine, isolation of infectious cases, provision of clean water supplies, proper disposal of sewage, vaccination and inoculation, etc. have provided the main contributions to the fight against disease. Though in the more advanced communities many diseases once rampant have virtually disappeared, except perhaps for merely sporadic cases, others like influenza, infective hepatitis and the common cold, not only continue to defy prevention but still lack specific cures. And in many countries the once declining venereal diseases are again increasing. All methods of study are therefore welcome, whether clinical, biological, ecological or mathematical.

It is, of course, with the last of these approaches that this book is primarily concerned, though it should be emphasized straight away that such methods are not entirely independent of other disciplines. Thus clinical questions of diagnosis, prognosis and efficacy of treatment often depend on the statistical interpretation of appropriate data. Advice to patients and their immediate contacts is considerably influenced by current views as to when a patient is infectious and by what is known about variations in the incubation period. The cogency of many epidemiological arguments about, for instance, the possibility of virulence changing with time, or even the existence of infectiousness itself, may well depend on whether the effects apparently observed could in fact be due merely to non-significant chance fluctuations. Again, we may be interested in developing mathematical models because of the light they shed on some aspect of the biological mechanism at work, such as the life-cycle of the parasite involved. Alternatively, we can use these models to study the large-scale population phenomena of immediate relevance to any social and public health measures that might be advocated or undertaken. In particular, we want to know more about the transmission and spread of infectious disease, about trying to predict the course of an epidemic, and about the recognition of threshold densities of population which must be surpassed before a flare-up is likely.

In the context of endemic disease we require to know more about how the endemic level is related to factors which can be controlled by public health intervention. We need to develop models that will assist the decision-making process by helping to evaluate the consequences of choosing one of the alternative strategies available. Thus, mathematical models of the dynamics of a communicable disease can have a direct bearing on the choice of an immunization program, the optimal allocation of scarce resources, or the best combination of control or eradication techniques.

In all these matters mathematical and statistical investigations have an essential part to play. They originated in the rudimentary medical statistics of Graunt and Petty, who studied the London Bills of Mortality in the 17th century. In the latter half of the 18th century Daniel Bernoulli used a mathematical method to evaluate the effectiveness of the variolation technique against smallpox. But progress was slow, though the great sanitary revolution of the mid-19th century, followed by the rise of bacteriology in its second half, had by 1900 created the conditions required for further theoretical developments of the kind treated in this book. The growing availability of mortality statistics served to bring into sharper focus the problems facing public health authorities, while the new discoveries of bacteriology suggested suitable models for more exact mathematical investigation. Since the turn of the century there has been continued and accelerated progress in this field. Although it may never be possible to attain the kind of fine-drawn elaboration of theory now available in physics, the advancement already achieved by mathematical investigation in biological subjects such as evolution and genetics is extremely encouraging.

Most, but not quite all, of the earlier work on infectious disease from about 1900 to 1930 was essentially deterministic in character, that is, it did not take into account the probability aspects of the processes studied. These latter aspects can be of considerable importance in epidemic theory, even with large populations. The deficiency was beginning to be made good from about 1930 onwards by the idea of using chains of binomial distributions to represent successive crops of new cases. As a result of developments in the 1940's in the handling of stochastic processes further progress became possible. In subsequent years new ways have been found of dealing with the very variable phenomena that occur in practice. With small groups like individual families it is possible to obtain fairly homogeneous data from large numbers of such units. Analysis of epidemic patterns observed on the basis of specific mathematical models then permits both numerical estimation of parameters of epidemiological importance, such as chance of infection or length of incubation period, and statistical tests of how reliably hypothesis and observation agree. With large groups like whole communities the problems are more difficult, especially if we try to take account of spatial as well as temporal patterns of events; nevertheless, appreciable success has been achieved. The stochastic versions give much more satisfactory explanations than the older deterministic models of such observed phenomena as *undamped* epidemic waves in recurrent outbreaks, and critical community sizes for the existence of fade-out effects.

A wide range of models has now become available which can be adapted to a variety of different practical circumstances, depending on the disease involved, the community being studied, the kind of epidemiological or administrative questions being asked, etc.

The purpose of this book is to give a fairly wide coverage of the mathematical theory of the spread of infectious disease as it stands at present. Although purely mathematical points will be dealt with if they are essential to the main argument, or if they seem likely to be of use in future developments, the main emphasis will be on the biometrical, epidemiological, and public health aspects of the theory. Whereas some investigations are pursued in order to gain insight into the general character of epidemic processes, others are concerned with statistical methods of analysing specific kinds of observational data.

Those readers who are primarily mathematicians or statisticians should find little difficulty anywhere. At the same time it is hoped that much of the book will also be of interest and value to mathematically inclined biologists, epidemiologists, medical research workers and public health experts. Since these may not all wish to study the theory in detail, an attempt has been made in each chapter both to explain the general methods of investigation adopted and to make clear the practical consequences that follow. Where possible, worked examples are provided to facilitate applications by the reader to fresh data. This is particularly important where statistical estimation of parameters is involved and goodness-of-fit tests are to be performed. It is common nowadays for scientific workers who are not primarily mathematicians to acquire mastery of specific techniques like maximum-likelihood scoring. Since this latter procedure is frequently required in analysing actual data, full details are given of the appropriate scores and information functions wherever they are needed.

It should be noted, however, that the great advances made in recent years in the development of computerized methods often enable much of the labour of maximum-likelihood estimation to be bypassed. When a high-speed computer is accessible and suitable optimization programs are available, it will usually be far simpler and quicker to specify the likelihood as an explicit function, and then use the computer to find the parameter values that make the likelihood a maximum.

The new edition of this book presents the material covered in three main parts. Part 1 deals with general orientation, including the present introduction, a brief historical outline, a chapter on basic epidemiological principles, and a discussion of various methodological concepts. Under the latter heading are included such topics as the role of mathematical modelling, the effect of modern computer methods on estimation techniques and simulation, and the growing awareness of the importance of systems approaches to practical applications, especially those involving public health interventions.

Part 2 covers what may be called "general theory". This is primarily mathematical in content, with an emphasis on providing, hopefully, insight into epidemiological mechanisms and phenomena, as well as reviewing a number of investigatory techniques which may be of practical importance. Thus some of the topics of epidemiological relevance are: simple and general epidemics, recurrent epidemics and epidemicity, discrete-time models, spatial models, carrier models, and host—vector models. At the same time, special attention is given to deterministic and stochastic approaches, approximating systems, asymptotic methods, simulation studies, estimation procedures, model modification and development, etc. The last chapter of Part 2 is devoted to a review of the practical implications of the general theory.

In Part 3 we deal primarily with specific applications, utilizing, where possible, data on individual diseases. The broad topics covered are the detection of infectiousness, use of chain-binomial models (measles), the measurement of latent, infectious and incubation periods (measles, infectious hepatitis, small-pox), simple multistate models (tuberculosis, tetanus, typhoid, cholera), parasitic diseases (malaria, schistosomiasis), interference models (chickenpox/yaws, polio viruses), geographical spread (influenza), immunization programs (small-pox), and public health control. The diseases just mentioned in parentheses are some of those to which applications have been made in recent years. It is evident that since the first edition of this book in 1957, considerable advances have occurred in the direction of harnessing the mathematical theory of epidemics to the urgent needs of the world, first in achieving a better understanding of the underlying mechanisms of both epidemic and endemic phenomena, and secondly in helping to develop improved methods of control.

Nevertheless, an enormous amount of developmental work is required. We should resist any inclination to concentrate on matters of purely academic mathematical interest, and should subordinate theoretical investigations to those areas where fresh insight could have practical consequences. When one considers the huge number and variety of infectious diseases that afflict mankind, and how relatively little mathematical work has so far been undertaken in respect of most of them, it is clear that there is a vast field of research available to those who have the interest and ability to tackle these problems. The writer believes that mathematical investigations of the type described in this book have, if pursued in close cooperation with clinical and epidemiological research workers, and with public health authorities, a unique contribution to make to the alleviation and prevention of untold human misery.

2

Historical outline

In this chapter it is proposed to give a short historical account of the development of mathematical theories of the spread of epidemic diseases. It is hoped
that this will enable the detailed mathematical discussions appearing later to be
seen in perspective, and that a broad view will facilitate the choice of problems
for further research. Some readers may prefer to go straight on to the mathematics and return to this chapter later. There is no reason why this should not
be done, though the remaining chapters should probably be taken in the order
in which they appear, except perhaps by those readers who are to some extent
already acquainted with the subject.

2.1 The beginnings

Recorded accounts of epidemic outbreaks and speculation as to possible
causes go back at least as far as the ancient Greeks, e.g. the *Epidemics* of
Hippocrates (459–377 B.C.), but genuine progress in epidemiology was hardly
forthcoming until the 19th century. The spectacular rise of bacteriological
science in the second half of that century, due to the researches of Pasteur
(1822–95) and Koch (1843–1910), was perhaps the outstanding feature of
the commencement of modern scientific achievement in this field. Nevertheless,
some progress had already been made on a less fundamental level in the statistical appraisal of records showing the incidence and locality of known cases
of disease. Indeed, men like John Graunt (1620–74) and William Petty (1623–
87) had in the 17th century paid considerable attention to the London Bills
of Mortality. Their work may be taken to mark the beginning of vital and
medical statistics and the understanding of large-scale phenomena connected
with disease and mortality, but the time was not yet ripe for anything approach-
ing a connected theory of epidemics. In the first place, the requisite mathematical techniques were themselves only then in process of development, and
in the second place there were no sufficiently precise hypotheses about the
spread of disease suitable for expression in mathematical terms. Although a
good start was being made in the field of physics, particularly mechanics and

astronomy, nearly 200 years passed before any real progress was achieved in the biological sphere. It is true that as early as 1546 Fracastorius had postulated a living principle of contagion, which could be spread from person to person. And in 1760 Daniel Bernoulli used a mathematical method to evaluate the effectiveness of the technique of variolation against smallpox, with a view to influencing public health policy. However, it was not until an unmistakable physical basis for the cause of infectious disease had been established in the second half of the 19th century that the stage was set for the development of adequate mathematical theories of large-scale phenomena, as opposed to purely empirical descriptions.

Even before the fundamental advances in the new science of bacteriology, extremely valuable work was going on in the field of what we now call social medicine. By studying the temporal and spatial pattern of cholera cases, John Snow showed in 1855 that the disease was being spread by the contamination of water supplies. In particular there was the celebrated affair of the Broad Street Pump. Later, in 1873, William Budd established a similar manner of spread for typhoid. Parallel to these detailed investigations were the broader studies of statistical returns made by William Farr (1840), who hoped to discover empirical laws underlying the waxing and waning of epidemic outbreaks. These attempts and their later developments are described in the next section.

2.2   Curve fitting and prediction

Apart from the highly successful *ad hoc* studies made by men like Snow and Budd, we have the more deliberate investigation of pooled statistical returns by Farr. His work was very much in the spirit of Graunt and Petty, but was mathematically more sophisticated. In the *Second Report of the Registrar-General of England and Wales,* Farr (1840) effectively fitted a normal curve to smoothed quarterly data on deaths from smallpox, assuming the constancy of "second ratios" of successive pairs of frequencies. Later, in 1866 (letter to London *Daily News,* 17th February, quoted by Brownlee, 1915b), he attempted to use a similar method, based this time on the constancy of third ratios, to predict the course of an outbreak of rinderpest amongst cattle. The curve was fitted to four rising successive monthly totals and extrapolated values used for prediction. Although observed and predicted curves were both bell-shaped, agreement in detail was not very good. Similar curve-fitting methods used by Evans (1875) on the smallpox outbreak of 1871–2 also met with little real success.

More intensive studies of the same type were later undertaken by Brownlee (1906), who fitted various Pearson curves to epidemic data on many diseases occurring at different times and places. Further investigations of this type were reported in a series of papers (Brownlee, 1909 to 1918). These were all largely of an empirical nature, although to some extent related to the current ideas of Hamer (1906), mentioned in the next section, which involved the use of a specific *a priori* model. Such methods, if successful, would be extremely useful to public health authorities, but they have now been largely abandoned because of their intrinsic inaccuracy. All the same, we may still hope that the development of alternative lines of investigation will eventually permit some kind of predictions to be made, even if these should be more or less vague probability statements.

2.3 Deterministic models

By the end of the 19th century the general mechanism of epidemic spread, as revealed by bacteriological research, and the long familiarity with epidemiological data together made possible developments of a new kind. Hamer (1906) considered that the course of an epidemic must depend *inter alia* on the number of susceptibles and the contact-rate between susceptibles and infectious individuals. The simple mathematical assumptions used by Hamer are basic to all subsequent deterministic theories, and indeed appear in probability versions as well, in suitably modified form. Moreover, by using these ideas in a simple way, Hamer could deduce the existence of periodic recurrences. This was taken up again later by Soper (1929), as mentioned below.

In the meantime Ross (1911 and later) was working with a more structured mathematical model taking into account a whole set of basic parameters describing various aspects of the transmission of malaria. He also developed a more general theory which he called "*a priori* pathometry". It is important to notice that although Ross employed the idea of chance or probability in formulating his basic equations, these were actually still deterministic in character. This means that, for such a model, the future state of the epidemic process can be determined precisely when we are given the initial numbers of susceptibles and infectious individuals, together with the attack-, recovery-, birth- and death-rates. For the first time it was possible to use a well-organized mathematical theory as a genuine research tool in epidemiology. Deductions from the theory, possibly unforeseen and unexpected, could now be tested out in practice.

More elaborate mathematical studies of the same general type were later undertaken by Kermack and McKendrick (1927 to 1939). A greater degree of generality was introduced, including variable rates of infection, recovery, etc. These authors also considered the problem of endemic disease and related their findings (see also McKendrick, 1940) to experimental mouse epidemics. The most outstanding result obtained was, however, the celebrated Threshold Theorem, according to which the introduction of infectious cases into a community of susceptibles would not give rise to an epidemic outbreak if the density of susceptibles were below a certain critical value. If, on the other hand, the critical value were exceeded, then there would be an epidemic of magnitude sufficient to reduce the density of susceptibles as far below the threshold as it originally was above.

Further deterministic work specifically associated with measles was carried out by Soper (1929). Although his basic relationship was written as a difference equation, it was in essence very similar to the differential equations of other writers. The most important result here was the discovery that the basic assumptions entailed, so far as recurrent epidemics were concerned, a *damped* train of harmonic waves. Published data on measles, however, while exhibiting a marked oscillation in incidence from year to year, show no tendency to damping. Soper believed, wrongly, that allowance for an incubation period would remove the damping. It is the essential failure of such deterministic models to square with the facts that has led to their abandonment in many quarters and consequent replacement by corresponding probability, or stochastic, representations.

2.4   Stochastic models

As epidemiological data became more extensive and on occasion dealt with much smaller groups that those relevant to returns for large areas, the elements of chance and variation became ever more prominent. This was specially evident when small family or household groups were contemplated. The need for some kind of probability model was becoming increasingly necessary.

McKendrick (1926) was apparently the first to publish a genuinely stochastic treatment of an epidemic process. Whereas in deterministic models one takes the actual *number* of new cases in a short interval of time to be proportional to the numbers of both susceptibles and infectious cases, as well as to the length of the interval, McKendrick assumed that the *probability* of one new case in a short interval was proportional to the same quantity. This is a "continuous-infection" model and entails an individual being himself infectious from the instant he receives infection until the moment he dies, recovers, or is isolated. In the paper quoted, examples were given of probability distributions for the total number of cases in a household when infection was introduced from outside. This brilliant pioneering effort did not unfortunately attract much attention, and similar models were not again investigated until twenty years later. No doubt the absence of satisfactory methods of handling such models had much to do with this lapse, and it is curious to reflect that McKendrick himself subsequently embarked, with Kermack, on the series of deterministic investigations already mentioned.

An alternative probability treatment by Greenwood (1931) appearing five years later did, however, establish itself. Moreover, similar work was independently in progress in the United States, where in 1928 Lowell J. Reed and Wade Hampton Frost were already using the same kind of ideas in lectures and discussions (see Wilson and Burke, 1942; Abbey, 1952). This model assumed that the period of infectiousness was comparatively short and that the latent and incubation periods could be regarded as approximately constant. Starting with a single case in a closed group (or several simultaneously infectious cases), new cases would then occur in a series of stages or generations. We should, under suitable conditions, expect the cases occurring at any stage to have a binomial distribution depending on the numbers of susceptibles and infectious individuals present at the previous stage. We should thus have a chain of binomial distributions.

Greenwood's treatment is fully stochastic in the sense that once the probability element has been introduced, via the chance of contact adequate for an infectious person to transmit disease to a susceptible, it is retained all through the discussion. This allows one to calculate both the frequencies with which various types of chain appear and the distribution of total number of cases per household. The theoretical analyses of Reed and Frost seem to have been mainly deterministic, though in teaching they illustrated the probabilistic nature of epidemic processes by use of a mechanical model.

2.5 Developments during 1940–1957

It has been thought preferable to consider all developments after about 1940, and in particular after World War II, under a single heading, and not to separate sharply the deterministic and stochastic treatments. This is more in keeping with the modern approach which tends to regard deterministic treatments as approximately valid in certain circumstances, and at any rate worth examining first in any given situation. We then pass on to more precise (and usually mathematically more difficult) stochastic formulations, paying special attention to any striking features suggested by the deterministic model.

To some extent previous trends were continued. Thus deterministic discussions were carried further by a series of papers by Wilson (1945, 1947); Wilson and Burke (1942, 1943); Wilson and Worcester (1941a to 1945f) and D. G. Kendall (1956). Chain-binomial theory was extended by Greenwood (1946, 1949) and Bailey (1953b), and a re-examination of the Reed–Frost version with various extensions was undertaken by Abbey (1952).

Some of the most important developments followed from advances made in the early 1940's in the mathematical handling of stochastic processes. A renewed impetus was therefore given to study of the "continuous-infection" model originally introduced by McKendrick. Thus Bartlett (1946, 1949) developed a partial differential equation for the probability-generating function of two variables, which were the numbers of susceptibles and infectious persons at any instant. Several detailed results were then obtained by Bailey (1950, 1953a), both for this general case and the simpler one involving no removal. An interesting advance was the derivation by Whittle (1955) of a stochastic threshold theorem, in which a set of probability statements replaced the rigidly specified alternatives of Kermack and McKendrick's result.

Similar methods have also been highly successful in dealing with the problem of recurrent epidemics, especially in respect of the prominent position occupied by measles. As mentioned above, deterministic models of the Hamer–Soper type always involve appreciable damping of the epidemic waves, but this does not appear to be in agreement with observation. Subsequent work by Bartlett (1953, 1956, 1957) showed that if we adopt a stochastic model in the situation when recurrent epidemics may be expected then a much more realistic picture is obtained. Although no strict periodicity results, *undamped* outbreaks tend to be repeated at intervals having a certain probability distribution. In sufficiently small communities complete fade-out of infection may occur if fresh cases are not introduced, whereas in communities above a certain critical size it will merely happen that infection reaches a low level before building up again for a fresh outbreak. It is interesting to note that these conclusions are in broad agreement both with observed data and with the results of empirical investigations using Monte Carlo methods in conjunction with an electronic computer. This latter approach has also been used to study the behaviour of epidemic processes extended in space as well as time.

The continuous-infection model, which has generally been used for convenience in investigating large-scale phenomena, may in some cases be quite suitable for analysing household data. When dealing with this latter kind of material there is naturally more opportunity for testing the appropriateness of the mathematical model adopted. Thus with measles we find that chain-binomials are a better approximation to the truth than the continuous-infection model. Nevertheless, the picture is still far from satisfactory if we take the time-intervals between successive cases into account. Bailey (1956a,b) therefore attempted to develop a more elaborate model which involved a variable latent period after the receipt of infection followed by an extended infectious period when the disease can be transmitted to other susceptibles. The infectious period is supposed to be effectively terminated by the appearance of symptoms and consequent isolation of the patient. The development of such methods, entailing the estimation of parameters in appropriately chosen models followed by goodness-of-fit tests, clearly has an important bearing on elucidating the biological nature of epidemic processes.

2.6 Trends since 1957

It is convenient to describe further progress since 1957 in a separate section. That was the year of publication of the first edition of this book. The total number of references to mathematical work in the literature was at that time round about 100. Ten years later, an additional list of about the same size appeared in the review paper by Dietz (1967), bringing the total to approximately 200. Today, after the elapse of another eight years, the total is around 500. This is appreciably faster than exponential growth, and the breadth and variety of the coverage is now very extensive.

To review such a wealth of new material in a succinct manner would be very difficult, while to try to do justice to all individual authors would be impossible. However, it seems to the writer that the main trends of recent

years are as set out below, leaving the reader to fill in the details from the
more extensive coverage of the whole field in Parts 2 and 3.

To begin with, there have been several purely mathematical developments
in the treatment of the simple stochastic epidemic. A more closed expression
for the probability-generating function has been found by Bailey (1963), and
various approximations to the epidemic curve have been evolved by Williams
(1965a). A number of perturbation and diffusion approximations to the
moment-generating function have also been worked out by Bailey (1968), Weiss
(1970, 1971), and McNeil (1972). In addition, some departures from homogeneous mixing have been studied by Becker (1968), Severo (1969a,c), Kryscio
and Severo (1969), Kryscio (1972a), and McNeil (1972). Parameter-estimation
has been facilitated by the construction of algorithmic methods of computing
likelihoods by Severo (1967a) and Hill and Severo (1969).

The general stochastic epidemic has also come in for several new results.
More insight into the structure of the state probabilities has been provided by
the approaches of Gani (1965a, 1967), Siskind (1965), and Lynne Billard
(1973). The age-distribution of infectives has been studied by Sakino (1959,
1962c, 1963, 1967). Improved computational methods are supplied by the
algorithmic techniques of Severo (1967, 1969c). Improvements in obtaining
the distribution of total epidemic size have been given by Gani (1967) and
Williams (1970, 1971). The latter work leads directly to a new proof of the
Threshold Theorem. Branching process formulations have been looked at by
Bharucha-Reid (1958). An approximating stochastic system has been studied
by Ludwig (1973a); and a variety of new asymptotic approximations have
been derived by Violet Cane (1966), Daniels (1967, 1971), Downton (1967a),
Ridler-Rowe (1967), Nagaev and Startsev (1968, 1970), and Nagaev (1970,
1971). The theory of parameter estimation has been extended by Sally Ohlsen
(1964), Morgan (1965), and Bailey and Thomas (1971). Finally, a variety of
model modifications and extensions have also been developed. Thus Watson
(1972) has worked on the problem of several groups, and Severo (1969a) has
discussed generalizations of the mixing-rate. Small stochastic epidemics in large
populations were examined by Bailey (1964b) and Morgan (1964). Models
involving the direct removal of susceptibles have been studied by Sakino and
Hayashi (1959), and Sakino (1962b). A new departure was made by the investigation of problems dealing with the cost of epidemics, due to Becker (1970a),
Jerwood (1971), Gani (1973), Gani and Jerwood (1972), and Downton
(1972a,b).

In the area of recurrent epidemics and endemicity, previous work by Bartlett
was extended (Bartlett, 1957, 1960a,b,c, 1961, 1964, 1966, 1973), including
both analytical work and simulation studies, with special reference to the interpretation of real public health measles data. Ridler-Rowe (1967) has proved
some asymptotic results.

Previous to 1957, discrete-time models of chain-binomial type had been

subject to extensive statistical investigations, but no general theory existed.
This defect has begun to be remedied with the work of Gani (1969), and Gani
and Jerwood (1971), while approximating processes, valid when the changing
number of susceptibles can be neglected, have been studied by Bartoszyński
(1967, 1969, 1972). Ludwig has shown how chain-binomial models can legitimately be used to investigate certain more general models, provided that
attention is restricted to the final size of epidemic. Some asymptotic results
based on linearized stochastic equations have been given by Bartlett (1960a,c),
and have special relevance to the use of discrete-time analogues of continuous-
time processes in computerized simulation studies.

Some advances have been made in the solution of problems involving a
spatial distribution of individuals. Thus, detailed mathematical studies of
deterministic epidemics, largely in populations distributed along a line, have
been undertaken by D. G. Kendall (1965) and Mollison (1970, 1972a,b).
Approximating spatial systems ignoring the changing number of susceptibles
have been investigated by Neyman and Scott (1964); Bartoszyński, Łoś and
Wycech-Łoś (1965); and Bartoszyński (1969). Some results for a specialized
process over the positive quadrant of a square lattice were obtained by Morgan
and Welsh (1965). This approach was subsequently generalized by Hammersley
and Welsh (1965), and Hammersley (1966), in the format of percolation theory.
Computerized simulation studies of both simple and general epidemics over a
square lattice were carried out by Bailey (1967a). Finally, the simulation work
of Williams and Bjerknes (1971, 1972) on the growth of tumour cells in two
dimensions should be mentioned, because of the close analogy with two-
dimensional epidemic spread.

Another area which has received considerable attention in recent years is
that of models involving carriers, starting with the deterministic and stochastic
models of Weiss (1965). These were further developed by Dietz (1966) and
Downton (1967b). The case of time-dependent parameters was studied by
Dietz (1967) and the introduction of new carriers and susceptibles from outside
the population was incorporated in the model by Dietz and Downton (1968).
Downton (1968) also considered the creation of new carriers by cross-infection
from within the population, and a further analysis was made by Gillian Denton
(1972). Further work by Dietz (1969) dealt with a model having the immigration of susceptibles and the creation of new carriers by a birth process. A more
general model still was analysed by Becker (1970b). A large-population approximation was made by Pettigrew and Weiss (1967), involving both clinically
recognizable infectives and subclinically infected carriers, and a multigroup
model allowing for variations in susceptibility and infectiousness was investigated by Becker (1973).

The last area of general theory, as opposed to specific applications, is that
of host—vector and venereal disease models. Bartlett (1964, 1966) has extended
a simple version of the stochastic Threshold Theorem to the host and vector

situation, and Griffiths (1972a, 1973a) has investigated the properties of small stochastic epidemics in large populations using branching process representations in addition to the ordinary continuous-time theory.

The foregoing advances have all been of a primarily theoretical nature, although having in many cases an obvious relevance to practical problems. However, it is encouraging to be able to record a growing volume of applications that are more immediately related to epidemiological and public health needs.

First, in the attempt to test for the existence of infectious factors the pioneer work of Knox (1959, 1963a,b,c, 1964a,b, 1965) on space-time interactions triggered off a number of further investigations by Barton, David and Merrington (1965); Mustacchi, David and Fix (1965); Barton and David (1966); Barton, David, Fix, Merrington and Mustacchi (1967); Pike and Smith (1968); and Abe (1973). Other forms of epidemiologically significant clustering were examined by Ederer, Myers and Mantel (1964); Mustacchi (1965); Mantel (1967); and Larsen, Holmes and Heath (1973).

There have been relatively few new developments in chain-binomial modelling, but the modified models involving variable latent periods and extended infectious periods have been cast in a convenient computerized form by Bailey and Alff-Steinberger (1970) and applied to infectious hepatitis data. The model has also been used to evaluate family data on influenza by Owada, Sakamoto and Tanaka (1971).

A considerable amount of effort has been devoted in recent years to the elaboration of deterministic multistate models which attempt to be more realistic than the models so far investigated by purely mathematical methods. This epidemiological realism is usually paid for by mathematical intractability. Nevertheless, the use of computerized simulations has been extremely valuable in elucidating the properties of such models and in shedding light on proposed control strategies. Extensive studies of this type have been made in tuberculosis by Waaler, Geser and Andersen (1962); Brøgger (1967); Mahler and Piot (1966a,b); ReVelle (1967); ReVelle, Lynn and Feldmann (1967); Lynn and ReVelle (1968); Waaler (1968a,b); Waaler and Piot (1969, 1970); ReVelle and Male (1970); and Feldstein, Piot and Sundaresan (1973).

Similar applications have also been utilized for a number of other bacterial diseases, such as typhoid fever, tetanus and cholera, in the works of Cvjetanović, Grab and Uemura (1971); Cvjetanović, Grab, Uemura and Bytchenko (1972); Cvjetanović, Uemura, Grab and Sundaresan (1973); and Sundaresan, Grab, Uemura and Cvjetanović (1974).

Several potentially useful developments have been taking place in the vitally important sphere of parasitic disease. First, there is the now classical work of Macdonald (1957), posthumously collected together in Macdonald (1973). Field applications to malaria are described in Macdonald, Cuellar and Foll (1968). A new approach to the modelling of actual field data, taking account of the development of immunity in humans and the enormous seasonal variations occurring in mosquito populations, was undertaken by Dietz (1971) who used a primarily deterministic approach. An improved and modified model is described by Dietz, Molineaux and Thomas (1974), which involves a simpler immunity structure and contains explicit allowance for superinfection. This model was used to estimate parameters from field data and carry out statistical goodness-of-fit tests.

Secondly, there is a growing literature on the modelling of schistosomiasis (bilharziasis). Preliminary biometrical investigations were carried out by Hairston (1962, 1965a,b) and Macdonald (1965a). Sexual mating functions have been dealt with by Leyton (1968), and stochastic models for age prevalence curves by Linhart (1968). The population dynamics of the parasites have been looked at stochastically by Tallis and Leyton (1969), and deterministically by Goffman and Warren (1970). In addition, there have been some highly intricate developments by Nåsell (1972), and Nåsell and Hirsch (1971, 1972, 1973a,b), which could nevertheless be of considerable practical importance.

Another area of some public health consequence is the interference and interaction phenomena that may occur between different disease organisms. There is, for example, the work of Gart (1968, 1971, 1972) on yaws and chickenpox; while Lila Elveback (1964 and onwards) and her co-workers have developed a series of six fundamental models of increasing complexity that can be used for the study by computerized simulations of the public health control of poliomyelitis by means of live polio vaccine, including the situation where the effect of the vaccine is inhibited by enterovirus infections. The chief references are Elveback, Fox and Varma (1964); Elveback and Varma (1965); Elveback, Ackerman, Young and Fox (1968); Elveback, Ackerman, Gatewood and Fox (1971); Elveback (1971); Ewy (1971); Gatewood, Ackerman, Ewy, Elveback and Fox (1971); and Ewy, Ackerman, Gatewood, Elveback and Fox (1972).

Although in relatively small communities some form of homogeneous mixing can be assumed, this is impossible for widely dispersed populations. A certain amount of theoretical work has been done on multigroup models, but the first practical applications have been made in the USSR to predicting the spread of influenza. These models, originating with the work of Baroyan and Rvachev (1967), describe deterministically the spread of influenza between major cities in the USSR. Within any given city the transmission of disease is described in terms of restricted homogeneous mixing, but contacts between cities are represented on a migration basis, the latter being derived empirically from real transportation data. Several writers have contributed to the subsequent development of these concepts, notably Rvachev (1968b); Baroyan and Rvachev (1968); Baroyan, Genchikov, Rvachev and Shashkov (1969); Baroyan, Basilevsky, Ermakov, Frank, Rvachev and Shashkov (1970); Baroyan, Rvachev, Basilevksy, Ermakov, Frank, Rvachev and Shashkov (1971); and Rvachev (1971, 1972). It is of considerable interest to learn that verifiable predictions were obtained from a computerized analysis. Two additional papers by Rvachev (1967, 1968a) relate infectious processes in the organism to epidemic structure.

As the possibilities for epidemiological applications have increased in scope, so the implications for public health intervention and control have received more explicit attention. Thus the design of optimal immunization programs, especially in relation to the prevention of smallpox by vaccination, has been discussed by Becker (1972). More and more emphasis has been placed on the use of formal control theory methods by a series of writers, including Taylor (1968); Jacquette (1970); Sanders (1971); Gupta and Rink (1971); Gupta (1972); Abakuks (1973); Gupta and Rink (1973); Hethcote and Waltman (1973); and Morton and Wickwire (1974). The extent to which such sophisticated control-theoretic approaches can be assimilated to actual decision-making processes is a matter which is of considerable practical importance and which needs a good deal of further investigation.

3

Epidemiological principles

In this chapter it is proposed to give a short account of the main epidemiological concepts that appear to be of importance in discussing mathematical models of the order of complexity used in this book. For biologically more detailed accounts, especially those dealing with clinical and medical aspects, the reader should consult some of the many excellent textbooks available. It is, however, worth mentioning here a few comparatively non-technical books, such as the monumental history by Creighton (1965), or the very readable general expositions of Greenwood (1935), Pickles (1939), Geddes Smith (1943), Winslow (1943), Hare (1954), and Burnet and White (1972). The special coverage of parasitic diseases by Lapage (1963) is also useful. These should help the non-medical reader to obtain a clearer picture of the general behaviour of epidemic and endemic diseases in groups of individuals. For more quantitative discussions, Peller (1967) is worth consulting. In many fields of biological science it is possible to pursue the statistical theory of macroscopic processes more or less independently of the "fine structure" involved. To a great extent this is also true of the general mathematical theory of infectious disease spread, but in special applications, particularly where features like incubation periods and the occurrence of clinical symptoms are concerned, or the complicated processes of parasitic diseases are involved, more attention has to be paid to the biological details.

We are concerned in this book only with diseases that are infectious in the sense of being capable of transmission at some stage in the life-cycle of the appropriate organism from an infected host to an uninfected susceptible, with or without the agency of an intermediate insect or animal vector. There is much variation in the literature in the precise meaning attached to such terms as "infectious", "infective" and "contagious". Attention should also be drawn to the fact that, in American as opposed to English usage, "contagious" is often employed instead of "infectious". Again, the term "communicable disease" is very widely used nowadays in a similar context.

We shall now turn to an account of the salient features of the biological process underlying the spread of many infectious diseases. A regular cycle of events is involved and it is immaterial at what point we start the description. Suppose we consider an individual who has been exposed to infection, i.e. who has received infectious material by some means such as direct physical contact with an infectious person, breathing in infectious organisms, or eating contaminated food, etc. It may be that the individual concerned is resistant to a greater or lesser degree, according to the extent to which his own biological and biochemical defences can deal with the incoming organisms. This resistance or *immunity* may or may not have been acquired in response to previous exposure. On the other hand, the invading organisms may gain a foothold and proceed to embark on their usual course of development. In general we envisage the elapse of a *latent period* during which this development takes place purely internally, without the emission of any kind of infectious material. When the latent period ends, the infected person is in a position to communicate infectious organisms to other susceptibles, who in their turn become the scene of similar events. We shall call an actively infectious individual an *infective*, and the period during which organisms are discharged, the *infectious period*. At some stage in the individual's history of infection recognizable symptoms will occur. With acute infections this is commonly a signal for isolating the case from the community until he dies or recovers. If symptoms occur before the infectious period commences, adequate isolation will arrest the spread of disease. It is therefore presumably more common for symptoms to occur some time after the onset of infectiousness. If they occur during the infectious period, the relevant period of time for the transmission of disease is from the end of the latent period to removal from circulation, since we can usually ignore the small chance of further contacts after isolation. On the other hand, symptoms may not occur until after the infectious period is over. In this case there will be little direct evidence as to the latter's length and time of occurrence.

The time elapsing between the receipt of infection and the appearance of symptoms is normally called the *incubation period*, and the period from the observation of symptoms in one case to the observation of symptoms in a second case directly infected from the first is the *serial interval* (see Hope Simpson, 1948, for further discussion of various terms used). Thus the serial interval is the observable epidemiological unit, and it reflects to some extent the life cycle of the infectious organism. Nevertheless, it cannot be readily related to the mechanism of transfer, and for this some breakdown of the incubation period, such as that suggested above, seems to be required. When symptoms occur either during or immediately after the end of the infectious period, the incubation period is exactly equal to the sum of the latent period and the part of the infectious period during which the patient is still a danger to others.

In a very sophisticated mathematical treatment we should attempt to use the joint probability distribution for the lengths of latent and infectious periods and the time, measured from a suitable point, to the appearance of symptoms. Since this degree of generality presents formidable difficulties, most biometrical investigations undertaken so far have adopted various simplifying assumptions. Thus in the chain-binomial models of Reed, Frost and Greenwood the infectious period is contracted to a point, while the latent period is regarded as approximately constant. In the modification developed by Bailey the latent period has a roughly normal frequency distribution and the infectious period is extended in time, but of constant length. Again, the continuous-infection model of McKendrick and Bartlett entails a zero latent period and a negative exponential distribution for the infectious period. Various concessions of this sort have to be made to mathematical tractability, but with a suitably chosen model it is often possible to retain what seem to be the most important features of the mode of transmission of the disease in question.

Whether or not an infective actually communicates his disease to susceptibles in his vicinity is plainly a matter of chance. The magnitude of this chance may depend on the virulence of the organisms, the extent to which they are discharged, the natural resistance of the susceptibles, the degree of the latter's proximity to the infective, and so on. In the simple chain-binomial model all this is subsumed under the single concept of "adequate contact". It is supposed, for the group of individuals concerned, that at any given instant there is a certain chance of contact between any two individuals sufficient for the transmission of disease if one is an infective and one a susceptible. When there are several infectives in a group, a given susceptible will remain free of disease only if he happens to escape adequate contact with any of them.

With continuous-infection models a suitable analogous assumption is that the chance of *one* new case in a very short interval of time is jointly proportional to the length of the interval, the number of susceptibles and the number of infectives. Such ideas readily lead to mathematical equations describing the whole process. So far as possible we try to use probability models leading to specifications of the joint probability distribution of susceptibles and infectives at any instant. In spite of the mathematical difficulties of stochastic treatments, one can hardly avoid them for dealing with small groups, where large statistical fluctuations are likely to occur. When groups are sufficiently large, however, we can try to make use of deterministic approximations, but some caution is needed in doing this.

Models based on the foregoing assumptions usually imply that in the community considered all susceptibles and infectives mix together homogeneously. As a first approximation this is most nearly realized in small household groups, but is clearly at variance with the observed facts of social behaviour in a large town. The consequences of this limitation have not yet been fully explored, but the difficulty should always be borne in mind when one is trying to deal with processes in large communities.

One or two problems connected with immunity are also worth mentioning in this survey of the epidemiological features most relevant to present mathematical theory. In the first place it is common knowledge that some diseases, e.g. measles, usually confer life-long immunity from further attack. If records are available of all previous attacks of such a disease suffered by the individuals in a community, then we can reasonably assume that the unattacked represent the whole group of susceptibles. In practice, however, we may have to rely on general information and patients' own reports. It is possible therefore that immunizing attacks may have been forgotten. Similarly, the immunity thought to have been acquired by a previous history of disease may have been lost. Such complications can be allowed for in the mathematical analysis of household data, provided there are sufficient data of the right kind.

More difficult is the question of *carriers*. These are individuals who, although apparently healthy themselves, harbour infection which can be transmitted to others. For any disease in which carriers are at all common, appreciable modification of existing methods of analysing household data would be required. The treatment of large populations is also affected, but some general theory is now available. The trouble with a disease like poliomyelitis is that carriers far outnumber overt cases, so very few examples of multiple infection in households are available. The present types of analysis seem therefore to be rather uninformative.

We have so far in this chapter been thinking mainly in terms of case-to-case transmission of disease, though we have not actually excluded the possibility that infection might also be derived indirectly through contaminated food or liquids, rather than directly by contact with an infective. An important departure from this comparatively simple picture occurs with diseases like malaria that involve an intermediate host, or *vector*. The parasite responsible for this type of infection is obliged to spend part of its life-cycle inhabiting the vector, so that the normal path of transmission is from man, in his infectious phase, to vector, and subsequently from vector back to man. There are therefore two populations, each with its own set of susceptibles and infectives. Further biological details, essential to the modelling of malaria, are described in Chapter 17. In general, parasitic diseases are liable to be very complicated and to require individual attention.

The above outline contains the main epidemiological characteristics that have so far been considered for inclusion in mathematical models. Many important factors in infectious disease do not lead directly to macroscopic phenomena in relative isolation from other factors. We cannot subsequently expect to disentangle all aspects by purely statistical methods. Nevertheless, the judicious use of the types of inquiry described in this book should shed light on some factors, and should therefore, especially in concert with other methods of investigation, be able to contribute to epidemiological advances as well as to public health control.

4
Methodological aspects

Before embarking on the detailed mathematical discussions, to which the remainder of this book is devoted, it may be worth considering briefly a number of methodological aspects, concentrating more on the general philosophical implications, rather than on looking at technical details.

To begin with, it seems probable that most readers will feel that the use of mathematical theory in the attempt to describe, understand, and control epidemic or endemic disease requires no special justification. In some form or other, such theory is simply a normal adjunct of the scientific method. However, questions do arise as to what kind of mathematical work is worth undertaking, what is most likely to have fruitful applications to practical epidemiological and public health problems, or what may provide general insight into the basic mechanisms of epidemic spread. Of course, there are no hard-and-fast answers to such questions; it all depends on personal inclinations and points of view. Some mathematicians may prefer to concentrate on abstract discussions that exhibit great formal elegance and logical rigour. It is the personal conviction of the writer that such activities are not only largely a waste of time, but can be positively harmful by diverting mathematical skill away from more applied work that could be of positive benefit to mankind. A decision has therefore been made to discuss in Part 2 of this book a range of general theoretical investigations which have some bearing on practical issues, and to face in Part 3 the problems confronting epidemiologists and public health authorities when specific diseases have to be dealt with. The lessons to be learned from the general theory of Part 2 are reviewed in Chapter 12.

Given that some form of quantitative modelling is called for, one of the first questions to be answered is the choice between a deterministic or a stochastic approach. In the first flush of excitement over the development of new methods of handling stochastic processes in the 1940's and 1950's the mathematician's first choice was always to go for stochastic modelling, since it was more interesting; and in any case there were plenty of examples, such as the analysis of family data, for which deterministic models would be virtually meaningless. Nowadays a somewhat more balanced judgement is possible. When numbers of susceptibles and infectives are both large and mixing is reasonably homogeneous, a deterministic treatment is likely to be fairly satisfactory as a first approximation, though even here it may be difficult to account for large-scale phenomena, like the regularly observed recurrent outbreaks of measles, without recourse to some form of probability analysis.

Again, valuable work has been done in the modelling of tuberculosis and malaria, for example, using purely deterministic methods. And in the case of malaria it has proved possible to proceed to the stage of parameter estimation and goodness-of-fit testing in relation to actual field data. On the other hand, the investigation of fine-structure models involving latent periods and infectious periods with a view to estimating relevant parameters seems inevitably to entail the stochastic analysis of data drawn from relatively small groups.

In fact, of course, the type of modelling that is suitable and valid depends on circumstances. But we must not forget that though practical requirements often seem to determine a particular, possibly quite simple, approach, the validity of this approach may have to be established by a good deal of careful mathematical investigation or computer simulation, and the complexities of these necessary validations may considerably exceed those of the original formulations.

The above general comments on modelling are naturally not confined to the study of epidemics, but apply to the scientific analysis of any phenomena which involve appreciable statistical variation when sufficiently small units are investigated, but which tend to show more regular behaviour when averaging occurs over large numbers of units.

It goes almost without saying that the kind of modelling activities that can be undertaken also depend very critically on the computing facilities that are available. Thus, if the results of mathematical investigations can be put into simple closed forms, perhaps utilizing extensively tabulated higher mathematical functions, the computational work required to exhibit conclusions in numerical terms can often be performed on now old-fashioned desk machines with the minimum of effort.

However, one of the most laborious jobs the biometrician is called upon to do is the efficient estimation of several parameters in a model for which no explicit formulae for maximum-likelihood estimates are available. The use of a maximum-likelihood scoring technique is, of course, well known, and is used extensively in this book where the statistical analysis of actual data is described. Even so, the amount of work entailed can be almost prohibitively high, as with the estimation of latent and infectious periods for the model described in Chapter 15, when the maximum-likelihood scores and information functions all have complicated formulae and several iterations may be required to reach stability.

This kind of calculation has been revolutionized in recent years by the availability of computerized optimization programs. All we have to do in general is to write down a single formula for the overall likelihood, and use the optimization program to compute the parameter values which make the likelihood a maximum. A well-designed program will produce all the relevant standard errors as well, quite automatically. The computational time can sometimes be reduced from weeks to minutes in complicated examples (see Section 15.7). Such methods also work well for even more complex situations in which a single formula for the likelihood is not available, though an algorithm for calculating it can be specified (e.g. Section 6.8).

It would have been possible to rewrite all the maximum-likelihood scoring applications appearing in the first edition in the new format. But this would have been a disadvantage for those who did not have immediate access to a computerized optimization procedure, and who were prepared to carry out the calculations required on a desk machine.

Moreover, it is possible that yet another computational revolution is taking place. The advent of cheap *electronic* desk and pocket computers is causing many people to do in their own offices what they previously requested from sophisticated computing services. Indeed, the latter are often so hamstrung by technical complications and administrative delays, that the direct use of cheap and simple electronic equipment is highly attractive. In some circumstances, therefore, one might prefer to return to the earlier well-tried methods of maximum-likelihood scoring because they could be effected quite expeditiously and independently of bureaucratic complications.

Similar considerations also apply to the use of computerized simulations. Many full-scale simulation runs inevitably need the resources of a large computer, but the development work may be better carried out on a smaller machine, especially the programmable type of electronic desk computer that will operate in an interactive mode. Thus the type of computing facilities available may influence quite strongly the structure of the models themselves and the uses to which they can be put.

This leads on quite naturally to the consideration of yet another kind of modelling activity that has received increasing emphasis in recent years, namely the approach of system dynamics. When one confines attention to the now more or less classical modelling of single infectious diseases, no new principles are involved. Of course, new mathematical methods may be evolved or new ways of handling computer analysis may be devised, and this would increase the efficiency of the approach. However, with a growing awareness of the practical need for applications to public health decision-making, has come the realization that, in many developing countries, not only may there be several serious interacting diseases to be dealt with, but that the influence of many other factors such as health manpower, education, economics, agriculture, water resources, population growth, etc., must also be taken into account.

Multidisease models have as yet hardly been considered, though some interfacing with optimal-resource allocation modelling has been developed (see Chapter 16), and a start has been made on the investigation of disease prevention and control programs (Chapters 20 and 21). All this leads into the field which is the proper object of systems studies and policy analysis. The methodological implication for the kind of epidemiological modelling that we are primarily concerned with is that more emphasis should be placed on models that have some reasonable chance of being incorporated into a wider qualitative analysis directly geared to administrative and political decision-making. While such a development is at present very much in its infancy, this looks like being a major requirement in the near future. It follows that epidemic theory should certainly continue to search for new insights into the mechanisms of the population dynamics of infectious diseases, especially those of high priority in the world today, but that increased attention should be paid to formulating applied models that are sufficiently realistic to contribute directly to broad programs of intervention and control.

Part 2

General Theory

5

Simple epidemics

5.1 General notions

We shall first look at the simplest type of epidemic model in which infection spreads by contact between the members of a community, but in which there is no removal from circulation by death, recovery, or isolation. Ultimately, therefore, all susceptibles become infected. Although these assumptions are rather oversimplified for most practical purposes, they would in fact be approximately applicable to the sort of situation where (a) the disease was highly infectious but not sufficiently serious for cases to be withdrawn by death or isolation, and (b) no infective became clear of infection during the main part of the epidemic. This might well be the case for some of the milder infections of the upper respiratory tract, for example.

Any mathematical picture of the behaviour of an epidemic that attempts to be at all realistic in detail, e.g. specifying the number of new cases that will occur in a given short interval of time, must inevitably involve the use of probability concepts. When dealing with large numbers of both susceptibles and infectives we should expect the effect of statistical fluctuations on large-scale phenomena to be much reduced. In such circumstances it is not unreasonable to use as a first approximation a deterministic model, in which we assume that, for given numbers of susceptibles and infectives, and for a given attack-rate, certain definite numbers of new infectives will occur in any specified time. Although when the numbers of susceptibles and infectives are not both large it is unwise to press deterministic analyses very far, it is certainly worth while devoting some attention to them. We shall gain some insight into the mechanism of large-scale phenomena, and the results obtained will suggest various features worth examining more carefully when we come on to stochastic models. In the latter, probability distributions of the numbers of susceptibles or infectives occurring at any instant replace the point-values of deterministic treatments.

In general, the form of behaviour predicted by a stochastic model is likely to be very similar to that entailed by the corresponding deterministic version

31

when the numbers of susceptibles and infectives are both sufficiently large, but in other situations there may be important differences. Moreover, there is good reason to suppose that the assumption of homogeneous mixing is likely to be approximately valid for epidemics in only comparatively small groups. In such groups the probability element is of considerable importance, and we are accordingly obliged to take it into account. This is especially true if we investigate groups as small as individual households where statistical fluctuations may be very large. Even if we are mainly interested only in mean values we still require probability treatments. For although with some processes stochastic means are identical with the corresponding deterministic values, this is not in general true of epidemic processes.

Published epidemiological records often simply tell us the number of fresh notifications of disease each day or week. In fact we can use the concept of the *epidemic curve*, defined by the rate at which new cases are recognized, i.e. the rate of change with respect to time of the total number of removals. This curve (or, more accurately, the graph obtained by integrating it over units of one day or week, as the case may be) is the one we should naturally use to compare theory with observation. The corresponding stochastic analogue is the curve of the rate of change with respect to time of the stochastic mean of the total number of removals. When working with simple epidemics having no removal, it is convenient to define the epidemic curve in terms of the total number of cases instead of the total number of removals. Examination of actual data reveals *observed* epidemic curves that are at first sight unexpectedly smooth if we bear in mind the inherent statistical variation. However, it appears likely on reflection that this is due to the partial ironing out of fluctuations, both by summation over finite periods of time, e.g. in quoting so many new cases per day or week, and by summation over several relatively independent epidemics occurring simultaneously in distinct subgroups of the whole population.

With regard to the last point, it is well known that epidemics in a large population can often be broken down into smaller epidemics occurring in separate regional subdivisions. These smaller epidemics are in general not in phase but interact with each other to some extent. We could scarcely assume even a small town to be a single homogeneously mixing unit. Each individual is normally in close contact with only a small number of individuals, perhaps of order 10–50. The observed figures are therefore pooled data for several epidemics occurring simultaneously in small groups of associates. In reality such groups overlap and interact, but we can try using the concept of an *effective* number of independent groups, say k. The sort of model we have in mind is thus one involving k independent groups each of size n. For a set of small simple epidemics all approximately in phase, the coefficient of variation of the total number of infectives at any instant will be $k^{-\frac{1}{2}}$ times the coefficient of variation of any single group. As k increases, we therefore expect the curve for total number of infectives to approach in shape the curve of the stochastic mean for a group of size n. Similarly we should expect the overall epidemic curve to approach the curve for the rate of change with respect to time of the stochastic mean. This argument should give a rough method of comparing theory with observation, but there is in general considerable computational difficulty in deriving the required curves. Moreover, the assumption that the sub-epidemics are approximately in phase may often be rather unrealistic.

Apart from the attempt to obtain close correspondence between a theoretical model and actual processes, there is also the possibility of gaining insight into the mechanism of large-scale phenomena by studying simplified models having the right general characteristics.

So far as simple epidemics with no removal are concerned, the deterministic theory is relatively straightforward and is largely covered in Section 5.2. On the other hand, the simple stochastic epidemic, apparently first mentioned explicitly by Bartlett (1949), rapidly leads to complicated mathematical analysis. This is presumably due to the nonlinear character of the transition probabilities. Nevertheless, many mathematically interesting results are available, and an extensive literature has developed on this model alone. Sections 5.3 to 5.10 are devoted to an outline of the more tractable stochastic investigations.

It should be remembered, however, that the simple epidemic models are in general very oversimplified. Still, it is reasonable to deal with simpler problems first, in the expectation that the knowledge gained will prove to be capable of extension to more complicated, but more realistic, models in due course. This expectation is sometimes justified, but not as often as one might hope.

5.2 Deterministic model

In the simplest deterministic formulation we suppose that we have a homogeneously mixing group of individuals of total size $n + 1$, and that the epidemic is started off at time $t = 0$ by just one individual becoming infectious, the remaining n individuals all being susceptible, but as yet uninfected. In general, at time t, let us write x and y, regarded here as essentially continuous, for the numbers of susceptibles and infectives, respectively, so that $x + y = n + 1$. We next suppose, in accordance with the ideas already discussed, that the rate of occurrence of new infections is proportional to both the number of infectives and the number of susceptibles. Thus the actual number of new infections in the time-interval Δt can then be written as $\beta x y \Delta t$, where β is the infection-rate (or contact-rate). It follows that

$$\Delta x = -\beta x y \Delta t,$$

so that the process is described by the differential equation

$$\frac{dx}{dt} = -\beta x y = -\beta x(n - x + 1).$$

If we change the time-scale to $\tau = \beta t$, the basic differential equation becomes dimensionless so far as β is concerned. We thus have

$$\frac{dx}{d\tau} = -x(n-x+1), \tag{5.1}$$

with initial condition

$$x = n, \quad \tau = 0. \tag{5.2}$$

The solution of (5.1), subject to (5.2), is

$$x = \frac{n(n+1)}{n + e^{(n+1)\tau}}. \tag{5.3}$$

This implies that the number of infectives at time τ is

$$y = n - x + 1 = \frac{(n+1)e^{(n+1)\tau}}{n + e^{(n+1)\tau}}$$

$$= \frac{n+1}{1 + ne^{-(n+1)\tau}}. \tag{5.4}$$

We note in passing that the expression in (5.4) is one form of the well-known logistic function.

In practice we are often more interested in the *epidemic curve*, which gives the rate at which new infections accrue, i.e. $dy/d\tau = -dx/d\tau$. Calling this rate w, we see that

$$w = -\frac{dx}{d\tau} = xy = \frac{n(n+1)^2 \, e^{(n+1)\tau}}{\{n + e^{(n+1)\tau}\}^2}. \tag{5.5}$$

This epidemic curve attains its maximum when $\tau = (\log n)/(n+1)$. At this point $x = y = \frac{1}{2}(n+1)$, and $w = \frac{1}{4}(n+1)^2$. The function $w(\tau)$ is evidently symmetrical about the maximum ordinate.

Epidemic curves given by (5.5) are plotted for $n = 10$ and $n = 20$ in Fig. 5.1 and 5.2, where they are compared with the corresponding stochastic epidemic curves obtained in Section 5.5. It can be seen that both types of curves have their maxima in about the same place, but that the stochastic curves are asymmetrical and fall away more slowly.

There is no difficulty in generalizing the foregoing deterministic treatment to deal with an epidemic started by several infectious individuals. If the number of the latter is a, and if there are still n susceptibles to start with, we can readily obtain the more general version of (5.1) as

$$\frac{dx}{d\tau} = -x(n-x+a), \tag{5.6}$$

with initial condition, as before in (5.2),

$$x = n, \quad \tau = 0. \tag{5.7}$$

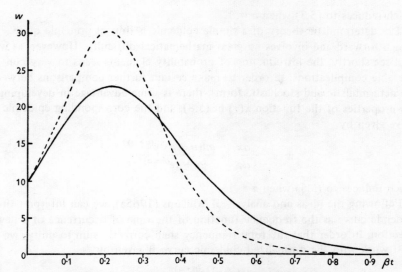

Fig. 5.1 Comparison of deterministic and stochastic epidemic curves for n = 10.
----- deterministic curve; ——— stochastic curve

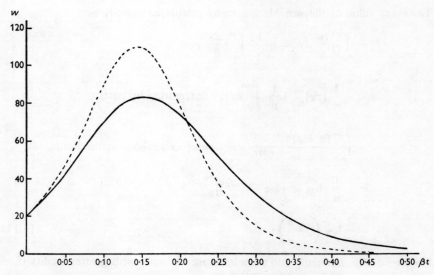

Fig. 5.2 Comparison of deterministic and stochastic epidemic curves for n = 20.
----- deterministic curve; ——— stochastic curve

The solution of (5.6) subject to (5.7) is

$$x = \frac{n(n+a)}{n + ae^{(n+a)\tau}},$$ (5.8)

which reduces to (5.3) when $a = 1$.

The deterministic theory of a simple epidemic is thus in principle quite straightforward and involves no great mathematical difficulty. However, as we shall see shortly, the introduction of probability elements leads to very considerable complications. In order to make certain further comparisons between the deterministic and stochastic forms, there is some advantage in developing the properties of the function $x(\tau)$ in (5.8), and the corresponding epidemic curve given by

$$w = -\frac{dx}{d\tau} = \frac{an(n+a)^2 e^{(n+a)\tau}}{\{n + ae^{(n+a)\tau}\}^2},$$
(5.9)

which reduces to (5.5) when $a = 1$.

Following the ideas and analysis of Williams (1965a), we can interpret the epidemic curve as the frequency function of the time of occurrence of a new infection. In order that the total frequency shall correctly sum to unity, we must work with the normalized epidemic curve W given by

$$W = \frac{w}{n} = \frac{a(n+a)^2 e^{(n+a)\tau}}{\{n + ae^{(n+a)\tau}\}^2}, \quad 0 \leqslant \tau < \infty.$$
(5.10)

The mean value of the variable τ is easily calculated directly as

$$\bar{\tau} = \int_0^\infty \frac{\tau w}{n} d\tau = -\frac{1}{n} \int_0^\infty \tau \frac{dx}{d\tau} d\tau$$

$$= -\frac{1}{n} [\tau x]_0^\infty + \frac{1}{n} \int_0^\infty x d\tau, \quad \text{integrating by parts,}$$

$$= \int_0^\infty \frac{(n+a)e^{-(n+a)\tau}}{a + ne^{-(n+a)\tau}} d\tau, \quad \text{since } \tau x \text{ vanishes at the limits,}$$

$$= -\frac{1}{n} \left[\log \{a + ne^{-(n+a)\tau}\} \right]_0^\infty$$

$$= \frac{1}{n} \log \left(1 + \frac{n}{a}\right).$$
(5.11)

More generally, moments and cumulants are obtained with greater facility if we transform τ to the variable T given by

$$T = (n+a)\tau - \log(n/a).$$
(5.12)

The frequency function in (5.10) can now be written as

$$f(T) = \left(1 + \frac{a}{n}\right) \frac{e^T}{(1 + e^T)^2}, \quad \log\left(\frac{a}{n}\right) \leqslant T < \infty.$$
(5.13)

The dominant behaviour as $n \to \infty$ and a remains finite is therefore represented by

$$f(T) = \tfrac{1}{4} \operatorname{sech}^2 T, \quad -\infty < T < \infty. \tag{5.14}$$

The moment-generating function of this distribution is

$$
\begin{aligned}
M(\theta) &= \int_{-\infty}^{\infty} \frac{e^{\theta T} e^T dT}{(1 + e^T)^2} \\
&= \int_0^1 x^{-\theta}(1-x)^\theta \, dx, \quad \text{putting } x = (1 + e^T)^{-1}, \\
&= B(1 - \theta, 1 + \theta) \\
&= \Gamma(1 - \theta) \, \Gamma(1 + \theta), \tag{5.15}
\end{aligned}
$$

and the cumulant-generating function is

$$K(\theta) = \log \Gamma(1 - \theta) + \log \Gamma(1 + \theta). \tag{5.16}$$

To obtain the cumulants of T we use the standard result, e.g. Erdélyi (1953, vol. 1, p. 45),

$$\log \Gamma(1 + \theta) = -\gamma\theta + \sum_{j=2}^{\infty} \frac{(-)^j}{j} \zeta(j)\theta^j, \tag{5.17}$$

where $\zeta(\nu)$ is Riemann's zeta-function. Substitution in (5.16) shows that

$$K(\theta) = \sum_{\nu=1}^{\infty} \frac{1}{\nu} \zeta(2\nu)\theta^{2\nu}, \tag{5.18}$$

where all odd powers of θ have vanished as expected, since $f(T)$ in (5.14) is clearly symmetrical about $T = 0$. The coefficient $\kappa_{2\nu}$ of $\theta^{2\nu}/(2\nu)!$ is thus

$$\kappa_{2\nu} = 2(2\nu - 1)! \, \zeta(2\nu). \tag{5.19}$$

In particular, the variance $\sigma^2 = \kappa_2 = \frac{\pi^2}{3}$, and the fourth cumulant $\kappa_4 = \frac{2\pi^4}{15}$. It follows that the usual measure of kurtosis is $\gamma_2 = \kappa_4/\kappa_2^2 = \frac{6}{5}$. The curve is leptokurtic, in agreement with its exponential tails. We may also note from (5.11) that $\bar{\tau} \to 0$ as $n \to \infty$, so that a consequence of homogeneous mixing is that the epidemic sweeps more rapidly through the population as n increases. However, this assumes a constant infection-rate. In fact, for large n we have $\bar{t} \sim (\log n)/\beta n$, since $\tau = \beta t$. To retain a biologically acceptable model we might make further assumptions about the limiting behaviour of β. Alternatively, modifications might be made in the basic model, as suggested by McNeil (1972). This proposal is discussed further in Section 5.10 below. See also the limitations introduced in Chapters 11, 16 and 17.

Finally, it is convenient to establish a partial differential equation for the moment-generating function of the proportion of susceptibles in the population given by

$$\xi = \frac{x}{n+a}. \tag{5.20}$$

This is of little importance in itself since we are here dealing with a deterministic process. But it will be useful to refer to later, when the equation obtained will be seen as the limiting form of its stochastic analogue.

Let us go back to (5.6) and (5.7), use the transformation in (5.20), and change the time-scale to $T = (n + a)\tau$. We quickly find

$$\frac{d\xi}{dT} = -\xi(1 - \xi), \tag{5.21}$$

with initial condition

$$\xi = \frac{n}{n+a}, \quad T = 0, \tag{5.22}$$

for which the solution is

$$\xi(T) = \frac{1}{1 + \gamma e^T}, \tag{5.23}$$

where

$$\gamma = a/n. \tag{5.24}$$

The moment-generating function of ξ at time T is simply $e^{\theta\xi}$, so that we can write

$$M_d(\theta, T) = e^{\xi\theta} = \exp\left(\frac{\theta}{1 + \gamma e^T}\right), \tag{5.25}$$

in which the suffix d on the left refers to "deterministic". It immediately follows from (5.25) that

$$\frac{\partial M_d}{\partial T} = \theta e^{\xi\theta} \frac{d\xi}{dT}, \quad \frac{\partial M_d}{\partial \theta} = \xi e^{\xi\theta}, \quad \frac{\partial^2 M_d}{\partial \theta^2} = \xi^2 e^{\xi\theta}. \tag{5.26}$$

Now multiplying (5.21) by $\theta e^{\xi\theta}$ and using (5.26) yields the required partial differential equation

$$\frac{\partial M_d}{\partial T} = \theta \left(\frac{\partial^2 M_d}{\partial \theta^2} - \frac{\partial M_d}{\partial \theta}\right), \tag{5.27}$$

with initial condition

$$M_d(\theta, 0) = e^{\theta/(1+\gamma)}. \tag{5.28}$$

5.3   Stochastic model

Let us now consider the simplest probability version of the deterministic model developed in the previous section. As before, we shall assume a homogeneously mixing group of $n + 1$ individuals, and suppose for simplicity that the epidemic starts at time $t = 0$ with one infective and n susceptibles. This time we must use random variables $X(t)$ and $Y(t)$ to represent the numbers of susceptibles and infectives, respectively, at time t, where $X(t) + Y(t) = n + 1$. Let us now consider contacts that are sufficient to transmit infection from an infective to a susceptible. Then the chance of a contact between any two *specified* individuals in an interval Δt is $\beta \Delta t + o(\Delta t)$, where β is the contact-rate. We shall assume β to be constant, but see Yang and Chiang (1972) for an investigation involving a time-dependent contact-rate $\beta(t)$. It follows that the chance of one new infection in the whole group in Δt is $\beta XY \Delta t$ to order Δt. It is convenient, as before, to change the time-scale to $\tau = \beta t$, so that the chance of $X(\tau)$ decreasing by one unit in Δt is $X(n - X + 1)\Delta \tau$ to order $\Delta \tau$. Thus the expression $X(n - X + 1)\Delta \tau$, for the probability of one new infection in $\Delta \tau$ in the stochastic model, is closely analogous to the expression $x(n - x + 1)\Delta \tau$, for the exact number of new infections in $\Delta \tau$ in the deterministic version.

We now write $p_r(\tau)$ for the probability that there are still r susceptibles remaining uninfected at time τ. It is easily seen that the probability of r susceptibles remaining at time $\tau + \Delta \tau$ can be expressed as

$$p_r(\tau + \Delta \tau) = (r + 1)(n - r)\Delta \tau p_{r+1}(\tau) + \{1 - r(n - r + 1)\Delta \tau\}p_r(\tau),$$

$$(5.29)$$

since there must have been either $r + 1$ susceptibles at τ followed by a new infection with probability $(r + 1)(n - r)\Delta \tau$, or r susceptibles at τ followed by no infection with probability $1 - r(n - r + 1)\Delta \tau$. Equation (5.29) immediately yields the system of state equations

$$\left. \begin{aligned} \frac{dp_r}{d\tau} &= (r + 1)(n - r)p_{r+1} - r(n - r + 1)p_r, \quad 0 \leqslant r \leqslant n - 1, \\ \frac{dp_n}{d\tau} &= -np_n, \end{aligned} \right\} \quad (5.30)$$

the initial condition being

$$p_n(0) = 1. \qquad (5.31)$$

Although the equations (5.30) are fairly simple in form, it is a remarkable fact that explicit solutions turn out to be rather awkward to handle. In principle we could solve them successively starting with the equation for p_n, but this is too cumbersome to be practicable. The best procedure is to use the

Laplace transform and its inverse with respect to time, given by

$$\phi^*(s) = \int_0^\infty e^{-s\tau}\phi(\tau)d\tau, \quad \mathbf{R}(s) > 0,$$

$$\phi(\tau) = \frac{1}{2\pi i}\int_{c-i\infty}^{c+i\infty} e^{s\tau}\phi^*(s)ds, \qquad\qquad\qquad (5.32)$$

where c is positive and greater than the real parts of all the singularities of $\phi^*(s)$.

Applying the transformation (5.32) to (5.30) and using (5.31) gives the recurrence relations

$$p_r^* = \frac{(r+1)(n-r)}{s+r(n-r+1)}p_{r+1}^*, \quad 0 \leqslant r \leqslant n-1,$$

and

$$p_n^* = \frac{1}{s+n}. \qquad\qquad\qquad\qquad\qquad (5.33)$$

An explicit solution for the transformed probabilities is thus readily obtained in the form

$$p_r^* = \frac{n!(n-r)!}{r!}\prod_{j=r}^n \{s+j(n-j+1)\}^{-1}, \quad 0 \leqslant r \leqslant n. \qquad (5.34)$$

In theory we need only invert (5.34) to derive $p_r(\tau)$. The right-hand side of (5.34) can be expressed as a sum of partial fractions containing terms like $\{s+j(n-j+1)\}^{-1}$ and $\{s+j(n-j+1)\}^{-2}$, the latter occurring when there are repeated factors, which happens if $r < \frac{1}{2}(n+1)$. The terms just mentioned lead to the inverses $e^{-j(n-j+1)\tau}$ and $\tau e^{-j(n-j+1)\tau}$, respectively. Unfortunately, the work involved in evaluating the partial fraction expansions and determining the various coefficients is very laborious, and the results are very inelegant when obtained (Bailey, 1957). Moreover, different formulae are required according to whether n is odd or even.

The main obstacle to an easy manipulation of the algebra is the presence of the repeated factors on the right of (5.34) when $r < \frac{1}{2}(n+1)$. This complication can be avoided by the following device. We consider a slightly modified model in which the chance of one new infection in $\Delta\tau$ is taken to be $r(N-r+1)\Delta\tau$ instead of $r(n-r+1)\Delta\tau$, where N is *not* an integer but may for convenience be thought of as only slightly different from n, i.e. $N = n + \epsilon$, for example. We find that we can proceed relatively easily and can at any stage recover results for the special case when $N = n$ simply by letting $\epsilon \to 0$.

It is easily verified that the state equations (5.30) are now replaced by

$$\frac{dp_r}{d\tau} = (r+1)(N-r)p_{r+1} - r(N-r+1)p_r, \quad 0 \leqslant r \leqslant n-1,$$

$$\frac{dp_n}{d\tau} = -n(N-n+1)p_n, \qquad\qquad\qquad\qquad (5.35)$$

with initial condition $p_n(0) = 1$, as before. The Laplace transforms of these equations are

$$\left.\begin{array}{l} p_r^* = \dfrac{(r+1)(N-r)}{s+r(N-r+1)} p_{r+1}^*, \quad 0 \leqslant r \leqslant n-1, \\[4mm] p_n^* = \dfrac{1}{s+n(N-n+1)}, \end{array}\right\} \qquad (5.36)$$

corresponding to (5.33). The explicit solution of (5.36) is therefore

$$p_r^* = \frac{n!(N-r)\ldots(N-n+1)}{r!} \prod_{j=r}^{n} \{s+j(N-j+1)\}^{-1}, \qquad (5.37)$$

corresponding to (5.34).

Since N is not an integer there are no repeated factors on the right of (5.37). We can therefore write p_r^* in the form

$$p_r^* = \sum_{j=r}^{n} \frac{c_{rj}}{s+j(N-j+1)}, \quad 0 \leqslant r \leqslant j \leqslant n, \qquad (5.38)$$

where
$$c_{rj} = \lim_{s \to -j(N-j+1)} \{s+j(N-j+1)\}p_r^*$$

$$= \frac{(-)^{j-r}(N-2j+1)n!(N-r)!}{r!(j-r)!(n-j)!(N-n)!(N-j-r+1)\ldots(N-j-n+1)}, \quad (5.39)$$

only a moderate amount of elementary algebra being required to obtain the result. The probabilities p_r themselves are, of course,

$$p_r = \sum_{j=r}^{n} c_{rj} e^{-j(N-j+1)\tau}, \quad 0 \leqslant r \leqslant j \leqslant n. \qquad (5.40)$$

To obtain the required inverse transform of (5.34) we have to let $N \to n$. Minor complications arise because one of the factors in the product $(N-j-r+1)\ldots(N-j-n+1)$ in the denominator of (5.39) may be ϵ, so that $c_{rj} \to \infty$ as $\epsilon \to 0$. However, by pairing off the terms involving c_{rj} and $c_{r,n-j+1}$, a finite limit is obtained,

In order to show some of the complexity entailed, we quote specific results for n even. First, if $r > \frac{1}{2}n$, we have

$$p_r = \sum_{j=1}^{n-r+1} c_{rj} e^{-j(n-j+1)\tau}, \quad r > \tfrac{1}{2}n, \qquad (5.41)$$

where
$$c_{rj} = \frac{(-)^{j-1}(n-2j+1)n!(n-r)!(r-j-1)!}{r!(j-1)!(n-j)!(n-r-j+1)!}. \qquad (5.42)$$

But if $r \leqslant \frac{1}{2}n$, there are repeated factors, and we must use

$$
\left.
\begin{aligned}
p_r &= \sum_{j=1}^{\frac{1}{2}n} c_{rj} e^{-j(n-j+1)\tau} + \sum_{j=r}^{\frac{1}{2}n} d_{rj}\tau e^{-j(n-j+1)\tau}, \quad 0 < r \leqslant \frac{1}{2}n, \\
\text{and} \qquad p_0 &= 1 + \sum_{j=1}^{\frac{1}{2}n} c_{0j} e^{-j(n-j+1)\tau} + \sum_{j=1}^{\frac{1}{2}n} d_{0j}\tau e^{-j(n-j+1)\tau},
\end{aligned}
\right\} \tag{5.43}
$$

where, if $j < r$, we still have the same value of c_{rj} given by (5.42), but if $j \geqslant r$ we have

$$
c_{rj} = \frac{(-)^r (n-2j+1)n!(n-r)!}{r!(j-1)!(n-j)!(n-r-j+1)!(j-r)!}
$$

$$
\times \left\{ \sum_{u=j}^{n-j} u^{-1} + \sum_{u=j-r+1}^{n-j-r+1} u^{-1} - \frac{2}{n-2j+1} \right\}, \quad j \geqslant r, \tag{5.44}
$$

subject to the proviso that when $r = 1$ the first summation in (5.44) does not arise, and the second is absent when $r = \frac{1}{2}n$, while

$$
d_{rj} = \frac{(-)^{r+1}(n-2j+1)^2 n!(n-r)!}{r!(j-1)!(n-j)!(n-j-r+1)!(j-r)!}. \tag{5.45}
$$

The corresponding formulae for the case of n odd entail some modification of the above results and are slightly more awkward in form. The exact numerical values of all the coefficients c_{rj} in the special case $n = 10$ are shown in Table 5.1.

The discussion in the present section should be sufficient to demonstrate the complexities inevitably arising in even the simplest type of stochastic epidemic process. These complexities appear to result largely from the introduction of transition probabilities that are quadratic functions of the basic random variable, rather than merely linear functions as with many of the commoner, and relatively tractable, birth-and-death processes. One possible way out of this difficulty, which is tractable at least asymptotically, is the suggestion of McNeil (1972) to modify the basic model so as to have a transition probability that is proportional to the square root of the product of the numbers of infectives and susceptibles. This idea is discussed further in section 5.10 below.

5.4   The probability-generating function

We saw in the last section how to obtain the individual state probabilities directly from the basic system of differential—difference equations. For some purposes, however, it is more convenient to work with the whole probability-generating function. This may be derived and handled in a variety of ways. First, we shall work with the modified model, for which the probability of one new infection in time-interval $\Delta\tau$ is $r(N - r + 1)\Delta\tau$, and use the explicit expressions for the transformed probabilities p_r^* appearing in (5.38). If the

Table 5.1 Probability distribution of number of susceptibles at time τ when $n = 10$. In any line corresponding to a particular probability, p_r, the tables give coefficients of terms appearing at the head of each column

Probabilities	$e^{-10\tau}$	$e^{-18\tau}$	$e^{-24\tau}$	$e^{-26\tau}$	$e^{-30\tau}$	$\tau e^{-30\tau}$	$\tau e^{-28\tau}$	$\tau e^{-24\tau}$	$\tau e^{-18\tau}$	$\tau e^{-10\tau}$	1
p_0	$408\frac{3}{14}$	$8\,697\frac{1}{2}$	$42\,589\frac{5}{7}$	$34\,740$	$-86\,436$	$-52\,920$	$-226\,800$	$-135\,000$	$-22\,050$	-810	1
p_1	$-489\frac{3}{14}$	$-17\,860\frac{1}{2}$	$-115\,714\frac{1}{7}$	$-119\,952$	$254\,016$	$158\,760$	$635\,040$	$324\,000$	$39\,690$	810	·
p_2	45	$10\,143$	$108\,000$	$155\,232$	$-273\,420$	$-176\,400$	$-635\,040$	$-252\,000$	$-17\,640$	·	·
p_3	15	-735	$-37\,500$	$-91\,140$	$129\,360$	$88\,200$	$264\,600$	$63\,000$	·	·	·
p_4	$7\frac{1}{2}$	$-157\frac{1}{2}$	$2\,250$	$22\,470$	$-24\,570$	$-18\,900$	$-37\,800$	·	·	·	·
p_5	$4\frac{1}{2}$	$-52\frac{1}{2}$	300	$-1\,260$	$1\,008$	$1\,260$	·	·	·	·	·
p_6	3	-21	60	-84	42	·	·	·	·	·	·
p_7	$2\frac{1}{7}$	-9	$12\frac{6}{7}$	-6	·	·	·	·	·	·	·
p_8	$1\frac{12}{28}$	$-3\frac{3}{7}$	$2\frac{1}{7}$	·	·	·	·	·	·	·	·
p_9	$1\frac{1}{4}$	$-1\frac{1}{4}$	·	·	·	·	·	·	·	·	·
p_{10}	1	·	·	·	·	·	·	·	·	·	·

required probability-generating function is

$$P(x, \tau) = \sum_{r=0}^{n} p_r(\tau) x^r,$$ (5.46)

then the transform is

$$P^*(x, s) = \sum_{r=0}^{n} p_r^*(s) x^r,$$

$$= \sum_{r=0}^{n} \sum_{j=r}^{n} \frac{c_{rj} x^r}{s + j(N-j+1)}, \text{ using (5.38),}$$

$$= \sum_{j=0}^{n} \sum_{r=0}^{j} \frac{c_{rj} x^r}{s + j(N-j+1)}, \text{ reversing the summations,}$$

$$= \sum_{j=0}^{n} \frac{1}{s + j(N-j+1)} \sum_{r=0}^{j} c_{rj} x^r.$$ (5.47)

It follows that $P(x, \tau)$ can be written as

$$P(x, \tau) = \sum_{j=0}^{n} e^{-j(N-j+1)\tau} G_j(x),$$ (5.48)

where

$$G_j(x) = \sum_{r=0}^{j} c_{rj} x^r.$$ (5.49)

If we can identify $G_j(x)$ as some well-known function then we immediately have a compact expression for $P(x, \tau)$. Fortunately, this can easily be seen to be the case. The ratio of the $(r + 1)$th and rth terms in (5.49) is, using (5.39),

$$\frac{c_{r+1,j}}{c_{rj}} x = \frac{(-j + r)(j - N - 1 + r)}{(-N + r)} x,$$ (5.50)

so that

$$G_j(x) = c_{0j} F(-j, j - N - 1; -N, x),$$ (5.51)

where $F(-j, j - N - 1; -N, x)$ is in fact a terminating hypergeometric series. We now put $c_{0j} \equiv c_j$. If $r = 0$ in (5.39), we have

$$c_j = \frac{(-)^j (N - 2j + 1) n! N!}{j!(n - j)!(N - n)!(N - j + 1)...(N - j - n + 1)},$$ (5.52)

and (5.48) becomes

$$P(x, \tau) = \sum_{j=0}^{n} c_j e^{-j(N-j+1)\tau} F(-j, j - N - 1; -N, x).$$ (5.53)

In particular, $c_0 = 1$, as expected, since $P(x, \tau) \to 1$ as $\tau \to \infty$.

As before, the special case $N = n$ is obtained by letting $\epsilon \to 0$. The problem of the c_j becoming infinite is solved by combining the terms for j and $n - j + 1$. No specially elegant result is obtained for the limiting form of $P(x, \tau)$ itself as $\epsilon \to 0$, but it can be used rather easily to derive an expression for the stochastic mean $\mu'_1(\tau)$. In general, it may be said that the greatest tractability is achieved with the device of using a non-integral N by retaining N until the latest possible stage, when we let $N \to n$. Thus, for the stochastic mean we have

$$\mu'_1(\tau) = \left[\frac{\partial P(x, \tau)}{\partial x} \right]_{x=1}$$

$$= \sum_{j=0}^{n} c_j e^{-j(N-j+1)\tau} \frac{(-j)(j-N-1)}{-N} F(-j+1, j-N; -N+1, 1)$$

$$= -\sum_{j=1}^{n} c_j e^{-j(N-j+1)\tau} \frac{\Gamma(N-j+2)\,\Gamma(j+1)}{\Gamma(N+1)}, \qquad (5.54)$$

using the standard result

$$F(-j+1, j-N; -N+1, 1) = \frac{\Gamma(N-j+1)\,\Gamma(j)}{\Gamma(N)}. \qquad (5.55)$$

Substituting in (5.54) the value of c_j given (5.52) yields the relatively simple expression

$$\mu'_1(\tau) = \sum_{j=1}^{n} \frac{(-)^{j+1}(N-2j+1)n!}{(n-j)!(N-n)...(N-n-j+1)} e^{-j(n-j+1)\tau}. \qquad (5.56)$$

This is the point at which to let $\epsilon \to 0$. The factor $N - n$ in the denominator on the right yields a coefficient in ϵ^{-1}, but combining the terms for j and $n - j + 1$ leads to a finite limit. We easily arrive at Haskey's formula

$$\mu'_1(\tau) = \sum_{j=1}^{} \frac{n!}{(n-j)!(j-1)!} \left\{ (n-2j+1)^2 \tau + 2 - (n-2j+1) \sum_{u=j}^{n-j} u^{-1} \right\} e^{-j(n-j+1)\tau},$$

$$(5.57)$$

where the upper limit of the main summation is $\frac{1}{2}n$ for n even; and $\frac{1}{2}(n + 1)$ for n odd with the introduction of a factor of $\frac{1}{2}$ into the term given by $j = \frac{1}{2}(n + 1)$. This result was originally obtained by Haskey (1954), who started with the transformed probabilities in (5.34) and then embarked on an extremely laborious, though highly skilful series of partial fraction expansions.

When $n = 10$, the explicit form of the stochastic mean is exactly

$$\mu'_1(\tau) = e^{-10\tau}(810\tau - 234\tfrac{17}{28}) + e^{-18\tau}(4410\tau - 902\tfrac{1}{4})$$

$$+ e^{-24\tau}(9000\tau - 1247\tfrac{1}{2}) + e^{-28\tau}(7560\tau + 126)$$

$$+ e^{-30\tau}(1260\tau + 2268). \qquad (5.58)$$

In Section 5.2 we defined the *epidemic curve* in a deterministic situation as the rate at which new infections accrue. The corresponding stochastic analogue in simple epidemics is the curve showing the rate of change with respect to time of the mean number of infectives that exist at any time. Thus we now have $w = d\mu'_1/d\tau$, and the special case of $n = 10$, (5.58) leads to the exact result

$$w(\tau) = e^{-10\tau}(8100\tau - 3156\tfrac{1}{14}) + e^{-18\tau}(79\,380\tau - 20\,650\tfrac{1}{2})$$
$$+ e^{-24\tau}(216\,000\tau - 38\,931\tfrac{3}{7}) + e^{-28\tau}(211\,680\tau - 4032)$$
$$+ e^{-30\tau}(37\,800\tau + 66\,780). \tag{5.59}$$

A similar *exact* expression for $\mu'_1(\tau)$ was also given by Bailey (1957) for $n = 20$ in the first edition of this book. There seems little point in reproducing this lengthy formula here, though it might occasionally be useful to compare with the results of approximating approaches. Haskey (1954) has investigated the case of $n = 30$ numerically, and has given coefficients of all terms occurring in the expression for the stochastic mean, as well as providing actual values of $w(\tau)$ for selected values of τ. (For the convenience of anyone referring to Haskey's original paper it should be mentioned that the last three entries in the third column of his Table 1 should all be negative, while the value of z (the same as our w) for $t = 0{\cdot}15$ in Table 2 should be 161.) Mansfield and Hensley (1960) have computed tables of $w(\tau)$ for $n = 5(1)40$. Actual graphs for $n = 5$ and 40 are presented by Dietz (1967) and compared with the corresponding deterministic curves.

It is of some interest to compare the epidemic curves for these stochastic models with the corresponding deterministic analogues. Fig. 5.1 and 5.2 show these comparisons for $n = 10$ and 20, respectively. It will be seen that while the deterministic curve is symmetrical about the maximum ordinate, the stochastic curve is asymmetrical and falls rather more slowly. Nevertheless the actual maxima do occur at approximately the same time.

When discussing some more general processes of the present type, Feller (1939) showed that, given certain definitions, the stochastic mean is always less than the corresponding deterministic value. Feller's conditions are satisfied in the present case, provided that we apply his arguments to the number of infectives instead of the number of susceptibles. Lest there be any confusion, it must be remembered that the graphs in Fig. 5.1 and 5.2 represent *rates of change* with respect to time of stochastic means.

To return to the probability-generating functions, we derived the formula in (5.53) for $P(x, \tau)$ for non-integral N using our knowledge of the explicit expression for the Laplace transforms p_r^* of the individual probabilities. Alternatively, we can derive a partial differential equation for $P(x, \tau)$ following the standard techniques for handling stochastic processes. Thus multiplying each equation in (5.30) by x^r and summing over the range $0 \leqslant r \leqslant n$ gives quite easily

$$\frac{\partial P}{\partial \tau} = (1-x)\left(n\frac{\partial P}{\partial x} - x\frac{\partial^2 P}{\partial x^2}\right), \tag{5.60}$$

with initial condition
$$P(x,0) = x^n. \tag{5.61}$$

The same procedure applied to (5.35) yields

$$\frac{\partial P}{\partial \tau} = (1-x)\left(N\frac{\partial P}{\partial x} - x\frac{\partial^2 P}{\partial x^2}\right), \tag{5.62}$$

with the same initial condition as (5.61).

Actually, equations like (5.60) and (5.62) can be written down more or less immediately from a specification of the transition probabilities, following the "random variable" technique of Bailey (1964a, Sec. 7.4). According to this, the required partial differential equation is

$$\frac{\partial P(x,\tau)}{\partial \tau} = \sum_{j\neq 0} (x^j - 1)f_j\left(x\frac{\partial}{\partial x}\right)P(x,\tau), \tag{5.63}$$

where the transition probabilities for the time-interval are given by

$$P\{\Delta X(\tau) = j \,|\, X(\tau)\} = f_j(X)\Delta\tau, \quad j \neq 0.$$

In the present case, the model with non-integral N has only one non-zero f_j, namely $f_{-1}(X) = X(N - X + 1)$. Substituting in (5.63) gives

$$\frac{\partial P}{\partial \tau} = (x^{-1}-1)\left(x\frac{\partial}{\partial x}\right)\left\{(N+1)-\left(x\frac{\partial}{\partial x}\right)\right\}P,$$

which reduces directly to (5.62).

Now equation (5.62) is a typical second-order partial differential equation for which we might expect to obtain a solution in terms of eigenfunctions by a standard method such as the separation of variables. Following Bailey (1963), we start by trying

$$P(x,\tau) = X(x)T(\tau), \tag{5.64}$$

where X is a function of x only, and T is a function of τ only. Substituting (5.64) in (5.62) gives

$$\frac{T'}{T} = \frac{N(1-x)X' - x(1-x)X''}{X} = -\lambda, \text{ say}, \tag{5.65}$$

where λ is some suitable constant independent of x and τ.

From the first and third elements of (5.65) we obtain

$$T = e^{-\lambda\tau}, \tag{5.66}$$

and from the second and third elements we have

$$x(1-x)X'' - N(1-x)X' - \lambda X = 0, \tag{5.67}$$

a solution of which is the hypergeometric function

$$X(x) = F(\alpha, \beta; \gamma, x), \tag{5.68}$$

where $\qquad\qquad \gamma = -N; \ \alpha + \beta = -N-1, \ \alpha\beta = \lambda. \tag{5.69}$

The eigenvalues λ are determined by the fact that the general solution has to be a polynomial of at most degree n in x. From this it follows that the hypergeometric series must terminate, and this requires that α, say, must be a negative integer subject to $\alpha + \beta = -N - 1$. The permissible eigenvalues are therefore

$$\lambda_j = j(N-j+1), \quad 0 \leqslant j \leqslant n. \tag{5.70}$$

A general solution can therefore be written as

$$P(x,\tau) = \sum_{j=0}^{n} d_j e^{-j(N-j+1)\tau} F(-j, j-N-1; -N, x). \tag{5.71}$$

This of course can be identified with the previous solution given in (5.53) with $d_j = c_j$, but in the present derivation the constants d_j still have to be determined.

It may be noted in passing that the use of a non-integral N makes the investigation more easily manageable, since all the eigenvalues λ_j are distinct, corresponding in fact to the $n + 1$ possible states of the system.

The d_j may be found from the initial condition. Thus, when $\tau = 0$ the d_j must satisfy

$$x^n = \sum_{j=0}^{n} d_j F(-j, j-N-1; -N, x). \tag{5.72}$$

The hypergeometric functions on the right of (5.72) obey certain orthogonality relations, which are best expressed in terms of the standard theory of Jacobi polynomials (see Erdélyi, 1953, vol. 2, Ch. 10). We can use

$$P_j^{\mu, \nu}(y) = \binom{j+\mu}{j} F\left(-j, j+\mu+\nu+1; \mu+1, \frac{1-y}{2}\right),$$

where we put $\mu = -N - 1, \nu = -1, y = 1 - 2x$. Admittedly, the standard results are restricted to $\mu > -1$, but it can be seen that coefficients calculated for the restricted range will also hold more generally. Thus (5.72) can be rewritten as

$$\sum_{j=0}^{n} d_n P_j^{\mu, \nu}(y) = \binom{j+\mu}{j} 2^{-n}(1-y)^n. \tag{5.73}$$

We now apply the following standard forms

$$\int_{-1}^{1} w(y)\, P_j^{\mu,\nu}(y)\, P_k^{\mu,\nu}(y)\, dy \;=\; \frac{2^{\mu+\nu+1}\,\Gamma(j+\mu+1)\,\Gamma(j+\nu+1)}{(2j+\mu+\nu+1)\, j!\, \Gamma(j+\mu+\nu+1)}, \quad k=j,$$

$$= 0, \quad k \neq j, \qquad\qquad (5.74)$$

and

$$\int_{-1}^{1} w(y)\, f(y)\, P_j^{\mu,\nu}(y)\, dy \;=\; \frac{1}{j!\,2^j} \int_{-1}^{1} f^{(j)}(y)\, w(y)(1-y^2)^j\, dy, \qquad (5.75)$$

where $w(y)$ is the appropriate weight-function $(1-y)^{\mu}(1+y)^{\nu}$. If we put $f(y) = 2^{-n}(1-y)^n$ in (5.75) we obtain

$$\int_{-1}^{1} w(y)\, 2^{-n}(1-y)^n\, P_j^{\mu,\nu}(y)\, dy \;=\; \frac{(-)^j n!}{2^{n+j} j!\,(n-j)!} \int_{-1}^{1} (1-y)^{n+\mu}(1+y)^{j+\nu}\, dy$$

$$= \frac{(-)^j 2^{\mu+\nu+1}\, n!\, \Gamma(n+\mu+1)\,\Gamma(j+\nu+1)}{j!\,(n-j)!\,\Gamma(n+j+\mu+\nu+2)}. \qquad (5.76)$$

All we now have to do is multiply (5.73) through by $w(y)\,P_j^{\mu,\nu}(y)$ and integrate from -1 to $+1$. Using (5.74) and (5.76) then gives

$$d_j = \frac{(-)^j n!\,(2j+\mu+\nu+1)(n+\mu)\dots(\mu+1)}{j!\,(n-j)!\,(n+j+\mu+\nu+1)\dots(j+\mu+\nu+1)}, \qquad (5.77)$$

after cancelling common factors, and replacing the ratios of gamma functions by the appropriate products. If we now put $\mu = -N-1$ and $\nu = -1$, we find that $d_j = c_j$, as given by (5.52).

5.5   The moment-generating function

Since we have already obtained a closed expression for the probability-generating function with non-integral N in (5.53), the moment-generating function can be derived immediately by substituting $x = e^{\theta}$ to give

$$M(\theta,\tau) = \sum_{j=0}^{n} c_j\, e^{-j(N-j+1)\tau}\, F(-j, j-N-1; -N, e^{\theta}), \qquad (5.78)$$

where c_j is defined as in (5.52). As before, the special case of $N = n$ is dealt with by letting $\epsilon \to 0$. Unfortunately, this does not appear to lead to the ready derivation of any new properties.

Alternatively, we obtained in (5.60) a simple partial differential equation for $P(x,\tau)$, and, again putting $x = e^{\theta}$, this leads directly to

$$\frac{\partial M}{\partial \tau} = (e^{-\theta} - 1)\left\{ (n+1)\frac{\partial M}{\partial \theta} - \frac{\partial^2 M}{\partial \theta^2} \right\}, \qquad (5.79)$$

the initial condition now being

$$M(\theta,0) = e^{n\theta}. \qquad (5.80)$$

The usual procedure of substituting the moment-generating function series expansion in terms of moments about the origin, given by

$$M(\theta,\tau) = 1 + \sum_{j=1}^{\infty} \mu_j'(\tau)\theta^j/j!,$$ (5.81)

into (5.79), and equating coefficients of θ^r, leads to the infinite set of equations

$$\frac{d\mu_r'}{d\tau} = \sum_{j=1}^{r} (-)^{r-j+1} \binom{r}{j-1} \{(n+1)\mu_j' - \mu_{j+1}'\}, \quad r \geqslant 1,$$ (5.82)

of which the first two are

$$\frac{d\mu_1'}{d\tau} = -\{(n+1)\mu_1' - \mu_2'\},$$ (5.83)

and

$$\frac{d\mu_2'}{d\tau} = +\{(n+1)\mu_1' - \mu_2'\} - 2\{(n+1)\mu_2' - \mu_3'\}.$$ (5.84)

It is clear that there is no way of solving such equations successively since the first one involves μ_2' as well as μ_1'. The origin of this difficulty is the one already alluded to at the end of Section 5.3, namely the use of transition probabilities that are quadratic, rather than linear, functions of the basic random variable.

Of course, if we already know μ_1', then we can use (5.83) to calculate μ_2', and hence the variance.

The possibility also exists in principle of developing a Taylor expansion for any moment μ_r' in powers of τ. Differentiating (5.82) $k-1$ times expresses $d^k\mu_r'/d\tau^k$ in terms of differential coefficients of order $k-1$, and these in turn can be expressed in terms of differential coefficients of order $k-2$, and so on. Ultimately, this process yields a linear function of a set of basic raw moments $\mu_p'(\tau)$, so that $[d^k\mu_r'/d\tau^k]_{\tau=0}$ can be put in terms of the $\mu_p'(0)$, where $\mu_p'(0) = n^p$. But no general method of handling the relevant recursions is so far available. The first four terms of the Taylor series for $\mu_1'(\tau)$ are found to be

$$\mu_1'(\tau) = n - n\tau - \frac{n(n-2)}{2!}\tau^2 - \frac{n(n^2 - 8n + 8)}{3!}\tau^3 - \dots.$$ (5.85)

This series hardly converges quickly enough for it to be of any computational importance, but it is possible that further investigation might lead to some more compact functional form than that already exhibited in (5.57).

Finally, as a prelude to obtaining in Section 5.8 some asymptotic results valid for large n, let us consider transforming the time τ and the random variable $X(\tau)$ in a manner analogous to that already used for the deterministic version in Section 5.2. Let us suppose, a little more generally, that the process starts at some time $\tau = 0$ with a infectives. Equation (5.79) is then replaced by

$$\frac{\partial M}{\partial \tau} = (e^{-\theta} - 1)\left\{(n+a)\frac{\partial M}{\partial \theta} - \frac{\partial^2 M}{\partial \theta^2}\right\}, \tag{5.86}$$

the initial condition remaining as $M(\theta, 0) = e^{n\theta}$. $\tag{5.87}$

As before, we change the time-scale to $T = (n+a)\tau$, and the random variable to

$$\Xi = \frac{X}{n+a}, \tag{5.88}$$

corresponding to (5.20). Evidently,

$$M_\Xi(\theta, \tau) = M_X\left(\frac{\theta}{n+a}, \tau\right).$$

Hence M_Ξ satisfies

$$\frac{\partial M}{\partial T} = (n+a)\{e^{-\theta/(n+a)} - 1\}\left(\frac{\partial M}{\partial \theta} - \frac{\partial^2 M}{\partial \theta^2}\right), \tag{5.89}$$

using (5.86) and (5.88). To first order in $(n+a)^{-1}$ we can write

$$\frac{\partial M_s}{\partial T} = \theta\left(1 - \frac{\theta}{2(n+a)}\right)\left(\frac{\partial^2 M_s}{\partial \theta^2} - \frac{\partial M_s}{\partial \theta}\right), \tag{5.90}$$

where we now use the suffix s to indicate "stochastic", the initial condition being

$$M_s(\theta, 0) = e^{\theta/(1+\gamma)}, \tag{5.91}$$

where $\gamma = a/n$, as in (5.24).

We can now compare the stochastic and deterministic partial differential equations. As $n \to \infty$, the equations in (5.89) or (5.90) pass over into the form already given in (5.27), the initial conditions in (5.28) and (5.91) remaining the same for all n.

5.6   The epidemic curve

In Section 5.2 we defined the epidemic curve for the deterministic model as the rate at which new infections occurred, and we described Williams' (1965a) approach of treating the suitably normalized epidemic curve as the frequency function of the time of occurrence of a new infection. Now, following the same approach in the stochastic version, also due to Williams, we consider that any set of infections occurring during the course of a single epidemic can be regarded as the statistical image of an underlying epidemic curve. Let k cases out of n occur in the interval $(\tau, \tau + d\tau)$, and let $f(\tau)$ be the frequency function for the time of occurrence of new cases. Then we can write

$$f(\tau)d\tau = E\left(\frac{k}{n}\right) = \frac{1}{n}\{\mu_1'(\tau + d\tau) - \mu'(\tau)\} = -\frac{1}{n}\frac{d\mu_1'}{d\tau}d\tau, \tag{5.92}$$

where $\mu_1'(\tau)$ is the average number of susceptibles at time τ.

It follows that a suitable procedure in the stochastic case is to define the epidemic curve as the rate of increase of the average number of infections existing at any time. That is, we can reasonably use as the basic, unnormalized, epidemic curve the function

$$w = -\frac{d\mu'_1}{d\tau},$$
(5.93)

where $\mu'_1(\tau)$ is given explicitly by Haskey's formula (5.57).

The normalized epidemic curve is then the function appearing in (5.92), namely,

$$W = \frac{w}{n} = -\frac{1}{n}\frac{d\mu'_1}{d\tau},$$
(5.94)

and this corresponds directly with the deterministic form shown in (5.10). An expression for the moment-generating function of this frequency distribution can now be found quite straightforwardly. It is most convenient to work first with Laplace transforms, as given by (5.32). We also need to generalize previous results slightly to allow for an initial number of infectives a. The probability of one new infective in $\Delta\tau$ is now $r(n-r+a)\Delta\tau$, but the initial condition so far as the number of susceptibles is concerned remains the same. It is easily verified that (5.33) is replaced by

$$\left.\begin{array}{l} p^*_r = \dfrac{(r+1)(n-r+a-1)}{s+r(n-r+a)} p^*_{r+1}, \quad 0 \leqslant r \leqslant n-1, \\[4mm] p^*_n = \dfrac{1}{s+na}, \end{array}\right\}$$
(5.95)

while (5.34) becomes

$$p^*_r = \frac{n!(n-r+a-1)!}{r!(a-1)!} \prod_{j=r}^{n} \{s+j(n-j+a)\}^{-1}, \quad 0 \leqslant r \leqslant n.$$
(5.96)

Next, we observe that the Laplace transform of W is

$$\begin{aligned} W^* &= \int_0^\infty e^{-s\tau} W d\tau \\ &= -\frac{1}{n}\int_0^\infty e^{-s\tau}\frac{d\mu'_1}{d\tau} d\tau, \text{ using (5.94),} \\ &= 1 - \frac{s}{n}\int_0^\infty e^{-s\tau}\mu'_1 d\tau, \end{aligned}$$
(5.97)

where we have integrated by parts and used the facts that $\mu'_1 = n$ when $\tau = 0$ and is exponentially small as $\tau \to \infty$. Since, by definition,

$$\mu'_1(\tau) = \sum_{r=0}^{n} r p_r(\tau),$$

we can write (5.97) as

$$W^* = 1 - \frac{s}{n} \sum_{r=1}^{n} r p_r^*$$

$$= 1 - \frac{s}{n} \sum_{r=1}^{n} \frac{1}{n-r+a} \prod_{j=r}^{n} \left\{ 1 + \frac{s}{j(n-j+a)} \right\}^{-1}, \quad \text{using (5.96),}$$

$$= 1 - \frac{s}{n} \sum_{r=a}^{n+a-1} \frac{1}{r} \prod_{j=n-r+a}^{n} \left\{ 1 + \frac{s}{j(n-j+a)} \right\}^{-1}, \qquad (5.98)$$

by an obvious substitution.

The moment-generating function of τ is accordingly

$$M(\theta) = 1 + \frac{\theta}{n} \sum_{r=a}^{n+a-1} \frac{1}{r} \prod_{j=n-r+a}^{n} \left\{ 1 - \frac{\theta}{j(n-j+a)} \right\}^{-1}. \qquad (5.99)$$

The mean value of the normalized stochastic epidemic curve is given by the coefficient of θ on the right of (5.99), and this can be written down immediately as

$$\bar{\tau} = \frac{1}{n} \sum_{r=a}^{n+a-1} \frac{1}{r}. \qquad (5.100)$$

This expression may be compared with the corresponding deterministic value given in (5.11). Although the two formulae are quite different in form, they are asymptotically equivalent for large n. Moreover it can be shown that the stochastic mean lags the deterministic mean by an amount inversely proportional to n.

Further moments may be obtained in the same way from (5.99) by picking out the coefficients of higher powers of θ, though this quickly becomes very cumbersome. Williams (*loc. cit.*) gives an explicit formula for the variance.

Let us now see what happens to the moment-generating function as $n \to \infty$. As with the deterministic discussion in Section 5.2, it is convenient to transform the time variable τ. On this occasion we use

$$U = (n+a)\tau - \log n = T - \log a, \qquad (5.101)$$

T being given by (5.12). The moment-generating function of U can therefore be obtained immediately from (5.99) as

$$M(\theta) = \frac{1}{n^\theta} \left[1 + \left(1 + \frac{a}{n} \right) \theta \sum_{r=a}^{n+a-1} \frac{1}{r} \prod_{j=n-r+a}^{n} \left\{ 1 - \frac{(n+a)\theta}{j(n-j+a)} \right\}^{-1} \right]. \qquad (5.102)$$

Since the sums and products involve terms whose *number* can be of order n, we must be careful not merely to suppress all terms of order n^{-1} when proceeding to the limit.

The terms like $1 - \dfrac{(n+a)\theta}{j(n-j+a)}$ on the right can be replaced by something more tractable if we note that

$$\left(1-\frac{\theta}{j}\right)\left(1-\frac{\theta}{n-j+a}\right) = 1-\frac{(n+a)\theta}{j(n-j+a)}+\frac{\theta^2}{j(n-j+a)}.$$

Hence, by a simple argument,

$$\frac{1-\dfrac{(n+a)\theta}{j(n-j+a)}}{\left(1-\dfrac{\theta}{j}\right)\left(1-\dfrac{\theta}{n-j+a}\right)} = 1+O\left(\frac{1}{j(n-j+a)}\right), \tag{5.103}$$

uniformly within any circle $|\theta| \leqslant \rho < 1$. It easily follows that the substitution

$$1-\frac{(n+a)\theta}{j(n-j+a)} \sim \left(1-\frac{\theta}{j}\right)\left(1-\frac{\theta}{n-j+a}\right)$$

in (5.102) introduces a relative error of at most $O\{\log n)/n\} \to 0$ as $n \to \infty$. Moreover if $\mathbf{R}(\theta) > 0$ then $n^\theta \to \infty$. The last $a-1$ terms in the summation can be ignored since they contribute only a finite amount to the total. Therefore, as $n \to \infty$, we can write asymptotically that

$$M(\theta) \sim \frac{\theta}{n^\theta}\sum_{r=a}^{n}\frac{1}{r}\prod_{j=n-r+a}^{n}\left(1-\frac{\theta}{j}\right)^{-1}\left(1-\frac{\theta}{n-j+a}\right)^{-1}$$

$$\sim \frac{\theta}{n^\theta}\sum_{r=a}^{n}\frac{1}{r}\prod_{j=1}^{a-1}\left(1-\frac{\theta}{j}\right)\prod_{j=1}^{n}\left(1-\frac{\theta}{j}\right)^{-1}\prod_{j=1}^{n-r+a-1}\left(1-\frac{\theta}{j}\right)\prod_{j=1}^{r}\left(1-\frac{\theta}{j}\right)^{-1}$$

$$\sim \frac{\theta}{n^\theta}\prod_{j=1}^{a-1}\left(1-\frac{\theta}{j}\right)\prod_{j=1}^{n}\left(1-\frac{\theta}{j}\right)^{-1}\sum_{r=a}^{n}\frac{1}{r}\prod_{j=1}^{n-r+a-1}\left(1-\frac{\theta}{j}\right)\prod_{j=1}^{r}\left(1-\frac{\theta}{j}\right)^{-1}$$

$$\tag{5.104}$$

When n is large the summation in (5.104) can be replaced by an integral. Suppose we make the substitution

$$r = nx, \quad 1 = ndx, \quad \frac{1}{r} = \frac{dx}{x}, \quad 0 \leqslant x \leqslant 1. \tag{5.105}$$

When n is large, so is r, except at the point $x = 0$, where the contribution to the result is negligible. In these circumstances we can use the standard result, e.g. Erdélyi (1953, vol. 1, p. 1),

$$\Gamma(1-\theta) = -\theta\Gamma(-\theta) = \lim_{n\to\infty}(-\theta)\frac{n!\,n^{-\theta}}{(-\theta)(1-\theta)\ldots(n-\theta)}$$

$$= \lim_{n\to\infty}\frac{n^{-\theta}}{(1-\theta)\ldots\left(1-\dfrac{\theta}{n}\right)}, \tag{5.106}$$

in conjunction with the substitution (5.105), to replace (5.104) by

$$M(\theta) \sim \theta\Gamma(1-\theta) \prod_{j=1}^{a-1} \left(1 - \frac{\theta}{j}\right) \int_0^1 x^\theta (1-x)^{-\theta} dx/x$$

$$= \theta\Gamma(1-\theta) \prod_{j=1}^{a-1} \left(1 - \frac{\theta}{j}\right) B(\theta, 1-\theta)$$

$$= \Gamma(1+\theta)\{\Gamma(1-\theta)\}^2 \prod_{j=1}^{a-1} \left(1 - \frac{\theta}{j}\right), \qquad (5.107)$$

using the familiar properties of the beta function.

We can now take logs of both sides of (5.107), and use the expansion (5.17) to obtain the cumulant-generating function. Equating powers of $\theta^\nu/\nu!$ then gives the νth cumulant κ_ν expressed by

$$\left.\begin{array}{l} \kappa_1 = \gamma - \displaystyle\sum_{r=1}^{a-1} \frac{1}{r}, \\[3mm] \kappa_\nu = (\nu-1)! \left[\{2 + (-)^\nu\}\, \zeta(\nu) - \displaystyle\sum_{r=1}^{a-1} \frac{1}{r^\nu}\right], \quad \nu \geqslant 2. \end{array}\right\} \qquad (5.108)$$

Remembering that we are working with the variable U, it is easily verified that, if we substitute the exact value of $\bar{\tau}$ given by (5.100) into (5.101) and then let $n \to \infty$, we obtain the quantity $\kappa_1 \equiv \kappa_1(U)$ appearing in (5.108), as expected.

Again, for large a, we can apply the result in (5.106), with a substituted for n, to the product on the right of (5.107), quickly obtaining the limiting form

$$M_U(\theta) \sim a^{-\theta}\Gamma(1-\theta)\,\Gamma(1+\theta), \qquad (5.109)$$

which is valid for large a and n, the suffix U indicating the relevant random variable. Since $T = U + \log a$, it follows that

$$\begin{aligned} M_T(\theta) &= e^{\theta \log a} M_U(\theta) \\ &= a^\theta M_U(\theta) \\ &\sim \Gamma(1-\theta)\,\Gamma(1+\theta), \end{aligned} \qquad (5.110)$$

which is identical with the limiting distribution given in (5.15) of the epidemic curve for the deterministic model (referred of course to time-scale T).

For small a the situation is very different, and becomes increasingly marked as a decreases. With $a = 1$, for example, the stochastic model yields a variance $\sigma^2 = \kappa_2 = \frac{1}{2}\pi^2$, which is $1\frac{1}{2}$ times the deterministic value. The skewness is now $\gamma_1 = \kappa_3/\kappa_2^{3/2} = 2\zeta(3)/\{3\zeta(2)\}^{3/2} = 0\cdot22$, compared with zero previously; while the kurtosis is now $\gamma_2 = \kappa_4/\kappa_2^2 = \frac{4}{5}$, which is $\frac{2}{3}$ of the value for the deterministic curve.

It is also possible to derive closed expressions for the distribution function and frequency function of the variable U. Since we already have an explicit form in (5.107) for the moment-generating function, we might expect to be able to derive the frequency function directly by inversion. Thus we can replace the product in (5.107) by gamma functions to give

$$M(\theta) \sim \Gamma(1 + \theta)\,\Gamma(1 - \theta)\,\Gamma(a - \theta)/\Gamma(a). \qquad (5.111)$$

If we now put $\theta = iz$ in (5.111) to yield the characteristic function $C(z)$, we should in principle be able to obtain the frequency function by simply finding the inverse Fourier transform of $C(z)$, evaluating the relevant complex integral in the usual way, using the calculus of residues. Unfortunately, no compact way of achieving the required result has yet been found. The following ingenious, though slightly intricate, argument is due to Williams (*loc. cit.*).

Let us write the frequency function of U as $f_a(U)$, distinguishing the initial number of infectives by the suffix a. The corresponding moment-generating function, given by (5.111), is $M_a(\theta)$. The general idea is to derive two different relationships between f_a and f_{a+1}, and then eliminate f_{a+1}. One of these is obtained directly from (5.111) simply replacing a by $a + 1$. Thus

$$M_{a+1}(\theta) = \left(1 - \frac{\theta}{a}\right)M_a(\theta). \qquad (5.112)$$

Inversion of (5.112) then gives

$$f_{a+1} = \left(1 + \frac{1}{a}\frac{d}{dU}\right)f_a. \qquad (5.113)$$

It is convenient to define a further function $G_a(U)$, which is the complement of the distribution function $F_a(U)$. Thus

$$F_a(U) = \int_{-\infty}^{U} f_a(v)\,dv; \quad G_a(U) = 1 - F_a(U) = \int_{U}^{\infty} f_a(v)\,dv. \quad (5.114)$$

Integrating (5.113) from U to ∞ leads immediately to the first relationship sought, namely

$$f_a = a(G_a - G_{a+1}). \qquad (5.115)$$

A second relationship is derived by considering $M_a(\theta - 1)$. First, we note from (5.111) that $M_a(\theta)$ converges in the infinite open strip $-1 < \mathbf{R}(\theta) < +1$. Also we see from (5.114) that

$$F_a \to 0 \text{ as } U \to -\infty; \quad G_a \to 0 \text{ as } U \to +\infty. \qquad (5.116)$$

If we then represent the moment-generating function transform operator by L, it is not difficult to deduce from (5.114) that $L(F_a)$ converges in the strip $-1 < \mathbf{R}(\theta) < 0$, and that $L(G_a)$ converges in $0 < \mathbf{R}(\theta) < +1$. Specifically, we obtain the results

and
$$L(F_a) = -M_a(\theta)/\theta, \quad -1 < \mathbf{R}(\theta) < 0, \qquad (5.117)$$
$$L(G_a) = M_a(\theta)/\theta, \quad 0 < \mathbf{R}(\theta) < +1. \qquad (5.118)$$

Now putting $\theta - 1$ for θ in (5.117) gives

$$L(e^{-U}F_a) = -\frac{M_a(\theta - 1)}{\theta - 1}, \quad 0 < \mathbf{R}(\theta) < 1$$

$$= a\, M_{a+1}(\theta)/\theta, \quad \text{using (5.111)},$$

$$= a\, L(G_a), \quad \text{from (5.118)}.$$

Hence the second relationship required is

$$e^{-U}F_a = a\, G_{a+1}. \tag{5.119}$$

Eliminating G_{a+1} between (5.115) and (5.119) yields the differential equation

$$\frac{dF_a}{dw} - \left(1 + \frac{a}{w}\right)F_a + \frac{a}{w} = 0, \tag{5.120}$$

where we have written $w = e^{-U}$, and have substituted $f_a = dF_a/dU$. Equation (5.120) can be integrated by elementary means, using the usual integrating factor $\{-(w + a \log w)\}$. This leads to the explicit solution

$$F_a = 1 - w^a e^w \int_w^\infty x^{-a} e^{-x} dx$$

$$= 1 - w e^w \int_1^\infty x^{-a} e^{-wx} dx$$

$$= 1 - w e^w E_a(w), \tag{5.121}$$

where $w = e^{-U}$, and $E_a(w)$ is a standard function closely related to the incomplete gamma function (see Abramowitz and Stegun, 1964, Ch. 5).

5.7 Duration times

Another interesting aspect of epidemic processes is the *duration time, T,* that is, the time that elapses before the epidemic ceases. In general, when removal from circulation is allowed, this will usually occur before the stock of susceptibles is exhausted. When the latter does occur, we say that the epidemic is *complete.* Otherwise, it is *incomplete.* In simple epidemics with no removal the process is always completed sooner or later. It is easily seen from, for example, equation (5.43) that all terms in $p_0(\tau)$ except the first tend to zero. Thus $p_0(\infty) = 1$.

A satisfactory explicit expression for the frequency distribution of the duration time is hard to obtain, but there is no difficulty in obtaining simple formulae for the cumulants. As we have already seen in Section 5.3, if there are r susceptibles and $n - r + 1$ infectives at time τ then the chance of one new infection in $\Delta\tau$ is $r(n - r + 1)\Delta\tau$. It follows that the time-interval τ_r between the occurrence of the rth infection and the $(r + 1)$th infection has the negative-exponential distribution given by

$$f(\tau_r) = r(n - r + 1)e^{-r(n-r+1)\tau_r}, \tag{5.122}$$

the moment-generating function being

$$M_r(\theta) = \left\{1 - \frac{\theta}{r(n-r+1)}\right\}^{-1}. \tag{5.123}$$

Since the τ_r are all independently distributed, it is clear that the moment-generating function of the duration time T, given by

$$T = \sum_{r=1}^{n} \tau_r, \tag{5.124}$$

is

$$M_T(\theta) = \prod_{r=1}^{n} \left\{1 - \frac{\theta}{r(n-r+1)}\right\}^{-1}. \tag{5.125}$$

Moreover, the νth cumulant κ_ν of T is simply the sum of the νth cumulants of the τ_r. Hence

$$\kappa_\nu = (\nu - 1)! \sum_{r=1}^{n} r^{-\nu}(n-r+1)^{-\nu}. \tag{5.126}$$

For desk computational purposes the easiest way of dealing with the latter expression is to expand by partial fractions to give terms involving inverse powers of natural numbers. Thus, following standard procedures, it is found that

$$\kappa_\nu = 2(\nu - 1)! \sum_{j=1}^{\nu} a_j S_j,$$

where

$$a_j = \binom{2\nu - j - 1}{\nu - 1} (n + 1)^{-2\nu + j}, \tag{5.127}$$

and

$$S_j = \sum_{u=1}^{n} u^{-j}.$$

For example,

$$\kappa_1 = \frac{2}{n+1} S_1, \quad \kappa_2 = \frac{4}{(n+1)^3} S_1 + \frac{2}{(n+1)^2} S_2, \quad \text{etc.} \tag{5.128}$$

A convenient further simplification can be made in terms of the polygamma functions $\psi(x)$, $\psi^{(1)}(x)$, $\psi^{(2)}(x)$, $\ldots$, which have been discussed and tabulated by Davis (1933, 1935) up to the hexagamma level, $\psi^{(4)}(x)$. We can use the well-known forms

$$S_1(n) = \psi(n + 1) - \psi(1),$$

$$S_j(n) = \frac{(-)^{j-1}}{(j-1)!} \{\psi^{(j-1)}(n + 1) - \psi^{(j-1)}(1)\}, \tag{5.129}$$

to express any κ_ν in terms of suitable polygamma functions.

Some exact values of κ_1, $\kappa_2^{\frac{1}{2}}$, γ_1, γ_2 and the coefficient of variation are shown in Table 5.2 for different values of n.

It is interesting to note that appreciable skewness and kurtosis persist even for infinite n. Moreover the coefficients γ_1 and γ_2 do not vary greatly over the range $10 \leqslant n \leqslant 80$. It is therefore worth considering the asymptotic form of the distribution as $n \to \infty$.

Table 5.2   *Some characteristics of the duration-time of a simple stochastic epidemic*

n	κ_1	$\kappa_2^{\frac{1}{2}} = \sigma$	γ_1	γ_2	C. of V. (%)
10	0·533	0·186	0·831	1·169	34·8
20	0·343	0·0938	0·774	1·081	27·4
40	0·209	0·0467	0·764	1·086	22·4
80	0·123	0·0231	0·771	1·114	18·9
∞	0·0	0·0	0·806	1·200	..

Asymptotically, we have $S_1(n) \sim \gamma + \log n$, where γ is Euler's constant, and $S_j(n) \sim \zeta(j), j > 1$, where $\zeta(j)$ is Riemann's zeta-function. Neglecting terms of relative order n^{-1}, we easily obtain, by substituting (5.129) in (5.127) and retaining the leading terms,

$$\left.\begin{aligned}
\kappa_1 &\sim \frac{2(\gamma + \log n)}{n + 1}, \\
\kappa_\nu &\sim \frac{2(\nu - 1)!}{n^\nu}\zeta(\nu), \quad \nu > 1.
\end{aligned}\right\} \tag{5.130}$$

The coefficient of variation, $\kappa_2^{\frac{1}{2}}/\kappa_1$, is thus asymptotically

$$\frac{\pi}{2\sqrt{3}(\log n)},$$

while the limiting values of γ_1 and γ_2 are

$$\lim_{n\to\infty} \gamma_1 = \frac{\sqrt{2}\zeta(3)}{\{\zeta(2)\}^{\frac{3}{2}}} = 0.806,$$

$$\lim_{n\to\infty} \gamma_2 = \frac{3\zeta(4)}{\{\zeta(2)\}^2} = 1.200.$$

It was first pointed out to me by D. G. Kendall (private communication, 1957) that a convenient closed form for the asymptotic distribution could be obtained by first using (5.130) to derive the cumulant-generating function for the variable $V = (n + 1)(T - \kappa_1)$, followed by inversion of the corresponding moment-generating function.

Actually it is simplest to work directly with the variable

$$W = (n + 1)T - 2\log n. \tag{5.131}$$

We can then write

$$\begin{aligned}
K_W(\theta) &\sim 2\gamma\theta + \sum_{\nu=2}^{\infty}(n + 1)^\nu \frac{2(\nu - 1)!}{n^\nu}\zeta(\nu)\frac{\theta^\nu}{\nu!} \\
&\to 2\gamma\theta + 2\sum_{\nu=2}^{\infty}\zeta(\nu)\theta^\nu/\nu
\end{aligned}$$

$$= 2\gamma\theta + 2 \sum_{\substack{v=2}}^{\infty} \lim_{k \to \infty} \sum_{j=1}^{k} \frac{1}{j^v} \frac{\theta^v}{v}$$

$$= 2\gamma\theta + 2 \lim_{k \to \infty} \sum_{j=1}^{k} \sum_{v=2}^{\infty} \frac{(\theta/j)^v}{v}$$

$$= 2\gamma\theta - 2 \lim_{k \to \infty} \sum_{j=1}^{k} \left\{ \frac{\theta}{j} + \log \left(1 - \frac{\theta}{j}\right) \right\}$$

$$= -2 \lim_{k \to \infty} \left\{ \log k^\theta \prod_{j=1}^{k} \left(1 - \frac{\theta}{j}\right) \right\},$$

using the usual definition of γ,

$$= 2 \log \Gamma(1 - \theta), \qquad (5.132)$$

using (5.106). Taking exponentials of (5.132) yields

$$M_W(\theta) \sim \{\Gamma(1 - \theta)\}^2. \qquad (5.133)$$

A more direct derivation can be obtained by going back to the result in (5.125). Using the transformation (5.131), we have immediately

$$M_W(\theta) = n^{-2\theta} \prod_{r=1}^{n} \left\{ 1 - \frac{(n + 1)\theta}{r(n - r + 1)} \right\}^{-1}$$

$$\sim n^{-2\theta} \prod_{r=1}^{n} \left(1 - \frac{\theta}{r}\right)^{-1} \left(1 - \frac{\theta}{n - r + 1}\right)^{-1},$$

using (5.103) with $a = 1$, as $n \to \infty$. Thus

$$M_W(\theta) \sim \left\{ n^{-\theta} \prod_{r=1}^{n} \left(1 - \frac{\theta}{r}\right)^{-1} \right\}^2$$

$$= \{\Gamma(1 - \theta)\}^2,$$

using (5.106), again recovering the result in (5.133). Inversion is more or less immediate using a standard form. For example, formula (17) on p. 349 of Erdélyi (1954), with the substitutions $\alpha = \beta = \frac{1}{2}$, $x = e^{-W}$, $s = -\theta$, shows that the required frequency distribution is

$$f(W) = 2e^{-W}K_0(2e^{-\frac{1}{2}W}), \quad -\infty < W < \infty, \qquad (5.134)$$

while the distribution function is

$$F(W) = 2e^{-\frac{1}{2}W}K_1(2e^{-\frac{1}{2}W}), \qquad (5.135)$$

where K_0 and K_1 are modified Bessel functions of the second kind. A more detailed and rigorous derivation of this result is given in D.G. Kendall (1957).

The limiting frequency function $f(W)$ has a mode at about $W = 0 \cdot 51$, and its asymmetry is illustrated by the fact that approximately 60 percent of the area under the curve lies to the right of the mode.

Generally speaking, Table 5.2 exhibits a quite considerable coefficient of variation, especially for groups whose size is less than about 40. Suppose, therefore, we envisage a more extended mathematical model involving epidemics (not necessarily simultaneous) in each of several idealized independent groups of only moderate size. It follows that quite substantial variation in epidemiological behaviour may be expected in the different groups, due only to statistical fluctuations. The practical implication is that, although it is tempting in practice to ascribe to unexpected findings such special causes as abnormal virulence or infectiousness, we should be particularly careful in the present context. A similar state of affairs will be found to exist in the more elaborate and realistic epidemic processes to be discussed later.

The results of this section can readily be extended to cover epidemics starting with a infectives, and to deal with the distribution of partial completion times, e.g. the time taken for the kth infection, say, to appear, where $a \leqslant k \leqslant n + a$. We simply start with the obvious generalization of (5.125), and can use either the exact approach starting with the partial fraction expansions of cumulants or the more direct method of proceeding with an asymptotic derivation. Störmer (1964) quotes, but does not prove, an asymptotic result for k and $n + a - k$ both large.

5.8 Perturbation and diffusion approximations

We have seen at the end of Section 5.2 that the moment-generating function $M_d(\theta, T)$ for the proportion ξ of susceptibles in the population at time $T = (n + a)\tau$ for the deterministic model satisfies the partial differential equation

$$\frac{\partial M_d}{\partial T} = \theta \left(\frac{\partial^2 M_d}{\partial \theta^2} - \frac{\partial M_d}{\partial \theta} \right), \tag{5.136}$$

with initial condition

$$M_d(\theta, 0) = e^{\theta/(1+\gamma)}, \tag{5.137}$$

where $\gamma = a/n$. Analogously, it appeared in Section 5.5 that the moment-generating function $M_s(\theta, T)$ for the proportion of susceptibles Ξ in the stochastic version satisfies the equation, to first order in N^{-1},

$$\frac{\partial M_s}{\partial T} = \theta \left(1 - \frac{\theta}{2N} \right) \left(\frac{\partial^2 M_s}{\partial \theta^2} - \frac{\partial M_s}{\partial \theta} \right), \tag{5.138}$$

with initial condition

$$M_s(\theta, 0) = e^{\theta/(1+\gamma)}, \tag{5.139}$$

where we are now writing

$$N = n + a. \tag{5.140}$$

As $N \to \infty$, equation (5.138) passes over into (5.136).

These results are now in a form suitable for the application of standard perturbation theory, provided that we can find a solution of (5.136) in terms of a basic eigenfunction expansion. The discussion turns out to be somewhat intricate, and for a full treatment of the details reference may be made to the paper by Bailey (1968). The essentials can be outlined as follows.

First, we try to solve (5.136) separating the variables. Substituting $M = q(\theta)e^{-\lambda T}$ in (5.136) gives

$$\theta \frac{d^2 q}{d\theta^2} - \theta \frac{dq}{d\theta} + \lambda q = 0, \tag{5.141}$$

where λ is any admissible eigenvalue, and q is the corresponding eigenfunction. Now (5.141) is a special case of the confluent hypergeometric equation, whose solution can be expressed in terms of Bateman's k-function. It is, however, algebraically more convenient to consider the more general equation

$$\theta \frac{d^2 q_j}{d\theta^2} + (1 + \alpha - \theta) \frac{dq_j}{d\theta} + \lambda_j q_j = 0, \tag{5.142}$$

whose solutions are given by

$$q_j = L_j^{(\alpha)}(\theta), \tag{5.143}$$

where $L_j^{(\alpha)}(\theta)$ is a generalized Laguerre polynomial, provided that the eigenvalues are non-negative integers, i.e.

$$\lambda_j = j, \quad j = 0, 1, 2, ..., \tag{5.144}$$

and $\alpha > -1$. Actually (5.142) only reduces to (5.141) if $\alpha = -1$. Some, but not all, useful properties of Laguerre polynomials also hold for $\alpha = -1$. The required standard results may be found in Abramowitz and Stegun (1964, Ch. 22) and Erdélyi (1953). We therefore proceed by temporarily replacing (5.136) by

$$\frac{\partial M}{\partial T} = \theta \frac{\partial^2 M}{\partial \theta^2} + (1 + \alpha - \theta) \frac{\partial M}{\partial \theta}, \tag{5.145}$$

since a separation of variables leads to (5.142). The initial condition (5.137) is retained unchanged. Appropriate mathematical operations are carried for a general α, and specific results obtained by letting $\alpha \to -1$ (usually as late as possible in the derivation).

It follows immediately that a formal solution of (5.145) is

$$M_d^{(\alpha)}(\theta, T) = \sum_{j=0}^{\infty} a_j e^{-\lambda_j T} q_j = \sum_{j=0}^{\infty} a_j e^{-jT} L_j^{(\alpha)}(\theta), \tag{5.146}$$

where the coefficients a_j can be determined from the initial condition. Thus

$$e^{\theta/(1+\gamma)} = \sum_{j=0}^{\infty} a_j q_j = \sum_{j=0}^{\infty} a_j L_j^{(\alpha)}(\theta). \qquad (5.147)$$

Using the basic orthogonality relationship for generalized Laguerre polynomials given by

$$\int_0^{\infty} e^{-\theta}\,\theta^{\alpha} L_j^{(\alpha)}(\theta)\, L_k^{(\alpha)}(\theta)\, d\theta = \delta_{jk}\frac{\Gamma(\alpha+j+1)}{j!}, \qquad (5.148)$$

we obtain straightaway

$$a_j = \frac{j!}{\Gamma(\alpha+j+1)}\int_0^{\infty} e^{-\gamma\theta/(1+\gamma)}\,\theta^{\alpha} L_j^{(\alpha)}(\theta)\, d\theta$$

$$= (1+\gamma^{-1})^{\alpha+1}(-\gamma)^{-j}, \qquad (5.149)$$

since the Laplace transform in the last line but one can be evaluated using a standard result, e.g. formula (28) on p. 174 of Erdélyi (1954) with θ, j and $\gamma/(1+\gamma)$ substituted for t, n and p, respectively.

If we put $z = -\gamma^{-1}e^{-T}$ in the Laguerre polynomial generating function

$$(1-z)^{-\alpha-1}\exp\left(\frac{\theta z}{z-1}\right) = \sum_{j=0}^{\infty} z^j L_j^{(\alpha)}(\theta), \qquad (5.150)$$

we see that $M_d^{(\alpha)}(\theta, T)$ in (5.146), subject to (5.149), can be put into the more compact form

$$M_d^{(\alpha)}(\theta, T) = \left\{\frac{(1+\gamma)e^T}{1+\gamma e^T}\right\}^{\alpha+1}\exp\left(\frac{\theta}{1+\gamma e^T}\right), \qquad (5.151)$$

which, when $\alpha = -1$, reduces to the solution of (5.136), $M_d(\theta, T) = \exp\{\theta/(1+\gamma e^T)\}$, already given in (5.25), and in fact specified in advance of the construction of the differential equation.

The advantage of the eigenfunction expansion in (5.146) is that, as already mentioned, we can appeal to standard perturbation theory. The next step, accordingly, is to replace the stochastic partial differential equation in (5.138) by the more general form involving α, given by

$$\frac{\partial M}{\partial T} = \left(1-\frac{\theta}{2N}\right)\left\{\theta\frac{\partial^2 M}{\partial\theta^2} + (1+\alpha-\theta)\frac{\partial M}{\partial\theta}\right\}, \qquad (5.152)$$

which is simply the perturbed form, to order N^{-1}, of (5.145).

Substituting $M = Q(\theta)e^{-\Lambda T}$ in (5.152) allows the variables to separate and leads to

$$\left(1-\frac{\theta}{2N}\right)\left\{\theta\frac{d^2 Q_j}{d\theta^2} + (1+\alpha-\theta)\frac{dQ_j}{d\theta}\right\} + \Lambda_j Q_j = 0, \qquad (5.153)$$

corresponding to (5.142). The general solution of (5.152), corresponding to (5.146), is therefore

$$M_s^{(\alpha)}(\theta, T) = \sum_{j=0}^{\infty} A_j e^{-\Lambda_j T} Q_j(\theta), \tag{5.154}$$

where A_j, Λ_j and Q_j are the perturbed forms of a_j, λ_j and q_j, respectively.

If we now write the differential operators on the right-hand sides of (5.145) and (5.152) as L_0 and L, respectively, we can put (5.142) and (5.153) in the form

$$L_0 q_j = -\lambda_j q_j, \quad L Q_j = -\Lambda_j Q_j. \tag{5.155}$$

Next, we assume that Λ_j, Q_j and L can be expressed to first order in N^{-1} as

$$\left. \begin{aligned} \Lambda_j &= \lambda_j + N^{-1} l_j, \\ Q_j &= q_j + N^{-1} r_j, \\ L &= L_0 + N^{-1} L_1. \end{aligned} \right\} \tag{5.156}$$

Substituting (5.156) in (5.155), assuming that the r_j can be expressed as linear functions of the q_j, and conveniently taking $A_j \equiv a_j$, allows all the unknowns to be computed, and leads eventually, after letting $\alpha \to -1$, to the result

$$\left. \begin{aligned} M_s(\theta, T) &= M_d(\theta, T) + N^{-1} \left\{ A(T) \frac{\partial^2}{\partial T^2} - B(T) \frac{\partial}{\partial T} \right\} M_d(\theta, T), \\ \end{aligned} \right.$$

where

$$A(T) = T + \frac{(e^T - 1)(1 + \gamma^2 e^T)}{2\gamma e^T},$$

and

$$B(T) = \frac{(e^T - 1)(1 - \gamma^2 e^T)}{2\gamma e^T}. \tag{5.157}$$

Equation (5.157) means that the stochastic moment-generating function can, to first order in N^{-1}, be expressed entirely in terms of the deterministic moment-generating function, which is a simple known function.

Equating coefficients of θ in (5.157) gives

$$m(T) = \xi(T) + N^{-1} \left\{ A(T) \frac{\partial^2}{\partial T^2} - B(T) \frac{\partial}{\partial T} \right\} \xi(T), \tag{5.158}$$

where $m(T)$ is the mean of the stochastic variable Ξ, and $\xi(T)$ is the deterministic proportion of susceptibles already given in (5.23) and repeated here for convenience, namely

$$\xi(\tau) = \frac{1}{1 + \gamma e^T}. \tag{5.159}$$

From (5.159) it easily follows that

$$\xi' = -\xi(1-\xi), \quad \xi'' = \xi(1-\xi)(1-2\xi), \quad \xi''' = -\xi(1-\xi)(1-6\xi+6\xi^2).$$
(5.160)

Substituting for ξ' and ξ'' in (5.158) gives

$$m(T) = \xi\left\{1 + \frac{(1-\xi)\{B+A(1-2\xi)\}}{N}\right\}.$$
(5.161)

The corresponding "reduced" epidemic curve, defined for Ξ and T as $Z = -dm/dT$, is obtained by differentiating (5.161) and using (5.160). We find, after a little reduction,

$$Z(T) = -\xi'\left\{1 - \frac{(A'+B'-A-B)+2\xi(3A+B-A')-6A\xi^2}{N}\right\}.$$
(5.162)

The chief implications of these approximations can be seen by recalling that in cases of interest a/N will be relatively small. Thus, although our approximations are valid for sufficiently large a and N, it is still legitimate to consider the possibility of small γ. In this event the leading terms of A, B, A' and B' are all $O(\gamma^{-1})$, i.e.

$$A, B \sim \frac{1-e^{-T}}{2\gamma}; \quad A', B' \sim \frac{e^{-T}}{2\gamma}.$$
(5.163)

Hence, substituting (5.163) in (5.161) and (5.162),

$$m(T) \sim \xi\left\{1 + \frac{(1-e^{-T})(1-\xi)^2}{a}\right\},$$
(5.164)

and

$$Z(T) \sim -\xi'\left\{1 - \frac{(1-\xi)\{(3\xi-1)+e^{-T}(2-3\xi)\}}{a}\right\}.$$
(5.165)

From (5.164) it can be seen that, under the specified conditions, the curve for the stochastic mean number of susceptibles lies wholly above the deterministic curve, as expected (see also Section 5.4), though the curves have the same end-points, since $1 - e^{-T} = 0$ when $T = 0$, and $\xi \to 0$ as $T \to \infty$. Also, to order N^{-1}, the stochastic and deterministic epidemic curves start at the same point, but the stochastic curve rises more slowly to begin with.

Now, the deterministic epidemic curve reaches its maximum when $e^{-T} = \gamma$ and $\xi = \frac{1}{2}$. At this point, and therefore beyond it as well, $e^{-T} = o(1)$, In this region, therefore, the asymptotic results in (5.164) and (5.165) simplify still further to

$$m(T) \sim \xi\left\{1 + \frac{(1-\xi)^2}{a}\right\},$$
(5.166)

and

$$Z(T) \sim -\xi' \left\{ 1 - \frac{(1-\xi)(3\xi-1)}{a} \right\}. \tag{5.167}$$

The deterministic and stochastic epidemic curves evidently reach their maxima at approximately the same time, but as $Z' \sim (16a)^{-1} > 0$ when $\xi = \frac{1}{2}$, the peak of the stochastic curve must occur slightly later. At the point where $\xi = \frac{1}{2}$ the ratio of the ordinates is

$$\frac{Z(T)}{-\xi'} \sim 1 - \frac{1}{4a}, \quad \xi = \frac{1}{2}. \tag{5.168}$$

The fact that this result is still approximately true for $a = 1$, $n = 10$, 20 (see Fig. 5.1 and 5.2) may be fortuitous.

After the maxima are reached, the deterministic curve falls more rapidly than the stochastic curve. The cross-over point occurs when $\xi = \frac{1}{3}$, i.e. when $T = \log(2/\gamma)$. When $a = 1$ this appears to be an underestimate, but the approximation is expected to be valid only for sufficiently large a.

The stochastic variance can also be approximated rather easily. Equating coefficients of θ in (5.138) shows that for the "reduced" variable Ξ we have

$$\frac{dm_1}{dT} = m_2 - m_1,$$

where m_1 and m_2 are the first and second moments about the origin. Thus the variance $\sigma^2(T)$ is given by

$$\sigma^2(T) = m^2 - m_1^2 = \frac{dm}{dT} + m - m^2 = -Z + m - m^2. \tag{5.169}$$

For small γ we can substitute from (5.164) and (5.165) to yield

$$\sigma^2(T) \sim a^{-1}\xi(1-\xi)^2 \{\xi + e^{-T}(1-\xi)\}. \tag{5.170}$$

Near the maximum of the epidemic curve and thereafter, when e^{-T} is small, we have

$$\sigma^2 \sim a^{-1}\xi^2(1-\xi)^2, \quad \sigma \sim a^{-\frac{1}{2}}\xi(1-\xi). \tag{5.171}$$

A general difficulty about this particular type of perturbation approach is that, if we wanted to improve the accuracy by including terms of order N^{-2}, we should have to modify equation (5.138) appropriately before embarking on the analysis. It would not be sufficient merely to develop a second-order approximation to (5.138) as it stands. The complexity of the work would thus be considerably increased.

An alternative approach, which appears to be more flexible, is that of Weiss (1970, 1971). This involves approximations to the moments, regarded as expansible in powers of N^{-1}. Going back to the discussion at the beginning of Section 5.5, let us generalize equation (5.82) to the case where the process starts with a infectives and n susceptibles. Writing, as in (5.140), $n + a = N$, and transforming the time variable to $T = Nt$, we easily find

$$\frac{d\mu_r'}{dT} = \sum_{k=1}^{r} (-)^{r-k+1} \binom{r}{j-1} (N\mu_k' - \mu_{k+1}'), \quad r \geqslant 1. \qquad (5.172)$$

We next introduce a normalized set of moments $\nu_r(T)$ defined by

$$\nu_r(T) = N^{-r}\mu_r'(T). \qquad (5.173)$$

Substitution in (5.172) gives

$$\frac{d\nu_r}{dT} = r(\nu_{r+1} - \nu_r) + \frac{1}{N} \sum_{k=0}^{r-2} (-)^k \binom{r}{k+2} N^{-k} (\nu_{r-k-1} - \nu_{r-k}), \qquad (5.174)$$

where we have picked out the leading term and reversed the order of summation. Now suppose that the moments can be expanded in inverse powers of N, e.g.

$$\nu_r = \nu_r^{(0)} + \frac{\nu_r^{(1)}}{N} + \frac{\nu_r^{(2)}}{N^2} + ..., \qquad (5.175)$$

where appropriate initial conditions are

$$\nu_r^{(0)}(0) = \xi^r(0) = (1+\gamma)^{-r}; \qquad \nu_r^{(j)}(0) \equiv 0, \quad j \geqslant 1, \qquad (5.176)$$

in conformity with (5.23) and (5.137). We proceed by substituting (5.175) into (5.174) and equating coefficients of N^{-j}. This gives

$$\frac{d\nu_r^{(j)}}{dT} = r(\nu_{r+1}^{(j)} - \nu_r^{(j)}) + G_r^{(j)}, \quad j \geqslant 0, \qquad (5.177)$$

where

$$G_r^{(0)}(\tau) \equiv 0,$$

and

$$\left. \begin{array}{l} \\ G_r^{(j)} = \sum_{k=0}^{j-1} (-)^k \binom{r}{k+2} (\nu_{r-k-1}^{(j-k-1)} - \nu_{r-k}^{(j-k-1)}), \quad j \geqslant 1, \end{array} \right\} \qquad (5.178)$$

In dealing with equation (5.177) we may suppose that $G_r^{(j)}$ is known, since it is a linear function of the quantities $\nu_s^{(l)}$, where $l \leqslant j - 1$, though there is one quantity for which $s = r$.

It is convenient to define

$$\nu_0^{(0)}(T) = 1; \qquad \nu_0^{(j)}(T) = 0, \quad j \geqslant 1, \qquad (5.179)$$

and to work with the new variables

$$\nu_r^{(j)}(T) = rU_r^{(j)}(T), \qquad G_r^{(j)}(T) = rH_r^{(j)}(T). \qquad (5.180)$$

We can now write (5.177) as

$$\frac{dU_r^{(j)}}{dT} = (r+1)U_{r+1}^{(j)} - rU_r^{(j)} + H_r^{(j)}, \quad r \geqslant 1, \tag{5.181}$$

where the $H_r^{(j)}$ may be supposed known.

If we now introduce the generating functions

$$U^{(j)}(s, T) = \sum_{r=1}^{\infty} U_r^{(j)} s^r, \quad H^{(j)}(s, T) = \sum_{r=1}^{\infty} H_r^{(j)} s^r, \tag{5.182}$$

the set of equations in (5.181) can be represented by

$$\frac{\partial U^{(j)}}{\partial T} = (1-s)\frac{\partial U^{(j)}}{\partial s} + H^{(j)} - U_1^{(j)}, \tag{5.183}$$

subject to the initial conditions

$$\left.\begin{array}{l} U^{(0)}(s, 0) = -\log\left(1 - \dfrac{s}{1+\gamma}\right), \\[2mm] U^{(j)}(s, 0) = 0, \quad j \geqslant 1. \end{array}\right\} \tag{5.184}$$

These conditions follow straightforwardly from putting $T = 0$ in (5.182) and using (5.180) and (5.176).

Equation (5.183) can be solved by the method of characteristics to give

$$\left.\begin{array}{l} U^{(0)}(s, T) = -\log\{1 - s\xi(T)\}, \\[2mm] U^{(j)}(s, T) = \displaystyle\int_0^T \{H^{(j)}(1 + (s-1)e^{-(T-x)}, x) - U_1^{(j)}(x)\}\, dx. \end{array}\right\} \tag{5.185}$$

Although $U_1^{(j)}(x)$ appears in the integrand, it can be found explicitly by differentiating with respect to s.

Now as $N \to \infty$ we have a purely deterministic result, as already noted. Hence

$$v_r^{(0)}(T) = \xi^r(T), \tag{5.186}$$

and this is the zero'th approximation. Next, we have

$$H_r^{(j)}(T) = G_r^{(1)}(T)/r, \quad \text{from (5.180),}$$

$$= \frac{1}{r}\binom{r}{2}(v_{r-1}^{(0)} - v_r^{(0)}), \quad \text{using (5.178),}$$

$$= \tfrac{1}{2}(r-1)(1-\xi)\xi^{r-1}, \tag{5.187}$$

substituting from (5.186). It follows from (5.182) that $H^{(1)}(s, T)$ can be written

$$H^{(1)}(s, T) = \frac{s^2\xi(1-\xi)}{2(1-s\xi)^2}. \tag{5.188}$$

We now substitute this value of $H^{(1)}(s, T)$ in (5.185) with $j = 1$. It turns out that the integral can be evaluated exactly, and then expanded in a power series in s. A fair amount of algebra is involved, but eventually we obtain

$$v_r^{(1)} = \tfrac{1}{2}r\gamma^{-1}(1 - \xi)^2 \{(r + 1)(1 - 2Te^{-T} - e^{-2T})\xi^r$$
$$+ 2r\,e^{-T}(T - 1 + e^{-T})\xi^{r-1} + (r - 1)e^{-T}(1 - e^{-T})\xi^{r-2}\}. \quad (5.189)$$

Thus we have derived the first approximation to all moments in a rather neat form, and further terms $v_r^{(j)}$, $j > 1$, can be derived from (5.180) and (5.185), straightforwardly if laboriously. When $r = 1$ it can be verified that $v_1^{(1)} = \xi(1 - \xi)\{B + A(1 - 2\xi)\}$, agreeing with the relevant term appearing in (5.161), as it should.

Another approach has been adopted by Daniels (1971) which involves seeking perturbation approximations to the cumulant-generating function. This provides further insight into the nature of the approximation and explains some of the difficulties in extending these methods to more general types of epidemic. Of course, in the simple epidemic application we obtain the same special results as already derived above.

Again, with an appropriate limiting procedure, a diffusion type of approximation can be obtained (McNeil, 1972). Further light is shed on some of the difficulties associated with homogeneous mixing, already referred to in connexion with the deterministic model in Section 5.2. This in turn leads to the consideration of a modified model discussed below in Section 5.10. Essentially, following McNeil, but changing the notation and some of the algebraic details, we first note that it is a little more convenient to work with the number of infectives Y as the random variable. The appropriate partial differential equation for the moment-generating function $M_Y(\theta)$, corresponding to (5.86), but now written for the original t-time with the contact-rate β appearing explicitly, is easily seen to be

$$\frac{\partial M_Y}{\partial t} = \beta(e^\theta - 1)\left(N\frac{\partial M_Y}{\partial \theta} - \frac{\partial^2 M_Y}{\partial \theta^2}\right), \quad (5.190)$$

with initial condition

$$M_Y(\theta, 0) = e^{a\theta}. \quad (5.191)$$

Let us put $\beta = \alpha/N$, and change the random variable from $Y(t)$ to $Z_N(t)$ given by

$$Z_N = \frac{Y - N\eta}{N^{\frac{1}{2}}}, \quad (5.192)$$

where, for the moment, η is an arbitrary function of t not involving N. Subsequently, we shall identify η with the deterministic proportion of infectives. It is also convenient to work with the characteristic function of Z_N, represented by $C_N(\theta) \equiv M_N(i\theta)$. It follows from (5.192) that

$$C_N(\theta) = \mathrm{E}\,\{\exp(i\theta Z_N)\} = \{\exp(-iN^{\frac{1}{2}}\theta\eta)\}M_Y(iN^{-\frac{1}{2}}\theta).$$

Hence

$$M_Y(iN^{-\frac{1}{2}}\theta) = e^{iN^{\frac{1}{2}}\theta\eta}C_N(\theta). \tag{5.193}$$

We next substitute $iN^{-\frac{1}{2}}\theta$ for θ, and $-iN^{-\frac{1}{2}}\partial/\partial\theta$ for $\partial/\partial\theta$, in (5.190), and use (5.193) to write the partial differential equation in terms of $C_N(\theta)$. Expanding in powers of N, and neglecting terms of order $N^{-\frac{1}{2}}$, then gives after a little algebra

$$\frac{\partial C_N}{\partial t} = iN^{\frac{1}{2}}\{\alpha\eta(1-\eta)-\eta'\}\theta C_N - \tfrac{1}{2}\alpha\eta(1-\eta)\theta^2 C_N + \alpha(1-2\eta)\theta\,\frac{\partial C_N}{\partial\theta}. \tag{5.194}$$

The limiting form of this equation will only remain valid as $N \to \infty$ if

$$\eta' = \alpha\eta(1-\eta). \tag{5.195}$$

But this is essentially the same as (5.21), having regard to the facts that $\eta = 1 - \xi$ and $T = \alpha t$. So that the function $\eta(t)$ appearing in (5.192) is simply the deterministic number of infectives at any time. With this identification, equation (5.194) becomes

$$\frac{\partial C}{\partial t} = -\tfrac{1}{2}\alpha\eta(1-\eta)\theta^2 C + \alpha(1-2\eta)\theta\,\frac{\partial C}{\partial\theta}, \tag{5.196}$$

where

$$C_N \to C \text{ as } N \to \infty.$$

Applying the usual inverse Fourier transform to (5.196) yields a partial differential equation for the limiting frequency function $f(x, t)$, namely

$$\frac{\partial f}{\partial t} = \tfrac{1}{2}\alpha\eta(1-\eta)\,\frac{\partial^2 f}{\partial x^2} - \alpha(1-2\eta)\,\frac{\partial(xf)}{\partial x}. \tag{5.197}$$

This is the forward Kolmogorov, or Fokker–Planck, diffusion equation corresponding to a non-stationary Ornstein–Uhlenbeck process, and it describes the behaviour of the random variable $Z(t) = \lim Z_N(t)$ as $N \to \infty$. The infinitesimal mean and variance of the process are $\alpha(1 - 2\eta)x$ and $\alpha\eta(1 - \eta)$, respectively.

Reference to (5.23) and (5.24) shows that $\eta = 1 - \xi \to 0$ for any T as $N \to \infty$, unless we are careful to ensure that the initial proportion of infectives $\eta(0) = a/N$ is bounded away from zero. There is then no loss of generality in assuming that $Z(0) = 0$, and that the Brownian motion characterized by (5.197) has zero mean. We can find the variance $v(t)$ of $Z(t)$ by substituting the characteristic function

$$C(\theta, t) = \exp(-\tfrac{1}{2}v\theta^2) \tag{5.198}$$

into equation (5.196). We obtain

$$\frac{dv}{dt} = \alpha\eta(1-\eta) + 2\alpha(1-2\eta)v, \tag{5.199}$$

subject to initial condition $v(0) = 0$. (5.200)

Equation (5.199) can be solved quite straightforwardly, using the explicit form of η given by

$$\eta(t) = \{1 + (c-1)e^{-\alpha t}\}^{-1}, \tag{5.201}$$

where $$c = 1/\eta(0), \tag{5.202}$$

to yield

$$v(t) = \frac{(c-1)e^{2\alpha t}\{e^{\alpha t} + 2(c-1)\alpha t + c(c-2) - (c-1)^2 e^{-\alpha t}\}}{(c-1+e^{\alpha t})^4}. \tag{5.203}$$

(This differs slightly from McNeil's formula (2.13). The latter appears to have a typographical error in the numerator.)

In conclusion therefore we may say that, if the contact-rate β is replaced by α/N, and if the limiting process is well-behaved, the distribution of $Y(t)$ is asymptotically normal as $N \to \infty$ with mean $N\eta(t)$ and variance $Nv(t)$. Further, if the Z_N process remains Markovian in the limit as $N \to \infty$, then the distributions of the Z_N converge to those of a non-stationary Ornstein–Uhlenbeck process with mean zero and variance $v(t)$. The trajectory of the epidemic process can thus be seen as an infinitesimal diffusion process superimposed on the purely deterministic curve. It will be noticed that the diffusion drift is positive to begin with, and remains so until half the population has been infected, after which it becomes negative.

For further development of the ideas involved in this kind of approximation, see McNeil and Schach (1973) and van Kampen (1973). There are, however, other powerful approaches such as the "principle of the diffusion of arbitrary constants", developed by Daley and D.G. Kendall (1965) and further elaborated by Barbour (1972). This technique allows one to find approximate analytical solutions of stochastic formulations using only integrals of the deterministic equations.

5.9   Estimation of infection-rate

Reference was made at the end of Section 5.7 to the considerable variations in epidemiological behaviour that could occur through purely statistical fluctuations. In order not to jump to unwarranted conclusions in interpreting actual data, if indeed such were available, it would be essential to carry out an appropriate statistical analysis, of which parameter estimation would be an essential ingredient. For example, when faced with data from two very different realizations of simple epidemic processes, one could estimate the contact-rate from

each batch of data separately and carry out an appropriate significance test to
see if there was any real evidence of a difference in contact-rates.

It seems unlikely that such an unstructured model as the simple epidemic
would often be applicable in practice, as already mentioned in the introductory
Section 5.1. But suppose that we had some kind of serological test that we
could use to determine whether an apparently healthy person in a well-defined
closed group was a susceptible or an infective. Then, if numbers were large
enough for the deterministic version to apply, we could try fitting the curves
of (5.3) or (5.8) in standard fashion to data giving the number of susceptibles
(or infectives) at a series of suitably chosen points in time.

In a genuinely deterministic situation standard errors would of course be
zero. In an approximately deterministic context the standard errors might be
expected to be small. But in smaller populations where probability fluctuations
in the model were appreciable we should have to consider a stochastic formulation.

Let us imagine that we had data recording the actual times at which the
susceptibles became infected. Appropriate methods of analysis have been
developed by Moran (1951a, 1953), and can be applied in the present context
as follows.

Since the simple epidemic is always completed sooner or later we can gain
no information about the infection-rate from the total size of epidemic. One
possibility is to use the times at which each fresh infection takes place, if these
are observable. This would give us a set of time-intervals between successive
infections, which would constitute the basic observations. Suppose the epidemic
starts with a infective and n susceptibles, and let the time-interval between the
occurrence of the $(k-1)$th and kth subsequent infections be t_k. Thus k runs
from 1 to n, and t_1 is the interval elapsing between the introduction of the a
infectives into the group and the occurrence of the first new infection.

Now at any instant in the interval between the occurrences of the $(k-1)$th
and kth infections there are $a + k - 1$ infectives and $n - k + 1$ susceptibles.
So that the chance of a new infection taking place in time dt_k is $\beta g_k dt_k$, where

$$g_k = (a + k - 1)(n - k + 1). \qquad (5.204)$$

The fact that infection in each interval takes place as a random Poisson process
implies the well-known fact that the distribution of the time-interval to the
next event is negative exponential. Hence the distribution of t_k is

$$dF = \beta g_k \exp(-\beta g_k t_k) dt_k, \quad 0 \leqslant t_k < \infty. \qquad (5.205)$$

Thus $2\beta g_k t_k$ is distributed like χ^2 with two degrees of freedom,

and
$$2\beta \sum_{k=1}^{n} g_k t_k$$

like χ^2 with $2n$ degrees of freedom. It follows that

$$\frac{1}{n} \sum_{k=1}^{n} g_k t_k$$

is a sufficient and unbiased estimate of β^{-1} with variance $\beta^{-2} n^{-1}$. (This is, moreover, an estimate having *minimum* variance.) Unless n is large, the precision of the estimate of β^{-1} from a single epidemic would be rather low as the coefficient of variation is $n^{-\frac{1}{2}}$. However, a familiar argument using the tails of the χ^2 distribution leads to confidence limits for β. Again, we can test the difference between estimates drawn from two different groups by means of a variance-ratio test, since $n^{-1} \Sigma gt$ is distributed like an estimated variance with $2n$ degrees of freedom based on a normal sample. With several groups we should resort to Bartlett's test for the homogeneity of variances.

If n were fairly small, as in the case of household data, then we might well have information from several such groups. As a rule the initial number of infectives in each group would be $a = 1$, and in that event the usual procedure of maximum-likelihood estimation leads to the estimate and variance

$$\hat{\beta} = N/S, \quad \text{var}(\hat{\beta}) = \hat{\beta}^2/N, \tag{5.206}$$

where
$$N = \sum_i n_i,$$

n_i being the number of susceptibles in the ith household; and $S = \Sigma g_k t_k$, the summation being over all intervals in all households.

Secondly, it might be that in continually sampling the population at predetermined points of time we could say exactly how many infectives and susceptibles there were. The data could thus consist of a set of ordered pairs (t_i, s_i), $i \geqslant 0$, where at time t_i we observed s_i infectives, and where $t_i < t_j$ for $i < j$. If we knew that the epidemic started with a infectives at $t_0 = 0$, the first pair in the set would be $(0, a)$. Otherwise we could choose the time origin at the first observation, e.g. $(0, s_0)$. In general, the probability of observing s_{i+1} infectives at time t_{i+1} given s_i at t_i is precisely the probability of observing s_{i+1} at time $t_{i+1} - t_i$ in a simple stochastic epidemic starting at time zero with s_i infectives and $N - s_i$ susceptibles, where N is the total size of the homogeneously mixing group.

The required probabilities can therefore be obtained by solving a set of differential–difference equations which are a simple extension of (5.30), namely

$$\left. \begin{array}{l} \dfrac{dp_r}{dt} = \beta(r + 1)(N - r - 1)p_{r+1} - \beta r(N - r)p_r, \quad 0 \leqslant r \leqslant N - s_i, \\[2mm] \text{with initial condition} \qquad p_{N-s_i}(0) = 1, \end{array} \right\} \tag{5.207}$$

and assuming $p_{N-s_i+1} \equiv 0$. We want of course to calculate explicitly the probability of $p_{N-s_{i+1}}(t_{i+1} - t_i)$. The product of all such conditional probabilities supplies the likelihood of the observed data for any given value of β, and this leads to the calculation of the maximum-likelihood value $\hat{\beta}$ by whatever numerical or computer technique seems appropriate.

It will be evident from the discussion of Section 5.3 that the algebraic complexities of this work could be enormous. However, some simplification of the required manipulations was introduced by Severo (1967a), who developed an iterative solution of the state probabilities, assuming an arbitrary initial distribution of the number of infectives. The reader should refer to this work and later papers by the same author for full details. Writing $p_{N-s,s}(t\,|\,a)$ for the probability that there are s infectives and $N - s$ susceptibles in the population at time $t \geq 0$, given that there were a infectives at time $t = 0$, Severo showed that for $s = a(1)N$ and $\tau = \beta t \geq 0$,

$$p_{N-s,s}(\tau\,|\,a) = \sum_{j=1}^{s+1} c(s + 1, j) \exp\{-(N-j+1)(j-1)\tau\}, \quad (5.208)$$

where

$$c(i,j) = \begin{cases} 0, & i < j \text{ or } i = j = 1, \\ -\sum_{u=1}^{i-1} c_1(i, u), & 1 < i = j \neq a + 1, \\ 1, & i = j = a + 1, \\ b(i, i-1)\{c_1(i-1, j)\delta(b_j - b_i) - c_2(i-1, j)\delta^2(b_j - b_i) \\ \quad + c_2(i-1, j)\delta(b_j - b_i)\tau\}, & i > j, \end{cases}$$

for $i, j = 1, ..., N + 1$. The functions c_1 and c_2 are defined recursively as the term independent of τ, and the coefficient of τ, respectively, in $c(i, j)$. In addition, $b(i, i - 1) = (N - i + 2)(i - 2)$, $b_i = -(N - i + 1)(i - 1)$, and $\delta(0) = \tau$; $\delta(x) = x^{-1}$, $x \neq 0$.

All this still appears to betray a considerable degree of algebraic intricacy, but it does lead to a manageable computational technique. Hill and Severo (1969) describe a convenient method of practical application to small groups and provide tables of the probability that at an arbitrary point of time there are $s = a(1)N$ infectives, given that at time zero there are $a = 1(1)N - 1$ infectives, for $2 \leq N \leq 10$. A number of auxiliary tabulations needed for the calculations are also included. For data within the limits of the tables the analysis can be carried out quite expeditiously. In dealing with larger groups, a possible procedure would be to calculate the individual conditional probabilities directly from (5.207) by means of numerical integration for any given value of β. This naturally lends itself to a completely computerized method of calculating the likelihood, and hence to finding the value $\hat{\beta}$ that maximizes the likelihood by using a computerized optimizing programme. A procedure of this kind is described below for estimating the two unknown parameters of the general stochastic epidemic in Section 6.8.

5.10 Nonhomogeneous mixing and other modifications

Both the deterministic model of Section 5.2 and the stochastic model introduced in Section 5.3 have assumed that the whole group of individuals concerned, comprising both susceptibles and infectives, is subject to homogeneous mixing. While this may be quite reasonable for small groups such as families, and some children's classrooms, there are doubts as to its applicability in larger groups.

One of the simplest modifications is to envisage two or more distinct groups, each group mixing homogeneously within itself as well as there being cross-infection between groups. This situation can become very complex. Rushton and Mautner (1955) discussed a deterministic model for many groups where there was infection but no removal, as in Section 5.2 above. Again, the simple stochastic epidemic was first extended to the case of two groups by Haskey (1957), although he obtained explicit analytic results only when the rates of infection within groups and between groups were all equal. The derivation of these results was subsequently considerably simplified by Becker (1968). The algebra is extremely complicated, and it seems likely that the general theoretical handling of several groups could be simplified by an extended use of the device already introduced in Section 5.3, where the chance of one new infection in $\Delta\tau$ was taken to be $r(N - r + 1)\Delta\tau$ instead of $r(n - r + 1)\Delta\tau$. It will be remembered that we assumed N to be non-integral, such that $N = n + \epsilon$, where eventually we let $\epsilon \to 0$.

Alternatively, the recursion methods of Severo (1967a) can be applied. These were later generalized by Severo (1969c), who showed in particular how applications could be made to the problem of stochastic cross-infection between several groups. Further results have recently been obtained by Kryscio (1972a). The interested reader should refer to these papers for details.

It was pointed out in Section 5.2 that one consequence of (5.11) is that the epidemic sweeps through a single group more rapidly as n increases. In fact, the mean of the normalized epidemic curve $\bar{\tau} \to 0$ as $n \to \infty$. A similar conclusion follows from the corresponding result in (5.100) for the stochastic model. Again, we see from (5.130) that the average duration time of a simple stochastic epidemic in τ-time is $\kappa_1 \sim 2(n + 1)^{-1} \log n$, for large n (and with $a = 1$ initially). Reintroducing the contact-rate β, the average duration time in t-time is $\kappa_1 \sim 2\beta^{-1}(n + 1)^{-1} \log n$. Thus, for fixed β, we have $\kappa_1 \to 0$ as $n \to \infty$. If, on the other hand, we use the rescaling adopted in the diffusion approximation of Section 5.8, that is $\beta = \alpha/n$, we have $\kappa_1 \sim 2\alpha^{-1} \log n \to \infty$ as $n \to \infty$. In any case the diffusion approximation does not easily lead to a treatment of duration-time since the deterministic proportion of infectives $\eta(t)$ never actually reaches unity.

There is clearly some difficulty in utilizing the basic model so as to obtain a satisfactory approximate representation of the epidemiological events in real time t as the group size becomes large.

All this suggests that there may be some advantage in modifying the basic model. Thus Severo (1969a) has suggested that the probability of one new infective in time Δt might be expressed as $\beta r^{1-b} s^a \Delta t$ instead of $\beta rs\Delta t$, where r and s are the numbers of susceptibles and infectives, respectively. Severo called the parameter a the *infection power*, and b the *safety-in-numbers power*. Departures from the classical values previously assumed, namely $a = 1$ and $b = 0$, can be made plausible by arguing as follows. A slowly developing epidemic might be due to a very small infection rate. But if it still develops slowly even when there are many infectives, then we might want the transition probability to be relatively independent of the number of infectives, i.e. a would then be small. This would happen, for example, if the rate of physical contact in a community were high but the transference of infection depended more on the susceptibility of a susceptible than on the infectiousness of an infective. The Greenwood, as opposed to the Reed–Frost, version of the chain-binomial model is an example of this idea (see Chapter 13). Conversely, a rapidly moving epidemic might be accounted for by a large infection rate. But if the existence of k infectives is in some sense more than k times as bad as having only one infective, then we might represent this situation by setting $a > 1$.

In a similar way we might suppose that the existence of large numbers of susceptibles would somewhat inhibit the ability of an infective to get around the community. A small value of b would tend to imply that there was greater safety in having more rather than fewer susceptibles, while b close to unity would mean that the chance of a given susceptible becoming infected was relatively independent of the number of susceptibles.

The difficulty with all these modifications is that it is not easy to relate non-classical values of a and b to any very precise mechanisms of infection transfer, although we might on occasion construct a model that was an empirically better fit to observed data. This whole subject obviously requires additional thought and investigation. For further discussion of the analytic consequences of the modified model the reader should consult Severo (1969a), Kryscio and Severo (1969), and Kryscio (1972a).

Another approach to modifying the classical model, which appeals to notions of geographical spread, although not incorporating this feature explicitly, has been suggested by McNeil (1972). This goes as follows.

Suppose that we have an infection spreading deterministically in a region such that the infected area is circular, and the rate of spread is proportional to the length of the boundary of the infected area, i.e.

$$\frac{d(\pi r^2)}{dt} \propto 2\pi r \propto (\pi r^2)^{\frac{1}{2}}. \tag{5.209}$$

If the population is spread uniformly over the region, the proportion of infectives $\eta(t)$ at time t then satisfies

$$\eta' \propto \eta^{\frac{1}{2}}. \tag{5.210}$$

This might be regarded as an analogue of the usual Malthusian type of population growth, for which

$$\eta' \propto \eta, \tag{5.211}$$

appropriately modified to account for geographical spread. The corresponding modification of (5.195), namely

$$\eta' = \alpha\eta(1-\eta), \tag{5.212}$$

would then be

$$\eta' \propto \{\eta(1-\eta)\}^{\frac{1}{2}}. \tag{5.213}$$

The upshot of these considerations is to try replacing the stochastic model first described at the beginning of Section 5.3 by one in which the chance of one new infection in time Δt is $\beta(XY)^{\frac{1}{2}}\Delta t$, instead of $\beta XY \Delta t$. This model is somewhat intractable to exact analysis, but a convenient limiting form can be obtained. We cannot derive a partial differential equation for the moment-generating function $M_Y(\theta)$ quite as simply as in our previous discussions. But, going back to first principles, we have

$$\frac{\partial M_Y}{\partial t} = \beta(e^\theta - 1) \, \mathrm{E}\{Y^{\frac{1}{2}}(N-Y)^{\frac{1}{2}}e^{\theta y}\}. \tag{5.214}$$

We now use the variable transformation (5.192) as in the previous diffusion approximation, but do *not* this time rescale the contact-rate β. Next, replace θ in (5.214) by $iN^{\frac{1}{2}}\theta$, use (5.193) to put M_Y in terms of C_N, and substitute for Y in terms of Z_N from (5.192). We then obtain, after a certain amount of straightforward algebra, and neglecting terms of order $N^{-\frac{1}{2}}$, the equation

$$\frac{\partial C_N}{dt} = iN^{\frac{1}{2}}\{\beta\eta^{\frac{1}{2}}(1-\eta)^{\frac{1}{2}} - \eta'\}\theta C_N - \tfrac{1}{2}\beta\eta^{\frac{1}{2}}(1-\eta)^{\frac{1}{2}}\theta^2 C_N$$

$$+ \frac{\beta(1-2\eta)}{2\eta^{\frac{1}{2}}(1-\eta)^{\frac{1}{2}}}\theta \, \frac{\partial C_N}{\partial\theta}. \tag{5.215}$$

The limiting form of this equation will remain valid as $N \to \infty$ if

$$\eta' = \beta\eta^{\frac{1}{2}}(1-\eta)^{\frac{1}{2}}. \tag{5.216}$$

This is the same as (5.123) with the appropriate constant inserted, and it is also the deterministic equation corresponding to the present stochastic model.

With this identification, the limiting form of equation (5.215) is

$$\frac{\partial C}{\partial t} = -\tfrac{1}{2}\beta\eta^{\frac{1}{2}}(1-\eta)^{\frac{1}{2}}\theta^2 C + \frac{\beta(1-2\eta)}{2\eta^{\frac{1}{2}}(1-\eta)^{\frac{1}{2}}}\,\theta\,\frac{\partial C}{\partial\theta}, \tag{5.217}$$

where $C_N \to C$ as $N \to \infty$, and η satisfies (5.216). In fact the explicit solution of (5.216) is immediately seen by elementary integration to be

$$\left.\begin{array}{l} \eta(t) = \sin^2\left(\tfrac{1}{2}\beta t + k\right), \quad 0 \leqslant t \leqslant (\pi - 2k)/\beta, \\[2mm] \quad\quad \eta(0) = \sin^2 k. \end{array}\right\} \tag{5.218}$$

where

So far as this solution is concerned, there is no problem in assuming that the initial proportion of infectives $\eta(0)$ is vanishingly small in the asymptotic theory, since the curve for $\eta(t)$ in (5.218) does not degenerate (as it does in the classical situation represented by the curve in (5.201)). However, for a satisfactory further development in the present case it is better not to assume that $\eta(0) = 0$.

The corresponding deterministic epidemic curve is evidently

$$z = \eta'(t) = \tfrac{1}{2}\beta\sin(\beta t + 2k), \quad 0 \leqslant t \leqslant (\pi - 2k)/\beta. \tag{5.219}$$

It is worth remarking that with the present modified model the deterministic epidemic is actually completed in time $(\pi - 2k)/\beta$. The epidemic curve itself is still symmetrical, but is now part of a sine curve.

Let us return to equation (5.217). We see that, analogously to the interpretation of (5.196), we again have a diffusion equation representing a non-stationary Ornstein–Uhlenbeck process, and describing the behaviour of the random variable $Z(t) = \lim Z_N(t)$ as $N \to \infty$. There is no loss of generality in assuming that $Z(0) = 0$, and that the Brownian motion characterized by (5.217) has zero mean. As before we can find the variance $v(t)$ of $Z(t)$ by substituting the characteristic function

$$C(\theta, t) = e^{-\frac{1}{2}v\theta^2} \tag{5.220}$$

in equation (5.217). We obtain

$$\frac{dv}{dt} = \beta\eta^{\frac{1}{2}}(1-\eta)^{\frac{1}{2}} + \frac{\beta(1-2\eta)}{\eta^{\frac{1}{2}}(1-\eta^{\frac{1}{2}})}\,v. \tag{5.221}$$

Replacing η in (5.221) by the value given in (5.218) yields

$$\frac{dv}{dt} = \tfrac{1}{2}\beta\sin(\beta t + 2k) + 2\beta v\cot(\beta t + 2k). \tag{5.222}$$

This can be solved by elementary means to give

$$v(t) = \sin^2(\beta t + 2k)\left\{H + \tfrac{1}{2}\log\tan(\tfrac{1}{2}\beta t + k)\right\}, \tag{5.223}$$

where H is an arbitrary constant to be determined from the initial conditions.

Thus if $v(0) = 0$, we have

$$H = -\tfrac{1}{2}\log \tan k. \tag{5.224}$$

We can therefore write the expression for the variance in the form

$$v(t) = \tfrac{1}{2}\sin^2(\beta t + 2k)\log\left\{\frac{\tan(\tfrac{1}{2}\beta t + k)}{\tan k}\right\}. \tag{5.225}$$

It is clear that $v(t)$ vanishes at the end of the epidemic interval when $t = (\pi - 2k)/\beta$, as expected.

Inspection of (5.225) shows that we cannot let $k \to 0$, as happens when $\eta(0) \to 0$. (It appears that McNeil's equation (4.7), equivalent to (5.220) above, should contain the additional constant.)

Finally, a limiting form for the duration time can be obtained quite easily using the kind of argument already employed at the beginning of Section 5.7. If there are r susceptibles and $N - r$ infectives at time t, the chance of one new infection in time Δt is $\beta r^{\frac{1}{2}}(N - r)^{\frac{1}{2}}\Delta t$ in the present case. Thus the frequency distribution of the time-interval t_r between the occurrence of the rth infection and the $(r + 1)$th infection is negative exponential with parameter $\beta r^{\frac{1}{2}}(N - r)^{\frac{1}{2}}$. The mean of this interval is $\beta^{-1}r^{-\frac{1}{2}}(N - r)^{-\frac{1}{2}}$, and the variance is $\beta^{-2}r^{-1}(N - r)^{-1}$. Thus the mean and variance of the duration time T, given by

$$T = \sum_{r=a}^{N-1} t_r, \tag{5.226}$$

can be expressed as

$$\bar{T} = \beta^{-1}\sum_{r=a}^{N-1} r^{-\frac{1}{2}}(N-r)^{-\frac{1}{2}}.$$

and

$$\operatorname{var} T = \beta^{-2}\sum_{r=a}^{N-1} r^{-1}(N-r)^{-1}.$$

For N large and a small, the first summation can be approximately represented by an integral in the usual way. The second summation, putting each term in partial fractions, is also straightforward to deal with. We quickly find

$$\bar{T} \sim \frac{\pi}{\beta}, \quad \operatorname{var} T \sim \frac{2\log N}{\beta^2 N}. \tag{5.227}$$

It follows that $T \to \pi/\beta$ in probability as $N \to \infty$.

Moreover, it can be shown that in the limit T is normally distributed. The νth cumulant of t_r is $\beta^{-\nu}r^{-\nu/2}(N - r)^{-\nu/2}$. Thus the νth cumulant of T is

$$\kappa_\nu = \beta^{-\nu}\sum_{r=a}^{N-1} r^{-\nu/2}(N-r)^{-\nu/2}. \tag{5.228}$$

For ν even, with $\nu = 2m$ say, comparison with (5.126) and (5.130) shows that

$$\kappa_{2m} \sim 2\beta^{-2m}\zeta(m)N^{-m}, \quad m > 1. \tag{5.229}$$

But for odd $\nu \geqslant 3$, we cannot use this argument and must proceed more directly. In fact, for *any* $\nu \geqslant 3$, we can write

$$
\begin{aligned}
\kappa_\nu &\sim \beta^{-\nu} \sum_{r=1}^{N-1} r^{-\nu/2}(N-r)^{-\nu/2} \\
&= \beta^{-\nu} N^{-\nu} \sum_{r=1}^{N-1} \left(\frac{r}{N}\right)^{-\nu/2} \left(1 - \frac{r}{N}\right)^{-\nu/2} \\
&= \beta^{-\nu} N^{-\nu} \sum_{r=1}^{N-1} \left\{\left(\frac{r}{N}\right)^{-\nu/2} + \left(1 - \frac{r}{N}\right)^{-\nu/2}\right\} \bigg/ f\!\left(\frac{r}{N}, \frac{\nu}{2}\right) \\
&= 2\beta^{-\nu} N^{-\nu/2} \sum_{r=1}^{N-1} r^{-\nu/2} \bigg/ f\!\left(\frac{r}{N}, \frac{\nu}{2}\right),
\end{aligned}
\tag{5.230}
$$

where
$$
f(x, \alpha) = x^\alpha + (1-x)^\alpha.
\tag{5.231}
$$

For given $\alpha > 0$, it is easy to show that $f(x, \alpha)$ is bounded in the range $0 \leqslant x \leqslant 1$. The summation is therefore asymptotically equal to $\zeta(\tfrac{1}{2}\nu)$ as $N \to \infty$. It follows that

$$
\kappa_\nu = O(\zeta(\tfrac{1}{2}\nu)N^{-\nu/2}), \quad \nu \geqslant 3.
\tag{5.232}
$$

This result is quite consistent with (5.229) but is less informative.

Let us now transform the duration-time to standard measure, e.g.

$$
W = \frac{T - \kappa_1}{\kappa_2^{1/2}}.
\tag{5.233}
$$

We see that the νth cumulant k_ν of W is

$$
k_\nu = \frac{\kappa_\nu}{\kappa_2^{\nu/2}} = O\!\left(\frac{N^{-\nu/2}}{(N^{-1}\log N)^{\nu/2}}\right) = O(\log N)^{-\nu/2} \to 0,
$$

as $N \to \infty$, valid for $\nu \geqslant 3$. It immediately follows that W is normally distributed with zero mean and unit standard deviation.

Finally, we mention the modification made by Grace Yang (1968; 1972a, b) in which a "mutation" parameter is introduced, so that new infectives also arise in a random way from the group of susceptibles. This leads of course to additional complications, but some new simplified methods of analysis have been devised.

6
General epidemics

6.1 General notions

We now turn to a more realistic and generally applicable representation of an epidemic. In addition to the essential ingredient of any epidemic process provided by the transfer of infection, we consider the possibility of removal of infectives from circulation by death or isolation. Both the latter events are subsumed under the single concept of removal. Basic parameters in the model are therefore the infection-rate and the removal-rate. This type of process is called "general" merely in the rather special sense of not being confined to infection only. There is in principle no limit to the extent to which ever more elaborate generalizations could take account of migration, loss of immunity, spatial distribution of cases, etc. However, the type of epidemic considered here does have characteristics which are sufficiently near to reality for useful results to be obtained.

Various important limitations are involved (though some of these are relaxed in the extensions considered in Section 6.9). For example, there is the assumption of an independent isolated group of given size, subject to homogeneous mixing. Again, it is assumed that when a susceptible is infected he immediately becomes infectious, i.e. there is no latent period. In the deterministic model infection and removal occur at certain specified density-dependent rates. It should however be noted that the supposition in the stochastic model that removal occurs as a random Poisson process implies that the infectious period (and incubation period) has a negative exponential distribution.

The above assumptions are mathematically convenient, and lead to theoretical descriptions of epidemic processes from which useful practical interpretations can be drawn. But at the same time we should not expect too close an agreement between theory and observation if data are examined in great detail.

Another aspect of the general model that is important in relation to practical interpretation and analysis of actual data is the following. Usually we do not know, and cannot observe, when a susceptible becomes infected. It is only when symptoms appear that the existence of the disease is recognized. If the

latter is at all serious the patient is then removed by isolation. This is the event
we can actually observe. The patient may subsequently die or he may recover,
when he is assumed, in the present discussion, to be immune to further infection. As the pattern of events after the recognition and isolation of a case is
not immediately relevant to the transmission of infection, it is not included in
the model.

In Section 6.2 we shall look at the deterministic model, noting in particular
the important Threshold Theorem first enunciated in approximate terms by
Kermack and McKendrick (1927), and the exact mathematical treatment given
by D.G. Kendall (1956). The remainder of the chapter is largely devoted to
discussion of the stochastic model, for which the literature has now become
very extensive. Section 6.4 deals with an analysis of the total size of the epidemic, and Section 6.5 presents the stochastic analogue of Kermack and
McKendrick's Threshold Theorem. Because of the relative intractability of the
general stochastic epidemic, approximation methods are of great importance.
Approximating stochastic systems are introduced in Section 6.6, and recent
work on asymptotic approximations is presented in Section 6.7. Section 6.8
discusses the estimation of parameters, including some recent developments.
Finally, a brief survey is given in Section 6.9 of the possibilities of relaxing
many of the restrictions previously employed so as to make the models more
realistic.

6.2   Deterministic model

Let us start by analysing the more general deterministic case, which entails
the removal of infectives from circulation by death or isolation in addition to
the mechanisms of infection already introduced for the simple deterministic
epidemic in Section 5.2.

Suppose we have a community of total size n, comprising, at time t, x susceptibles, y infectives in circulation, and z individuals who are isolated, dead, or
recovered and immune. Thus $x + y + z = n$. It will be realized that, so far as
transmission of disease is concerned, recovery is a comparatively unimportant
event that happens to some cases who have been isolated. As before, we have
β as the infection-rate, but now there is also the removal-rate γ to be taken
into account. In time Δt, therefore, there are $\beta xy\, \Delta t$ new infections and $\gamma y\, \Delta t$
removals. The basic differential equations are easily seen to be

$$\left. \begin{aligned} \frac{dx}{dt} &= -\beta xy, \\[2mm] \frac{dy}{dt} &= \beta xy - \gamma y, \\[2mm] \frac{dz}{dt} &= \gamma y. \end{aligned} \right\} \qquad (6.1)$$

It will be convenient in the sequel to make use of $\rho = \gamma/\beta$, the *relative removal-rate*. First, we shall consider an approximate method of examining these equations, and shall then go on to derive an exact solution.

At the start of the epidemic, when $t = 0$, let (x,y,z) take the values $(x_0,y_0,0)$. In particular, if y_0 is small, x_0 will be approximately equal to n. It follows from (6.1) that unless $\rho < x_0$ no epidemic can start to build up as this requires $[dy/dt]_{t=0} > 0$. The relative removal-rate, $\rho = x_0$, therefore gives a threshold density of susceptibles. A more precise discussion of this threshold behaviour will be given later. For the moment let us consider the approximate solution of (6.1) obtained by Kermack and McKendrick (1927). Eliminating y from the first and third of these equations by division gives, after integration,

$$x = x_0 e^{-z/\rho} \tag{6.2}$$

while the third equation can be written

$$\frac{dz}{dt} = \gamma(n - x - z), \tag{6.3}$$

using $x + y + z = n$. From (6.2) and (6.3) we obtain

$$\frac{dz}{dt} = \gamma(n - z - x_0 e^{-z/\rho}). \tag{6.4}$$

Direct solution of (6.4) to give z as a function of t does not appear possible, although an exact parametric form due to D. G. Kendall is available. This is discussed later. Here we consider the approximation that results from expanding the exponential factor in (6.4) as far as the term in z^2, giving

$$\frac{dz}{dt} = \gamma\left\{n - x_0 + \left(\frac{x_0}{\rho} - 1\right)z - \frac{x_0}{2\rho^2}z^2\right\}. \tag{6.5}$$

Although we are assuming that z/ρ is small, it is necessary to introduce the second-order terms as $(x_0/\rho) - 1$ may also be small. This will occur, for example, near the threshold, when $\rho = x_0$. Equation (6.5) is soluble by standard methods, and yields

$$z = \frac{\rho^2}{x_0}\left\{\frac{x_0}{\rho} - 1 + \alpha\tanh\left(\tfrac{1}{2}\alpha\gamma t - \phi\right)\right\},$$

where

$$\alpha = \left\{\left(\frac{x_0}{\rho} - 1\right)^2 + \frac{2x_0 y_0}{\rho^2}\right\}^{\frac{1}{2}}, \tag{6.6}$$

and

$$\phi = \tanh^{-1}\frac{1}{\alpha}\left(\frac{x_0}{\rho} - 1\right).$$

The epidemic curve is therefore

$$\frac{dz}{dt} = \frac{\gamma\alpha^2\rho^2}{2x_0}\operatorname{sech}^2\left(\tfrac{1}{2}\alpha\gamma t - \phi\right), \tag{6.7}$$

which is in general a symmetrical bell-shaped curve. It illustrates very well the common observation that in many actual epidemics the number of new cases reported each day climbs to a peak value and then dies away again. The deterministic model, moreover, exhibits this behaviour without recourse to variable rates of infection and removal, although these may well occur in practice as additional complications.

We next consider the total size of the epidemic, i.e. the total number of removals after the elapse of a very long, ideally infinite, period of time. If we let $t \to \infty$ in (6.6) we obtain

$$z_\infty = \frac{\rho^2}{x_0}\left(\frac{x_0}{\rho} - 1 + \alpha\right). \tag{6.8}$$

We can write this as

$$z_\infty \sim 2\rho\left(1 - \frac{\rho}{x_0}\right), \tag{6.9}$$

if $2x_0 y_0/\rho^2$ can be neglected compared with $\{(x_0/\rho) - 1\}^2$, since then α is approximately equal to $(x_0/\rho) - 1$. The approximate result (6.9) can also be derived by putting $dz/dt = 0$ and $x_0 \doteqdot n$ in (6.5). As we have already noted, there will be no true epidemic if $x_0 < \rho$. Suppose now that $x_0 > \rho$, and that we write

$$x_0 = \rho + \nu. \tag{6.10}$$

Substituting (6.10) in (6.9) shows that the total size of epidemic is approximately 2ν. The initial number of susceptibles, $\rho + \nu$, is thus reduced finally to $\rho - \nu$, i.e. to a value as far below the threshold, ρ, as it was originally above. This is Kermack and McKendrick's Threshold Theorem, which is clearly of considerable importance in understanding the mechanism underlying the absence or occurrence of outbreaks of epidemic disease. Similar results were obtained by Kermack and McKendrick for the more general case of variable infection- and removal-rates, and there is also an interesting extension to the situation where an intermediate host or vector is involved, as with malaria. This is discussed later in Section 11.2.

We now turn to a more mathematically precise treatment of the foregoing analysis based on the very elegant discussion of D. G. Kendall (1956). First, we examine the approximation used above by looking at the model for which it is an exact solution. Suppose, for the moment, we assume that the infection-rate is a function, $\beta(z)$, of z. Then (6.2) is replaced by

$$x = x_0 \exp\left\{-\frac{1}{\gamma}\int_0^z \beta(w)dw\right\}, \tag{6.11}$$

which, together with (6.3), gives

$$\frac{dz}{dt} = \gamma\left[n - z - x_0 \exp\left\{-\frac{1}{\gamma}\int_0^z \beta(w)dw\right\}\right]. \tag{6.12}$$

The equation (6.12) is the same as the approximation appearing in (6.5) when

$$\beta(z) = \frac{2\beta}{(1 - z/\rho) + (1 - z/\rho)^{-1}}. \tag{6.13}$$

Thus $\beta(0) = \beta$ and $\beta(z) < \beta$ when $0 < z < \rho$. Kermack and McKendrick's approximation therefore consistently underestimates the infection-rate and consequently the total size of epidemic as well. Moreover, if at any time $z > \rho$, the model will be quite unrealistic since we should then have a negative infection-rate. If the latter is to be kept within 10 per cent of its initial value we must have $z_\infty \leqslant 0.373\rho$.

Returning now to (6.4), we are led to consider the equation

$$n - z - x_0 \, e^{-z/\rho} = 0. \tag{6.14}$$

Let the unique negative and positive roots of (6.14) be $-\eta_1$ and η_2, respectively. We can therefore integrate (6.4) to give

$$t = \frac{1}{\gamma} \int_0^z \frac{dw}{n - w - x_0 \, e^{-w/\rho}}, \quad 0 \leqslant z < \eta_2, \tag{6.15}$$

which, when taken in conjunction with (6.4), gives a formal solution for the epidemic curve, dz/dt, in terms of a pair of parametric equations. The whole of the curve for $0 \leqslant t < \infty$ is involved since the integral in (6.15) diverges when $z \to \eta_2$, and therefore $z_\infty = \eta_2$. Unfortunately, the integral also diverges at the lower limit as $x_0 \to n$, so that in this case an infinite time elapses before the epidemic starts.

The latter difficulty is overcome by changing the origin to the point where $x = \rho$, which may be called the *centre* of the epidemic. Since

$$\frac{d}{dt}\left(\frac{dz}{dt}\right) = \gamma^2 y\left(\frac{x}{\rho} - 1\right), \tag{6.16}$$

as we find by differentiating (6.4) and substituting from (6.1) and (6.2), the peak of the epidemic curve occurs at the centre. From the third equation in (6.1) we see that the maximum number of infectives also occurs at the same time. We now write $x_0 = \rho$, and can still choose to take $z_0 = 0$, without loss of generality. The consequence of this is that the *numerical* value of $z(t)$ is the number of removals in $(0, t)$ for $t > 0$, and in $(t, 0)$ if $t < 0$. The corresponding parametric solution is thus

$$\left.\begin{aligned} t &= \frac{1}{\gamma} \int_0^z \frac{dw}{y_0 - w + \rho(1 - e^{-w/\rho})}, \\[2mm] \frac{dz}{dt} &= \gamma\{y_0 - z + \rho(1 - e^{-z/\rho})\}, \end{aligned}\right\} \tag{6.17}$$

where $-\infty < t < \infty$ and $-\zeta_1 < z < \zeta_2$, the quantities $-\zeta_1$ and ζ_2 now being the unique negative and positive roots, respectively, of

$$y_0 - \zeta + \rho(1 - e^{-\zeta/\rho}) = 0. \tag{6.18}$$

It will be seen that this way of looking at an epidemic has involved a certain change of attitude. Instead of regarding it as a continuous process starting at a specific point of time with x_0 susceptibles and y_0 infectives, we are considering the whole epidemic as an entity existing in the interval $-\infty < t < \infty$, with origin located for convenience at the point corresponding to the peak of the epidemic curve.

From (6.17) we see that $z_{-\infty} = -\zeta_1$ and $z_\infty = \zeta_2$, so that ζ_1 and ζ_2 are the numbers of removals occurring before and after the central point, the total size of the epidemic being $\zeta_1 + \zeta_2$. These will not in general be equal, so that here the epidemic curve is asymmetrical, in contrast to the Kermack and McKendrick approximation. We also have $y_{-\infty} = 0$, since $[dz/dt]_{t=-\infty} = 0$. Again, when $t = -\infty$, the total number, N, of susceptibles in the population is $N = \rho + y_0 + \zeta_1$, which is now the equivalent population size.

We next define the *intensity* of the epidemic as the proportion of the total number of susceptibles that finally contracts the disease, namely,

$$i = \frac{\zeta_1 + \zeta_2}{N}. \tag{6.19}$$

Thus we see that, when $t = -\infty$, the quantities (x, y, z) specifying the constitution of the population take the values $(N, 0, -\zeta_1)$, while at the other end of the time-scale when $t = \infty$ we have $(N - Ni, 0, Ni - \zeta_1)$. From the modified form of (6.2) applicable here, namely,

$$x = Ne^{-(z+\zeta_1)/\rho}, \tag{6.20}$$

it follows that

$$N - Ni = Ne^{-Ni/\rho}, \tag{6.21}$$

or

$$\frac{N}{\rho} = -\frac{\log(1-i)}{i}. \tag{6.22}$$

Table 6.1 gives the value of N/ρ for various values of i. (This table is similar to that given by Kendall, but the entries in the last three columns all contain an extra significant figure.) We can obtain further explicit information by considering the constitution of the population when $t = 0$, i.e. $(\rho, y_0, 0)$. This time (6.20) gives

$$\rho = Ne^{-\zeta_1/\rho}, \tag{6.23}$$

from which we obtain, in conjunction with (6.19),

$$\frac{\zeta_1}{\zeta_1 + \zeta_2} = \frac{\rho}{Ni} \log \frac{N}{\rho}. \tag{6.24}$$

This expression, also tabulated in Table 6.1, is the proportion of the total epidemic occurring before $t = 0$, and it is to some extent a measure of asymmetry in the epidemic curve. We can also calculate the number of infectives at $t = 0$ from $y_0 = N - \rho - \zeta_1$, i.e.

$$y_0 = N - \rho - \rho \log \frac{N}{\rho}, \tag{6.25}$$

while the peak height of the epidemic curve is simply γy_0.

Examination of this table reveals some very interesting characteristics of a general deterministic epidemic, and shows more accurately the nature of the threshold phenomena involved. As we have already noted, we must have $N > \rho$ for a mere trace of infection to cause an epidemic to build up. When the latter occurs, the number of susceptibles falls first to the threshold value, when the rate of cases notified is at its peak, and then continues to drop until it reaches the ultimate value $N(1 - i)$. If, for example, $N = 105$, $\rho = 100$, then we see from Table 6.1 that when $N/\rho = 1 \cdot 05$, $i \doteq 0 \cdot 09$. Thus 9 percent of the population will be affected by the disease, and the final number of susceptibles will

Table 6.1   *Some characteristics of a general deterministic epidemic*

Intensity of epidemic i	Ratio of population to threshold N/ρ	Percentage of population infectious at central epoch y_0/N	Percentage of removals occurring before central epoch $\zeta_1/(\zeta_1 + \zeta_2)$
0·00	1·000	0·00	50·0
0·10	1·054	0·13	49·5
0·20	1·116	0·56	49·1
0·30	1·189	1·33	48·5
0·40	1·277	2·55	47·9
0·50	1·386	4·30	47·1
0·60	1·527	6·79	46·2
0·70	1·720	10·33	45·0
0·80	2·012	15·55	43·4
0·90	2·558	24·20	40·8
0·95	3·153	31·87	38·3
0·98	3·992	40·27	35·4

be about 96. The approximate threshold theorem is therefore reasonably satisfactory. But if for the same value of ρ we took $N = 201$, so that the intensity was 0·80, then the final number of susceptibles would actually be about 40. In contrast with this, we should have obtained the value zero from the crude threshold theorem and 100 from the more accurate formula (6.9). From the last column of Table 6.1 we can see the degree of skewness exhibited by the epidemic curve. When N/ρ is as high as 4, nearly two-thirds of the removals occur after the peak, and this is in fact the type of asymmetry often found in actual notifications of infectious diseases.

While the general pattern of events portrayed in Table 6.1 applies to epidemics that exist over the whole interval $-\infty < t < \infty$, and are started up by a mere trace of infection, it is not difficult to deduce the consequences of introducing a non-zero number of infectives, a, into a population of susceptibles at some finite time. We can either re-work a modified form of the preceding analysis, or, alternatively, refer to a suitably chosen part of the process above. Suppose therefore that we envisage an epidemic starting with $x = N'$ and $y = a$. This can be regarded as a stage in the development of the process specified by (6.17), provided we take the corresponding value of z to be

$$- \zeta_1 - \rho \log (N'/N) = \rho \log (\rho/N'), \qquad (6.26)$$

using (6.20) and (6.23). It is then clear that with $a > 0$ we always have some kind of epidemic spread. If $\rho > N'$, the initial value of z is positive, and we are already past the centre. This means that the epidemic curve is J-shaped, and falls away to zero, corresponding to a minor outbreak only. If, on the other hand, $\rho < N'$, z is initially negative. In this case we are still in a pre-central phase, and there will be a true epidemic with a peaked epidemic curve. In either event the total number of secondary cases is evidently $N' - N(1 - i)$. For the purposes of calculation we need to know N in terms of N', a and ρ. This can be done by considering the total of x, y and z, which must remain constant and can be written as $N - \zeta_1$ or $N' + a + \rho \log (\rho/N')$, leading to the equation

$$N - \rho \log N = a + N' - \rho \log N'. \qquad (6.27)$$

These results suggest the sort of phenomena we should look for, though perhaps in a more diffuse form, when we come to examine the stochastic versions of these deterministic processes. This will be done in Section 6.3.

Certain extensions to equations (6.1), involving the removal of susceptibles and the arrival of fresh susceptibles and infectives, have been considered by Goffman (1965, 1966b). However, his main interest is in applications to the transmission and spread of ideas.

Again, Hammond and Tyrrell (1971) have used an alternative model, having a constant average duration of infection, to provide empirical descriptions of common-cold epidemics on Tristan da Cunha.

6.3 Stochastic model

We shall now consider the stochastic version of the general type of epidemic, with both infection and removal, already analysed deterministically in the previous section. It is quite easy to generalize the argument at the beginning of Section 5.3, where we dealt with the simple stochastic epidemic in terms of random variables $X(t)$ and $Y(t)$, representing the numbers of susceptibles and infectives, respectively. As before, we can write the chance of one new infection in Δt as $\beta XY \Delta t$, where β is the infection-rate. When this transition occurs, X decreases by one unit and Y increases by one unit. But this time we have the possibility of removal as well. The chance of one removal in Δt can be taken as $\gamma Y \Delta t$, where γ is the removal-rate. The variable Y decreases by one unit after the transition, but X remains unchanged. We can therefore argue as follows.

We suppose that at time $t = 0$ there are n susceptibles and a infectives. It is worth allowing for the possibility of more than one initial case, as we may want to apply this theory to household data where multiple introductions are not uncommon. We shall write $p_{rs}(t)$ for the probability that at time t there are r susceptibles still uninfected and s infectives in circulation. The chance of one new infection in time Δt is taken to be $\beta rs \Delta t$, and the chance of one removal $\gamma s \Delta t$. As mentioned above, this implies that the time-interval from the infection of any given susceptible to his eventual removal has a negative exponential distribution. As before, it is convenient to use the time-scale given by $\tau = \beta t$ instead of t. We now write $\gamma/\beta = \rho$, the ratio of removal-rate to infection-rate, which we shall call the *relative removal-rate*. The usual arguments about the relation between adjacent probability states lead to the differential–difference equations

$$\frac{dp_{rs}}{d\tau} = (r + 1)(s - 1)p_{r+1,s-1} - s(r + \rho)p_{rs} + \rho(s + 1)p_{r,s+1},$$

and

$$\frac{dp_{na}}{d\tau} = -a(n + \rho)p_{na}, \qquad\qquad\qquad (6.28)$$

where $$0 \leqslant r + s \leqslant n + a, \quad 0 \leqslant r \leqslant n, \quad 0 \leqslant s \leqslant n + a,$$

with initial condition $$p_{na}(0) = 1. \qquad\qquad\qquad (6.29)$$

It is worth noting here that if we introduce the probability-generating function, given by

$$P(z, w, \tau) = \sum_{r,s} p_{rs}(\tau) z^r w^s, \qquad\qquad (6.30)$$

this satisfies the partial differential equation

$$\frac{\partial P}{\partial \tau} = (w^2 - zw)\frac{\partial^2 P}{\partial z \partial w} + \rho(1 - w)\frac{\partial P}{\partial w}, \qquad\qquad (6.31)$$

with initial condition

$$P(z, w, 0) = z^n w^a, \qquad\qquad (6.32)$$

as may be shown by use of (6.28) or directly by a standard method (Bailey, 1964a, Sec. 7.4).

Use of the Laplace transformation appearing above in (5.32) replaces (6.28) by

$$(r + 1)(s - 1)q_{r+1,s-1} - \{s(r + \rho) + \lambda\}q_{rs} + \rho(s + 1)q_{r,s+1} = 0,$$

and

$$- \{a(n + \rho) + \lambda\}q_{na} + 1 = 0, \qquad (6.33)$$

subject to the same restrictions on the ranges of r and s as before, and where the q_{rs} are the Laplace transforms of the corresponding p_{rs}. Any q_{rs} whose suffixes fall outside the permitted ranges is taken to be identically zero. An exact calculation of the probabilities would be extremely laborious in all but the very simplest cases. It would, however, be quite straightforward as, starting with q_{na}, we could calculate all the q_{rs} in succession. Expansion in terms of partial fractions for λ, and application of the inverse Laplace transformation, would then exhibit each p_{rs} as the sum of exponential terms like $e^{-i(j+\rho)\tau}$.

No completely satisfactory way has yet been found of handling such expressions to yield individual probabilities, moments or cumulants, distribution of duration time, epidemic curves, etc. Nevertheless, certain possibilities for extensive manipulation do exist. Thus the recursive techniques of Severo (1967a, 1969c), already referred to in Sections 5.9 and 5.10, can be applied to the system of ordinary differential–difference equations in the state probabilities $p_{rs}(\tau)$ given in (6.28). The resulting algorithms can be used in practice to compute probabilities and likelihoods, for example, provided that the total population size is small.

The real difficulty, however, is to obtain an adequate degree of mathematical insight into the structure of the processes involved. An alternative approach adopted by Gani (1965a, 1967) and Siskind (1965) is to replace the expression in (6.30) for the probability-generating function by

$$P(z, w, \tau) = \sum_{r=0}^{n} z^r f_r(w, \tau), \tag{6.34}$$

where
$$f_r(w, \tau) = \sum_{s=0}^{n+a-r} w^s p_{rs}(\tau). \tag{6.35}$$

Substitution in the second-order partial differential equation (6.31) then leads to a set of linear first-order partial differential equations in the functions $f_r(w, \tau)$. Siskind (1965) solved this set of equations by direct recursive integration, leading eventually to formally explicit formulae for the individual probabilities $p_{rs}(\tau)$, the probability-generating function, the distribution of total epidemic size, and the distribution of extinction time for the process. Unfortunately, the amount of algebra required in these derivations is little short of heroic, and many of the results entail highly complicated formulae involving the use of multiple summation and product operators. One would of course like to have all this expressed more compactly in terms of known functions, but so far this has not proved feasible. A somewhat similar series of investigations were later carried out by Sakino (1968).

Gani (1965a), writing at the same time as Siskind, chose instead to work with the Laplace transforms (as in (5.32) above) of the $f_r(w, \tau)$ given by

$$F_r(w, \lambda) = \int_0^\infty e^{-\lambda\tau} f_r(w, \tau)d\tau, \quad \mathbf{R}(\lambda) > 0. \tag{6.36}$$

Using (6.32), the relevant set of linear first-order partial differential equations in the $F_r(w, \lambda)$ is easily found to be

$$\lambda F_r = w^2(r+1)\frac{\partial F_{r+1}}{\partial w} - \{(r+\rho)w - \rho\}\frac{\partial F_r}{\partial w}, \quad 0 \leqslant r \leqslant n-1,$$

$$\lambda F_n = w^a - \{(n+\rho)w - \rho\}\frac{\partial F_r}{\partial w}. \qquad\qquad\qquad (6.37)$$

These equations can also be integrated recursively. In some respects the work proceeds a little more easily than before, but the algebra is still very heavy and unwieldy to use in all but the simplest cases.

In his later paper, Gani (1967) proposed a simpler method of solution based on a matrix formulation of the problem. Suppose we take the equations in (6.37) in the reverse order given by $r = n, n-1, ..., 2, 1, 0$. Then they can be condensed in the matrix form

$$\mathbf{A}\frac{\partial \mathbf{F}}{\partial w} + \lambda \mathbf{F} = w^a \mathbf{E}, \qquad (6.38)$$

where $\mathbf{F}$ and $\mathbf{E}$ are $(n+1)$-rowed column vectors whose transposes are

$$\mathbf{F}' \equiv \{F_n, F_{n-1}, ..., F_0\}, \qquad \mathbf{E}' = \{1, 0, ..., 0\}, \qquad (6.39)$$

and $\mathbf{A}(w)$ is given by

$$\mathbf{A}(w) =$$

$$\begin{bmatrix}
(n+\rho)w - \rho & & & & \\
-nw^2 & (n-1+\rho)w - \rho & & & \\
& -(n-1)w^2 & (n-2+\rho)w - \rho & & \\
& ... & ... & ... & \\
& & -2w^2 & (1+\rho)w - \rho & \\
& & & -w^2 & \rho w - \rho
\end{bmatrix}$$

$$(6.40)$$

in which all empty positions are taken to be zero.

Now, using Taylor's Thorem, we can write

$$\mathbf{F}(w, \lambda) = \sum_{r=0}^{n+a} \mathbf{F}^{(r)}(0, \lambda)\frac{w^r}{r!}. \qquad (6.41)$$

This series must terminate with $r = n + a$ since w^{n+a} is the highest degree of w that can occur in the probability-generating function. From (6.38) it is possible ultimately to express all higher derivatives $\mathbf{F}^{(r)}(0, \lambda)$ in terms of $\mathbf{F}^{(0)}(0, \lambda) \equiv \mathbf{F}(0, \lambda)$.

After a certain amount of manipulation the required solution of (6.38) can be expressed in terms of the first $n + 1$ rows of the matrix equation

$$\begin{bmatrix} F(w,\lambda) \\ \int_0^w F(v,\lambda)dv \end{bmatrix} = \sum_{i=0}^{n+a+1} \frac{w^i}{i!} \left\{ \prod_{j=0}^{i-1} \mathbf{B}_j \right\} \mathbf{G} - \sum_{i=a+1}^{n+a+1} \frac{w^i}{i!} \frac{a!}{\rho} \left\{ \prod_{j=a+1}^{i-1} \mathbf{B}_j \right\} \mathbf{E}, \quad (6.42)$$

where
$$\mathbf{B}_j \equiv \begin{bmatrix} \frac{1}{\rho} \{ j\mathbf{A}^{(1)}(0) + \lambda \mathbf{I} \} & \frac{j(j-1)}{2\rho} \mathbf{A}^{(2)}(0) \\ \mathbf{I} & \mathbf{O} \end{bmatrix}, \quad (6.43)$$

$$\mathbf{G} \equiv \begin{bmatrix} F(0,\lambda) \\ \mathbf{O} \end{bmatrix}, \quad (6.44)$$

$$F(0,\lambda) = \left\{ \prod_{j=0}^{n+a} \mathbf{B}_j \right\}_{n+1}^{-1} \left[\frac{a!}{\rho} \left\{ \prod_{j=a+1}^{n+a} \mathbf{B}_j \right\}_{n+1} \mathbf{E} \right], \quad (6.45)$$

$\mathbf{I}$ is an $(n+1) \times (n+1)$ unit matrix, $\mathbf{O}$ is a zero vector or matrix of appropriate dimensions, $\mathbf{E}$ is a column vector of $2n+2$ elements of which the first is unity and the rest zero, the suffix $n+1$ indicates a truncated matrix involving the first $n+1$ rows and columns only, and we adopt the conventions that

$$\left. \begin{aligned} \prod_{j=h}^{k} \mathbf{B}_j &= \mathbf{I}, \quad h = k+1 \\ &= \mathbf{B}_k \mathbf{B}_{k-1} \dots \mathbf{B}_h, \quad h \leq k, \end{aligned} \right\} \quad (6.46)$$

the matrix multiplications being carried out in the order shown.

It should perhaps be pointed out that the matrix to be inverted in (6.45) is non-singular. By considering the structure of $\mathbf{A}^{(1)}(0)$ and $\mathbf{A}^{(2)}(0)$ it is not difficult to see that the matrix in question is triangular with non-zero eigenvalues for $\mathbf{R}(\lambda) > 0$.

For small values of a and n the algorithm arrived at above can be quite manageable. Gani gives an example with $a = 1$ and $n = 1$, and quotes J. Moreno as having successfully applied the method to higher values of a and n. Of course it will be noted that this yields the relevant $F_r(w, \lambda)$. To obtain the $f_r(w, \tau)$ we must invert the Laplace transforms, and then proceed via (6.35), (6.34) and (6.30) to obtain the probability-generating function and individual probabilities. This additional labour could be quite appreciable even in small groups, unless it can be systematized in some way. We shall return to some of the above results when discussing the distribution of the total epidemic size in the next section.

More recently, Lynne Billard (1973) has extended the Severo approach to yield formulae for the state probabilities which are simpler and less recursive than Severo's, and also to give expressions for the factorial moments of the number of susceptibles. Insight into the mathematical structure is enhanced, and the use of Laplace transforms is avoided, but a considerable number of multiple summations and products is still involved.

Which approach one prefers is probably very much a matter of individual taste. To the writer, however, the later work of Gani (1967) appears both to entail the simplest derivations and to exhibit the greatest degree of mathematical structure. At the same time the challenge to produce more compact results in terms of known functions still exists.

Mention should also be made of the work of Sakino (1959, 1962c, 1963, 1967) which investigates certain aspects of the age-distribution of infectives at time t, where age means the time elapsing for any individual since the point of infection. A full discussion of such problems would obviously lead to undertakings of even greater complexity than those described above.

6.4 Total size of epidemic

In spite of the difficulties just mentioned, useful results can be obtained if we attempt to investigate the distribution of the total size of epidemic, i.e. the value of $n - r$ for $t = \infty$, not counting the initial cases. Following Bailey (1953a) we may proceed as follows. As $t \to \infty$, all the terms in p_{rs} involving negative exponentials like $e^{-i(i+\rho)\tau}$ vanish, unless $i = 0$. The only term that remains is in fact equal to the coefficient of λ^{-1} in the expansion of q_{rs}. Since the epidemic ceases to involve fresh susceptibles as soon as $s = 0$, it easily follows that the probability P_w of an epidemic of total size w, not counting the initial a infectives, is given by

$$P_w = \lim_{t \to \infty} p_{n-w,0}, \quad 0 \leqslant w \leqslant n,$$
$$= \lim_{\lambda \to 0} \lambda q_{n-w,0},$$
$$= \lim_{\lambda \to 0} \rho q_{n-w,1},$$

putting $r = n - w$ and $s = 0$ in (6.33). Therefore

$$P_w = \rho f_{n-w,1}, \quad 0 \leqslant w \leqslant n, \tag{6.47}$$

where
$$f_{rs} = \lim_{\lambda \to 0} q_{rs}, \tag{6.48}$$
and
$$1 \leqslant r + s \leqslant n + a, \quad 0 \leqslant r \leqslant n, \quad 1 \leqslant s \leqslant n + a.$$

Putting $\lambda = 0$ in (6.33), and using the definition of f_{rs} in (6.48), gives the equations satisfied by the latter quantities, namely

$$(r+1)(s-1)f_{r+1,s-1} - s(r+\rho)f_{rs} + \rho(s+1)f_{r,s+1} = 0,$$
and
$$-a(n+\rho)f_{na} + 1 = 0, \tag{6.49}$$

the limits for r and s being the same as those appearing in (6.48). A convenient simplification of these equations is obtained by putting

$$f_{rs} = \frac{n!(r+\rho-1)! \, \rho^{n+a-r-s}}{sr!(n+\rho)!} g_{rs}. \tag{6.50}$$

Substitution in (6.49) then gives the recurrence formulae

$$g_{r+1,s-1} - g_{rs} + (r + \rho)^{-1} g_{r,s+1} = 0,$$

and $$g_{na} = 1.$$ (6.51)

One way of dealing with this is to solve partially so as to express g_{rs} as a linear function of $g_{r+1, i}$, $i = s - 1, ..., n + a - r - 1$. The expressions required are easily found to be

$$g_{rs} = \sum_{i=s-1}^{n+a-r-1} (r + \rho)^{s-i-1} g_{r+1,i}, \quad s \geqslant 2,$$

$$g_{r1} = (r + \rho)^{-1} g_{r2},$$

$$g_{na} = 1.$$ (6.52)

There is little difficulty in using (6.52) for computational purposes with small values of n, but it has the disadvantage of entailing the calculation of all the g_{rs}, whereas we are really concerned only with the g_{r1}.

An alternative method of some interest involves the solution of (6.51) using the set of generating functions

$$G_r(x) = \sum_{s=1}^{n+a-r} g_{rs}x^{s+1}, \quad 0 \leqslant r \leqslant n,$$ (6.53)

so as to yield a system of equations containing the g_{r1}, and hence the P_w, only. This can be done most readily by adapting somewhat a slightly more general method used by Whittle (1955) in the same context. Multiplying the first equation in (6.51) by x^{s+2} and summing over s leads to

$$G_r(x) = \frac{x^2}{x - (r + \rho)^{-1}} \{G_{r+1}(x) - (r + \rho)^{-1} g_{r1}\}, \quad 0 \leqslant r \leqslant n,$$ (6.54)

where, for the sake of uniformity, we introduce the *definition*

$$G_{n+1}(x) = x^a.$$ (6.55)

Since $G_r(x)$ is a polynomial, the denominator on the right-hand side of (6.54) must be a factor of the expression inside the braces. This is the most crucial step in the argument, giving immediately

$$g_{r1} = (r + \rho)G_{r+1}\left(\frac{1}{r + \rho}\right).$$ (6.56)

We now make repeated application of the recurrence relation in (6.54), with $x = (r + \rho)^{-1}$, to the right-hand side of (6.56). This leads finally, after a certain amount of elementary algebra and use of (6.47) and (6.50), to the set of equations

$$\sum_{w=0}^{j} \binom{n-w}{n-j}\left(\frac{n-j+\rho}{\rho}\right)^{w} P_w = \binom{n}{j}\left(\frac{n-j+\rho}{\rho}\right)^{-a}, \quad 0 \leqslant j \leqslant n,$$ (6.57)

in the required probabilities P_w.

An explicit expression for P_w can be obtained in partitional terms by an argument suggested to the author by Dr F. G. Foster. (See also Foster (1955) for a further discussion of the type of equations investigated by Whittle, and referred to above.) We regard the progress of the epidemic in terms of the succession of population states represented by the points (r, s). The process is thus seen as a random walk starting from the point (n, a) and ending at one of the points $(n - w, 0)$, $0 \leqslant w \leqslant n$, with an absorbing barrier along the line $s = 0$. The transitional probabilities are

$$\Pr\{(r, s) \to (r - 1, s + 1)\} = \frac{r}{r + \rho},$$

and $\qquad\qquad \Pr\{(r, s) \to (r, s - 1)\} = \frac{\rho}{r + \rho}.$ $\qquad\qquad$ (6.58)

The formula required can be written down more or less directly by considering the sum of probabilities of all possible paths from (n, a) to $(n - w, 0)$. One way of doing this is to take all paths to the point $(n - w, 1)$ which do not go below the line $s = 1$, followed by the final step to $(n - w, 0)$ with probability $\rho/(n + \rho - w)$. We thus obtain

$$P_w = \frac{n!\rho^{a+w}}{(n - w)!(n + \rho) \dots (n + \rho - w)}$$

$$\times \sum_{\alpha} (n + \rho)^{-\alpha_0} (n + \rho - 1)^{-\alpha_1} \dots (n + \rho - w)^{-\alpha_w}, \qquad (6.59)$$

where the summation is over all compositions of $a + w - 1$ into $w + 1$ parts such that

$$0 \leqslant \sum_{j=0}^{i} \alpha_j \leqslant a + i - 1$$

for $0 \leqslant i \leqslant w - 1$, and $1 \leqslant \alpha_w \leqslant a + w - 1$. If n were large, difficulties might arise from the partitional nature of the summation owing to uncertainty as to whether all relevant terms had been included.

It was recently pointed out by Williams (1970, 1971) that an appreciable simplification could be achieved by replacing the two-dimensional quantities P_w, seen as functions of w and n, by a one-dimensional function as follows. If we divide through equation (6.57) by the quantity on its right, we obtain

$$\sum_{w=0}^{j} \binom{j}{w} \left(1 - \frac{j}{n + \rho}\right)^{w+1} \left(1 + \frac{n}{\rho}\right)^{w+1} P_w \Big/ \binom{n}{w} = 1. \qquad (6.60)$$

From the form of these equations we can see that the transformation

$$f_w = \left(1 + \frac{n}{\rho}\right)^{w+1} P_w \Big/ \binom{n}{w} \qquad (6.61)$$

leads to a set of equations in the one-dimensional f_w, which will be expressible as functions of $n + \rho$. Writing

$$x = (n + \rho)^{-1}, \qquad (6.62)$$

and substituting (6.61) in (6.60), gives

$$\sum_{w=0}^{j} \binom{j}{w} (1-jx)^{w+1} f_w(x) = 1, \quad j \geq 0. \tag{6.63}$$

These equations constitute an infinite set, which is triangular in form and relatively easy to solve successively, starting with $f_0(x) = 1$, $f_1(x) = x/(1-x)^2$, etc. Using (6.61), we can easily recover the P_w.

The calculation of total epidemic size can also be approached using the methods of Gani (1967) described in the last section. It follows from the definition of $F_r(w, \lambda)$ in (6.36) that

$$F_r(0,\lambda) = \int_0^\infty e^{-\lambda\tau} f_r(0,\tau) d\tau$$

$$= \int_0^\infty e^{-\lambda\tau} p_{r0}(\tau) d\tau, \quad \text{using (6.35),}$$

$$= q_{r0}, \tag{6.64}$$

by the definition following (6.33). Hence, as in the first paragraph of this section,

$$P_w = \lim_{t\to\infty} p_{n-w,0}, \quad 0 \leq w \leq n,$$

$$= \lim_{\lambda\to 0} \lambda q_{n-w,0}$$

$$= \lim_{\lambda\to 0} \lambda F_{n-w}(0,\lambda), \quad \text{using (6.64).} \tag{6.65}$$

Let us now write $\mathbf{P}$ for the column vector whose transpose is $\mathbf{P}' = \{P_0, P_1, ..., P_n\}$. Using (6.39) and (6.65), we see that

$$\mathbf{P} = \lim_{\lambda\to 0} \lambda \mathbf{F}(0,\lambda)$$

$$= a! \left\{ \prod_{j=1}^{n+a} \mathbf{B}_j(0) \right\}_{n+1}^{-1} \left\{ \prod_{j=a+1}^{n+a} \mathbf{B}_j(0) \right\}_{n+1} \mathbf{E}, \tag{6.66}$$

where we have substituted from (6.45), noting that

$$\mathbf{B}_0(\lambda) = \begin{bmatrix} \dfrac{\lambda}{\rho} \mathbf{I} & \mathbf{O} \\[2mm] \mathbf{I} & \mathbf{O} \end{bmatrix}.$$

A convenient aspect of (6.66) is that it allows us to compute the vector of probabilities of total epidemic size in terms of a set of direct matrix operations. Gani illustrates the method for the simple case $a = 1$, $n = 1$, and it is evident that computer calculations for more general values of a and n would be quite straightforward. For very small a and n there is no obvious advantage over direct solution of the equations in (6.63), but for large a or n the Gani method may well be superior, since all the matrices $\mathbf{B}_j(0)$ are very simple in form. It should be remembered, however, that the equations in (6.63) are triangular in form, and their solution presents no great numerical problem.

Table 6.2 *Probabilities, P_w, and maximum-likelihood scores for ρ, for $a = 1$ and $n = 1, 2, 3, 4$ and 5*

$n = 1$: $\quad P_0 = \rho/(\rho+1) \quad \hat{\rho} = a_0/a_1 \quad I_\rho = N/\rho(\rho+1)^2$

$\qquad\quad P_1 = 1/(\rho+1)$

$n = 2$: $\quad P_0 = \rho/(\rho+2)$

$\qquad\quad P_1 = 2\rho^2/(\rho+2)(\rho+1)^2$

$\qquad\quad P_2 = 2(2\rho+1)/(\rho+2)(\rho+1)^2$

$$S(\rho) = \frac{a_0 + 2a_1}{\rho} + \frac{2a_2}{2\rho+1} - \frac{2(a_1+a_2)}{\rho+1} - \frac{N}{\rho+2}$$

$n = 3$: $\quad P_0 = \rho/(\rho+3)$

$\qquad\quad P_1 = 3\rho^2/(\rho+3)(\rho+2)^2$

$\qquad\quad P_2 = 6\rho^3(2\rho+3)/(\rho+3)(\rho+2)^2(\rho+1)^3$

$\qquad\quad P_3 = 6(5\rho^3 + 12\rho^2 + 8\rho + 2)/(\rho+3)(\rho+2)^2(\rho+1)^3$

$$S(\rho) = \frac{a_0 + 2a_1 + 3a_2}{\rho} + \frac{2a_2}{2\rho+3} + \frac{(15\rho^2 + 24\rho + 8)\,a_3}{5\rho^3 + 12\rho^2 + 8\rho + 2} - \frac{3(a_2+a_3)}{\rho+1} - \frac{2(a_1+a_2+a_3)}{\rho+2} - \frac{N}{\rho+3}$$

$n = 4$: $\quad P_0 = \rho/(\rho+4)$

$\qquad\quad P_1 = 4\rho^2/(\rho+4)(\rho+3)^2$

$\qquad\quad P_2 = 12\rho^3(2\rho+5)/(\rho+4)(\rho+3)^2(\rho+2)^3$

$\qquad\quad P_3 = 24\rho^4(5\rho^3 + 27\rho^2 + 47\rho + 27)/(\rho+4)(\rho+3)^2(\rho+2)^3(\rho+1)^4$

$\qquad\quad P_4 = 24(14\rho^6 + 93\rho^5 + 235\rho^4 + 293\rho^3 + 197\rho^2 + 74\rho + 12)/(\rho+4)(\rho+3)^2(\rho+2)^3(\rho+1)^4$

$$S(\rho) = \frac{a_0 + 2a_1 + 3a_2 + 4a_3}{\rho} + \frac{2a_2}{2\rho+5} + \frac{(15\rho^2 + 54\rho + 47)\,a_3}{5\rho^3 + 27\rho^2 + 47\rho + 27}$$
$$+ \frac{(84\rho^5 + 465\rho^4 + 940\rho^3 + 879\rho^2 + 394\rho + 74)\,a_4}{14\rho^6 + 93\rho^5 + 235\rho^4 + 293\rho^3 + 197\rho^2 + 74\rho + 12}$$
$$- \frac{4(a_3+a_4)}{\rho+1} - \frac{3(a_2+a_3+a_4)}{\rho+2} - \frac{2(a_1+a_2+a_3+a_4)}{\rho+3} - \frac{N}{\rho+4}$$

$n = 5$: $\quad P_0 = \rho/(\rho+5)$

$\qquad\quad P_1 = 5\rho^2/(\rho+5)(\rho+4)^2$

$\qquad\quad P_2 = 20\rho^3(2\rho+7)/(\rho+5)(\rho+4)^2(\rho+3)^3$

$\qquad\quad P_3 = 60\rho^4(5\rho^3 + 42\rho^2 + 116\rho + 106)/(\rho+5)(\rho+4)^2(\rho+3)^3(\rho+2)^4$

$$P_4 = \frac{120\rho^5(14\rho^6 + 177\rho^5 + 910\rho^4 + 2443\rho^3 + 3626\rho^2 + 2836\rho + 918)}{(\rho+5)(\rho+4)^2(\rho+3)^3(\rho+2)^4(\rho+1)^5}$$

$$P_5 = \frac{120(42\rho^{10} + 596\rho^9 + 3604\rho^8 + 12{,}240\rho^7 + 25{,}941\rho^6 + 36{,}144\rho^5 + 34{,}061\rho^4 + 21{,}952\rho^3 + 9456\rho^2 + 2448\rho + 288)}{(\rho+5)(\rho+4)^2(\rho+3)^3(\rho+2)^4(\rho+1)^5}$$

$$S(\rho) = \frac{a_0 + 2a_1 + 3a_2 + 4a_3 + 5a_4}{\rho} + \frac{2a_2}{2\rho+7} + \frac{(15\rho^2 + 84\rho + 116)\,a_3}{5\rho^3 + 42\rho^2 + 116\rho + 106}$$
$$+ \frac{(84\rho^5 + 885\rho^4 + 3640\rho^3 + 7329\rho^2 + 7252\rho + 2836)\,a_4}{14\rho^6 + 177\rho^5 + 910\rho^4 + 2443\rho^3 + 3626\rho^2 + 2836\rho + 918}$$
$$+ \frac{(420\rho^9 + 5364\rho^8 + 28{,}832\rho^7 + 85{,}680\rho^6 + 155{,}646\rho^5 + 180{,}720\rho^4 + 136{,}244\rho^3 + 65{,}856\rho^2 + 18{,}912\rho + 2448)\,a_5}{42\rho^{10} + 596\rho^9 + 3604\rho^8 + 12{,}240\rho^7 + 25{,}941\rho^6 + 36{,}144\rho^5 + 34{,}061\rho^4 + 21{,}952\rho^3 + 9456\rho^2 + 2448\rho + 288}$$
$$- \frac{5(a_4+a_5)}{\rho+1} - \frac{4(a_3+a_4+a_5)}{\rho+2} - \frac{3(a_2+a_3+a_4+a_5)}{\rho+3}$$
$$- \frac{2(a_1+a_2+a_3+a_4+a_5)}{\rho+4} - \frac{N}{\rho+5}$$

Some actual values of P_w, expressed as functions of ρ, are given in Table 6.2 for $a = 1$ and $n = 1, 2, 3, 4,$ and 5. Formulae to facilitate the maximum-likelihood estimation of ρ are also given, but this will be described more fully when the whole question of estimating ρ from observed household distributions is taken up again in Section 6.8.

It is worth mentioning here that the first published account of an epidemic model of this sort appeared as early as 1926 in a paper by McKendrick. Unfortunately, McKendrick was considerably ahead of his time and the research attracted little attention. Nevertheless, his treatment of the probability model was fully stochastic, though lacking the now available techniques of investigation. In particular, McKendrick gave the probability distributions for total size of epidemic for the two cases $a = 1$, $\rho = 2$, $n = 4$ and 5, remarking on the U-shaped distributions obtained. A more extensive set of results are shown in Fig. 6.1, 6.2 and 6.3, for $a = 1$, $n = 10$, 20 and 40, over suitable ranges of values of ρ. All the probabilities used here were originally calculated using equations (6.47), (6.50) and (6.51). It is immediately clear from the diagrams that when the relative removal-rate ρ is large the epidemic tends to be small, and conversely. At first sight one is impressed by the fairly gradual transition between the two extremes, and a similar continuous change can be observed in the drop in average size of epidemic with increasing ρ shown in Table 6.3. Nevertheless, as pointed out by D. G. Kendall (discussion to Bailey, 1955, and Kendall, 1956), for $n \leqslant \rho$ the

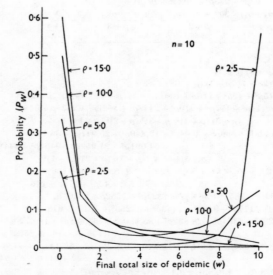

Fig. 6.1   Diagram showing the probability of the final total size of the epidemic for groups of ten susceptibles, starting with the introduction of one new infectious case

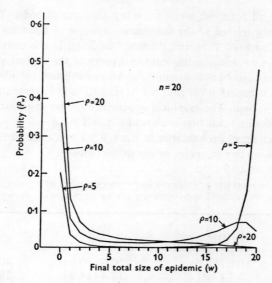

Fig. 6.2 Diagram showing the probability of the final total size of the epidemic for groups of twenty susceptibles, starting with the introduction of one new infectious case

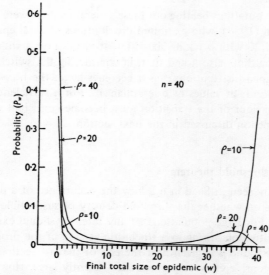

Fig. 6.3 Diagram showing the probability of the final total size of the epidemic for groups of forty susceptibles, starting with the introduction of one new infectious case

distributions are all J-shaped, while for $n > \rho$ they are bimodal. This state of affairs is obviously related to the stochastic analogue of Kermack and McKendrick's Threshold Theorem, discussed in detail in the next section. There is not, however, a necessarily discontinuous jump at the critical value $n = \rho$ from one type of distribution to another. An unpublished calculation by the writer for the just supercritical case $a = 1$, $n = 40$, $\rho = 39$, reveals a distribution still markedly J-shaped. The graphical appearance of the distribution is in fact hardly distinguishable from that shown in Fig. 6.3 for $a = 1$, $n = 40$, $\rho = 40$, although the very small probabilities in the tail for epidemic sizes of 38, 39 and 40 do show relative increases of about 50 percent.

Table 6.3   *Average total size of epidemic $\bar{w}$, for various values of ρ and n, with $a = 1$. The values for Kendall's approximating stochastic system are shown in brackets*

ρ/n	n		
	10	20	40
0	10·0 (10·0)	20·0 (20·0)	40·0 (40·0)
0·25	7·1 (7·5)	14·4 (14·9)	29·1 (29·6)
0·50	4·3 (4·8)	8·0 (8·8)	15·3 (16·8)
0·75	2·7 (3·8)	4·3 (5·1)	6·9 (7·4)
1·00	1·9 —	2·6 —	3·6 —
1·25	1·4 (4)	1·8 (4)	2·2 (4)
1·50	1·1 (2)	1·3 (2)	1·5 (2)

Additional computations bearing out these general features were made by Spicer and Lipton (1958), who exhibited distributions of total epidemic size for $n = 5$, 10 and 20 with ρ taking six different values over a wide range in each case. These authors also noted that, in considering the switchover from J-shaped to U-shaped distributions, "as n becomes larger the transition is much less abrupt and occurs at values of ρ less than n". For n sufficiently large, however, the behaviour of the transition must become consistent with the threshold phenomenon discussed in the next section.

6.5   Stochastic threshold theorem

We have already seen in Section 6.2 how the occurrence of a deterministic epidemic depends on whether the threshold density of susceptibles is actually exceeded or not. For large populations, at any rate, we should expect to find some analogous situation arising in a stochastic version of the process. A hint of what might be found was given near the end of the last section, but the population sizes considered were perhaps insufficiently large. However, as pointed out by Bartlett (1955, p. 129), when n is large, the population of infectives is approximately subject to a birth-and-death process with birth- and death-rates βn and γ, respectively. Now the chance of ultimate extinction for such a process is $(\rho/n)^a$ if $\rho < n$, and unity if $\rho \geqslant n$, where we write $\rho = \gamma/\beta$, as before. Thus in the latter case we might expect only a small outbreak, but in the former either a minor outbreak or a major build-up. Although the absence of explicit general expressions for the probability distribution of total size of epidemic makes an exact analysis difficult, an ingenious method of investigating limiting behaviour more fully has been found by Whittle (1955), and is the basis of the following discussion.

We concentrate attention on calculating the probability that an epidemic of not more than a given *intensity* (cf. Section 6.2) shall take place. If π_i is the chance that not more than a proportion i of the n susceptibles are eventually attacked, then

$$\pi_i = \sum_{w=0}^{ni} P_w, \qquad (6.67)$$

where the P_w are given by (6.57) or (6.59), or by (6.61) and (6.63). Suppose we now compare the process under consideration, for which the chance of one new infection in time Δt is $\beta rs \, \Delta t$, with two other processes for which the corresponding chances are $\beta ns \, \Delta t$ and $\beta n (1 - i)s \, \Delta t$. Then it is intuitively clear that, so far as epidemics of not more than ni new cases are concerned, the true process lies uniformly between the other two, in the sense that the probabilities of given epidemic size are intermediate. The advantage of this procedure is that the two new processes, one "fast" and one "slow", are fairly straightforward birth-and-death processes for which explicit solutions are available.

A direct method of procedure is first to consider a process for which the chance of one new infection in time Δt is $As \, \Delta t$, substituting the special values of A, i.e. βn and $\beta n (1 - i)$, later. Thus we have a birth-and-death process for the *population of infectives*, with constant birth- and death-rates, A and γ. We must, however, introduce the restriction that no new births occur if the cumulative population size, $u = a + w$, i.e. the total number of individuals who have ever been infected, reaches $n + a$. The value of $u - a$ as $t \to \infty$ gives the total size of epidemic as previously defined. It is easily seen that so far as epidemic sizes, given by $a \leqslant u_\infty \leqslant n + a - 1$, are concerned, the probabilities for these states of the restricted process are exactly the same as those for the corresponding states in the unrestricted process, for which u may take any value. The balance of probability, to make up a total of unity, is then assigned to the state $u_\infty = n + a$. We can therefore obtain a solution by first considering the unrestricted process, for which the standard approach already used above (cf. Kendall, 1948a) readily leads to the partial differential equation

$$\left. \begin{aligned} \frac{\partial P}{\partial t} &= \{Ayx^2 - (A + \gamma)x + \gamma\}\frac{\partial P}{\partial x}, \\[2pt] \text{where} \qquad P(x, y, t) &= \Sigma p_{su}x^s y^u, \end{aligned} \right\} \qquad (6\!:\!68)$$

and the boundary condition is

$$P(x, y, 0) = x^a y^a. \tag{6.69}$$

Auxiliary equations for (6.68) are

$$\frac{dP}{0} = \frac{dt}{1} = \frac{dx}{Ayx^2 - (A + \gamma)x + \gamma} = \frac{dy}{0}, \tag{6.70}$$

from which we can obtain the independent integrals

$$\left.\begin{array}{r} P = \text{const.,} \\ y = \text{const.,} \\ \dfrac{x - \xi}{\eta - x} e^{-Ay(\eta - \xi)t} = \text{const.,} \end{array}\right\} \tag{6.71}$$

where $\xi(y)$ and $\eta(y)$ are the roots of the quadratic in x

$$Ayx^2 - (A + \gamma)x + \gamma = 0, \tag{6.72}$$

chosen so that $0 < \xi < 1 < \eta$ when $y < 1$. The general solution is then

$$P = \Psi\left\{y, \frac{x - \xi}{\eta - x} e^{-Ay(\eta - \xi)t}\right\}. \tag{6.73}$$

The form of the arbitrary function Ψ is determined from the boundary condition (6.69). We find

$$P(x, y, t) = y^a \left\{\frac{\xi(\eta - x) + \eta(x - \xi)e^{-Ay(\eta - \xi)t}}{(\eta - x) + (x - \xi)e^{-Ay(\eta - \xi)t}}\right\}^a, \tag{6.74}$$

from which the limiting distribution of u is obtained as

$$P(1, y, \infty) = y^a \xi^a$$

$$= \left(\frac{A + \gamma}{2A}\right)^a \{1 - (1 - ky)^{\frac{1}{2}}\}^a, \tag{6.75}$$

where

$$k = \frac{4A\gamma}{(A + \gamma)^2}, \tag{6.76}$$

and the positive square root is taken in (6.75). We can expand (6.75) in powers of y using Lagrange's expansion for $\psi(\zeta) \equiv \zeta^a$, where $\zeta = 1 - (1 - ky)^{\frac{1}{2}}$ is the root of $\zeta^2 - 2\zeta + ky = 0$ that vanishes when $y = 0$. This gives the following probabilities for the variable $w = u - a$,

$$\left.\begin{array}{l} P_w(A) = \dfrac{a(2w + a - 1)!}{w!(w + a)!} \dfrac{A^w \gamma^{w+a}}{(A + \gamma)^{2w+a}}, \quad 0 \leqslant w \leqslant n - 1, \\[3mm] P_n(A) = 1 - \displaystyle\sum_{w=0}^{n-1} P_w(A). \end{array}\right\} \tag{6.77}$$

Although the solution of the general process for unrestricted cumulative population size given by (6.74) has been derived on the assumption of almost certain ultimate extinction, for which we must have $\gamma \geqslant A$, it is easily seen that the solution of the restricted process given by (6.77) will in fact be valid for any γ or A.

It is worth observing here that (6.77) can also be obtained, as was done by Whittle, by writing down the basic set of differential–difference equations for the probabilities, and using the method of solution employed in Section 6.3 to deal with equation (6.28). The simplest recurrence relation obtainable is like (6.51), but without the factor $(r+\rho)^{-1}$. Subsequent analysis along similar lines leads to a set of simultaneous equations corresponding to (6.57). The difficulty is that we then have to depend on spotting the solution, to be verified subsequently by induction.

Returning now to the "fast" and "slow" processes, with A put equal to βn and $\beta n(1-i)$, respectively, we see that

$$\sum_0^{ni} P_w(\beta n) \leqslant \pi_i \equiv \sum_0^{ni} P_w \leqslant \sum_0^{ni} P_w(\beta n - \beta ni). \tag{6.78}$$

Let us consider the partial sum

$$\sum_0^{ni} P_w(A)$$

as n becomes large. From (6.77) we have, using (6.76),

$$\frac{P_{w+1}(A)}{P_w(A)} = \frac{(2w+a+1)(2w+a)}{(w+1)(w+a+1)} \frac{A\gamma}{(A+\gamma)^2}$$

$$= k\left\{1 - \frac{3}{2w} + O\left(\frac{1}{w^2}\right)\right\}. \tag{6.79}$$

Since k can never exceed unity, it follows from the ratio test that

$$\sum_0^{\infty} P_w(A)$$

converges and has the value

$$\sum_0^{\infty} P_w(A) = \left\{\frac{A+\gamma-|A-\gamma|}{2A}\right\}^a$$

$$= [\min\{\gamma/A, 1\}]^a. \tag{6.80}$$

Applying this result to (6.78) gives, for sufficiently large n,

$$[\min\{\rho/n, 1\}]^a \leqslant \pi_i \leqslant [\min\{\rho/n(1-i), 1\}]^a, \tag{6.81}$$

writing $\rho = \gamma/\beta$, as before.

Three main cases follow from (6.81), namely,

$$\left.\begin{array}{ll} \text{(i)} \ \rho < n(1-i), & \left(\dfrac{\rho}{n}\right)^{a} \leqslant \pi_i \leqslant \left\{\dfrac{\rho}{n(1-i)}\right\}^{a}; \\[4mm] \text{(ii)} \ n(1-i) \leqslant \rho < n, & \left(\dfrac{\rho}{n}\right)^{a} \leqslant \pi_i \leqslant 1; \\[4mm] \text{(iii)} \ n \leqslant \rho, & \pi_i = 1. \end{array}\right\} \quad (6.82)$$

The statements appearing in (6.82) constitute Whittle's Stochastic Threshold Theorem. This is the stochastic analogue of the deterministic threshold results already discussed in Section 6.2. Whittle's theorem may be interpreted by saying that if $\rho \geqslant n$, there is zero probability of an epidemic exceeding any pre-assigned intensity i; while if $\rho < n$, the probability of an epidemic is approximately $1 - (\rho/n)^{a}$, for small i.

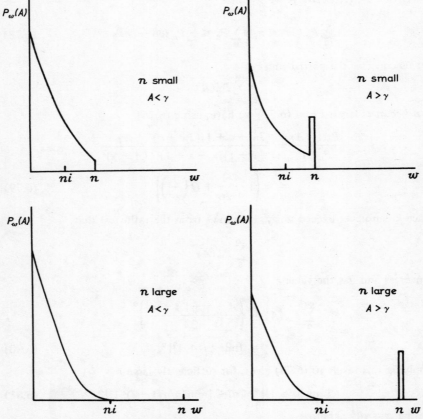

Fig. 6.4   General appearance of the frequency distribution P_w for total size of epidemic, on the assumption of a constant infection-rate

Further light is shed on the behaviour of the process by considering the general shape of the distribution in (6.77). In any case $P_w(A)$ diminishes, after a certain point, with increasing w, for $w \leqslant n - 1$, and will tend to zero if n is sufficiently large. If $\gamma \geqslant A$, the sum of the probabilities up to the point ni will tend to unity. But if $\gamma < A$, the sum will tend to the value $1 - (\gamma/A)^a$, so that $P_n(A)$ must equal $(\gamma/A)^a$. The general appearance of the frequency distribution for large and small n and $\gamma \lessgtr A$ (i.e. $\rho \lessgtr n$, if i is small) is shown in Fig. 6.4. These results, applicable to modified processes with *constant* infection-rates, exhibit clear-cut behaviour. True epidemic processes with varying rates may be expected to show the same general characteristics in a more continuous form. Indeed such a conclusion is very much in harmony with the comments made by D. G. Kendall (near end of Section 6.4) on the exact distributions for $a = 1$ and $n = 10, 20, 40$ already presented in Fig. 6.1, 6.2 and 6.3. It appears that if $\rho > n$ there is likely to be only a minor outbreak, but if $\rho < n$ we can expect *either* a minor outbreak *or* a major epidemic, intermediate situations being relatively improbable.

Recently, a more direct, algebraic proof of the threshold theorem for large n has been obtained by Williams (1970, 1971) working from his own result previously exhibited in (6.63). He showed, after a fair amount of ingenious but lengthy algebra (Williams, 1970), that P_w could be asymptotically represented, as $n \to \infty$, by

$$P_w \sim \frac{(2w)!}{w!(w+1)!} \frac{\theta^{w+1}}{(1+\theta)^{2w+1}},$$

(6.83)

where

$$\theta = \rho/n,$$

(6.84)

θ being the relative removal rate per susceptible. The elegant simplicity of the result in (6.83) suggests that it should be obtainable more immediately from the theory already discussed in Section 6.4. And in fact we can proceed in a fairly elementary way as follows.

From (6.47) and (6.50), we have, with $a = 1$,

$$
\begin{aligned}
P_w &= \frac{n!(n+\rho-w-1)!\rho^{w+1}}{(n-w)!(n+\rho)!} g_{n-w,1} \\
&= \frac{n(n-1)\ldots(n-w+1)\rho^{w+1}}{(n+\rho)(n+\rho-1)\ldots(n+\rho-w)} g_{n-w,1} \\
&= \frac{\left(1-\frac{1}{n}\right)\ldots\left(1-\frac{w-1}{n}\right)}{\left(1-\frac{1}{n+\rho}\right)\ldots\left(1-\frac{w}{n+\rho}\right)} \frac{n^w \rho^{w+1}}{(n+\rho)^{w+1}} g_{n-w,1} \\
&\sim \frac{n^w \rho^{w+1}}{(n+\rho)^{w+1}} g_{n-w,1}, \quad \text{as } n \to \infty \text{ with fixed } w, \\
&= \frac{n^w \theta^{w+1}}{(1+\theta)^{w+1}} g_{n-w,1},
\end{aligned}
$$

(6.85)

using (6.84), and where the $g_{n-w,1}$ are given by the solution of (6.51). Now, for any given w, we are concerned with the quantities g_{rs} for which $n - w \leqslant r \leqslant n$, that is $0 \leqslant n - r \leqslant w$. The factor $(r + \rho)^{-1}$ on the left of (6.51) can be written

$$(r + \rho)^{-1} = (n + \rho)^{-1} \left\{ 1 - \frac{n - r}{n + \rho} \right\}^{-1} = x, \qquad (6.86)$$

to first order in $x = (n + \rho)^{-1}$, as defined in (6.62), over the relevant range of $n - r$.

We can therefore replace (6.51) asymptotically by

$$g_{r+1,s-1} - g_{rs} + x g_{r,s+1} = 0,$$

and
$$g_{n1} = 1. \qquad (6.87)$$

Next, let us make the substitution

$$g_{rs} = a_{rs} x^{n-r-s+1}. \qquad (6.88)$$

Equations (6.87) then become

$$a_{rs} = a_{r+1,s-1} + a_{r,s+1},$$

and
$$a_{n1} = 1, \qquad (6.89)$$

where of course all a_{rs} outside the relevant ranges of subscripts, $0 \leqslant r \leqslant n$, $1 \leqslant s \leqslant n + 1$, $1 \leqslant r + s \leqslant n + 1$, as in (6.48) with $a = 1$, are identically zero.

Noting that $x = (n + \rho)^{-1} = n^{-1}(1 + \theta)^{-1}$, we can combine (6.85) and (6.88) to give

$$P_w \sim \frac{a_{n-w,1} \theta^{w+1}}{(1 + \theta)^{2w+1}}, \qquad (6.90)$$

where $a_{n-w,1}$ can be computed from the first $w + 1$ equations of the triangular set given by (6.89).

Values of $a_{n-w,1}$, starting with $w - 1$, are $1, 2, 5, 14, 52, \dots$. Suspecting a factorial in the denominator, we look at $w! \, a_{n-w,1}$. The resulting numbers in this series factorize to give $1, 4, 5.6, 6.7.8, 7.8.9.10, \dots$. We immediately surmise that

$$a_{n-w,1} = \frac{(2w)!}{w! \, (w + 1)!}, \qquad (6.91)$$

which with (6.90) gives the result already quoted in (6.83).

An elementary proof of the correctness of (6.91) is easy to obtain. Given this value of $a_{n-w,1}$, we can use (6.89) to construct $a_{n-w,2}$, $a_{n-w,3}$, etc. Examination of the ratios of successive terms in this series (actually four are sufficient) quickly suggests that the general term is

$$a_{n-w,j} = \frac{j(2w-j+1)!}{(w+1)!(w-j+1)!}.$$

(6.92)

It is readily verified that this satisfies (6.89) and is thus the general solution required.

Now

$$P(\theta) = \sum_{w=0}^{\infty} P_w$$

(6.93)

is the probability that the total number of cases is of *finite* size. Thus if $P(\theta) = 1$, there can be no true epidemic for the limiting case of $n \to \infty$. But if $P(\theta) < 1$, the distribution is defective, with the missing probability of $1 - \theta$ corresponding to a true epidemic running through the whole population.

Using (6.83), we have

$$P(\theta) = \sum_{w=0}^{\infty} \frac{(2w)!}{w!(w+1)!} \frac{\theta^{w+1}}{(1+\theta)^{2w+1}}$$

$$= \frac{\theta}{1+\theta} \sum_{w=0}^{\infty} \frac{(2w)!}{w!(w+1)!} y^w,$$

(6.94)

where

$$y = \frac{\theta}{(1+\theta)^2}.$$

(6.95)

The coefficients in the series on the right of (6.94) immediately recall a binomial expansion with index $\frac{1}{2}$. It is easily seen that the series in fact sums to

$$\sum_{w=0}^{\infty} \frac{(2w)!}{w!(w+1)!} y^w = \frac{1-(1-4y)^{\frac{1}{2}}}{2y}$$

(6.96)

Substituting (6.96) in (6.94), and using (6.95), gives

$$P(\theta) = \tfrac{1}{2}(1+\theta - |1-\theta|),$$

(6.97)

the modulus of $1 - \theta$ appearing since we have to take the positive square root of $(1-4y)^{\frac{1}{2}}$. Thus we finally have

$$\begin{aligned} P(\theta) &= \theta, \quad \theta < 1, \\ &= 1, \quad \theta \geqslant 1. \end{aligned}$$

(6.98)

(We can also derive these expressions algebraically by noting that the terms in (6.94) are a special case of (6.77) and (6.80) with $a = 1$, $A = 1$, $\gamma = \theta$.)

The results in (6.98) constitute Williams' version of the threshold theorem, namely that when the relative removal rate per susceptible θ is greater than or equal to unity there is no true epidemic, while if it is less than unity a true epidemic can occur with probability $1 - \theta$.

6.6   Approximating stochastic systems

Whittle's Stochastic Threshold Theorem developed in the previous section was derived not by analytical approximation to the true process but by considering more tractable stochastic models closely resembling the true process in its most important aspects. This idea of an approximating stochastic system has also been used by D. G. Kendall (1956) to investigate the same problem in two slightly different ways. His first argument runs as follows.

Starting from the rough ideas at the beginning of the last section, where we saw that the population of infectives could initially be regarded as subject to an ordinary birth-and-death process, we consider the approximate stochastic system specified by:

Case (i)   If $\rho \geqslant n$, when ultimate extinction is certain (i.e. has probability one), we take the population to be controlled by a simple birth-and-death process with birth- and death-rates βn and γ, respectively.

Case (ii)   If $p < n$, when the chance of extinction is $(\rho/n)^a$, we stipulate two modes of behaviour A and B, such that

$$\Pr\{A\} = (\rho/n)^a, \quad \Pr\{B\} = 1 - (\rho/n)^a. \tag{6.99}$$

In mode A we suppose the process to behave like Case (i) *subject to the additional requirement of ultimate extinction*, while in mode B we merely use the corresponding deterministic model.

The precise nature of mode A is settled very simply, since, as shown by W. A. O'N. Waugh (1958), a birth-and-death process with birth- and death-rates λ and μ, where $\lambda > \mu$, coincides when subject to the requirement of ultimate extinction with an unrestricted process having birth- and death-rates μ and λ.

Now when $\rho \geqslant n$, the average cumulative population size, including the initial a cases, is $a\rho/(\rho - n)$. We can derive this result directly from (6.75), since it is given by $[\partial P/\partial y]_{y=1}$ with A set equal to βn. The average size of epidemic is therefore given by

Case (i): $$\overline{w} = \frac{a\rho}{\rho - n} - a = \frac{an}{\rho - n}, \quad \rho \geqslant n. \tag{6.100}$$

We evidently cannot expect the approximating model to be realistic when $\rho = n$ and $\overline{w} = \infty$. If, on the other hand, $\rho < n$, we have

Case (ii): $$\overline{w} = \left(\frac{\rho}{n}\right)^a \frac{a\rho}{n - \rho} + \left\{1 - \left(\frac{\rho}{n}\right)^a\right\}(\zeta - a), \quad \rho < n, \tag{6.101}$$

where ζ, the total number of cases in the deterministic process, is the unique positive root of

$$a - \zeta + n(1 - e^{-\zeta/\rho}) = 0, \tag{6.102}$$

which is obtained by straightforward application of equation (6.2), noticing that, for the process considered here, (x, y, z) is $(n, a, 0)$ at $t = 0$, and $(n - \zeta + a, 0, \zeta)$ at $t = \infty$. The values of $\bar{w}$ for the approximating stochastic system are compared in Table 6.3 with the exact quantities, for various values of ρ/n when $n = 10, 20, 40$, and $a = 1$. There is a sufficiently encouraging amount of agreement here between the approximate and exact calculations, especially for $\rho < n$, to warrant further investigation into approximations of this type.

Some additional support for Kendall's approximating system was obtained from a small Monte Carlo experiment which he carried out involving twenty artificial realizations of a process with $n = 20$, $a = 1$ and $\beta = 1$, $\gamma = 10$, $\rho = 10$. The sample is of course rather small, but nevertheless some very interesting results were obtained. For example, with $(\rho/n)^a = \frac{1}{2}$, we expect equal numbers of the two modes of behaviour A and B. In fact, the numbers observed were 11 and 9 respectively. Again, the distribution of total epidemic size agreed closely with the theoretical values on which the graph for $\rho = 10$ in Fig. 6.1 is based. Grouping the values of w into the classes $0-2$, $3-17$ and $18-20$, so as to bring out the effect of the peaks at either end of the range, the expected numbers are 9.0, 7.2 and 3.8, compared with observed values of 9, 5 and 6, respectively. The goodness-of-fit χ^2 with 2 degrees of freedom is 1.95, which gives quite adequate agreement.

Another comparison between the Monte Carlo results and the approximating system can be made by considering the average number of infectives at various times. This is done in Fig. 6.5. The continuous curve represents the stochastic mean of the approximating system, for which we use Case (ii), since $\rho/n = 0.5$; and the linked circles show the corresponding Monte Carlo values accumulated over intervals of $\Delta t = 0.05$. The close agreement obtained, at any rate so far as post-peak behaviour is concerned, is most encouraging and suggests that further approximations of this type should be investigated. We are also interested in the epidemic curve obtained from the Monte Carlo experiment, and this is shown in Fig. 6.6. The values given by the linked circles indicate the average number of new removals in successive intervals of $\Delta t = 0.05$. It is unfortunate that we do not yet have available a theoretical curve with which to compare this empirical one.

The second approach discussed by Kendall is more akin to Whittle's method of bounding a stochastic epidemic from above and from below by two modified systems, in each of which the population of infectives has a constant and extreme birth-rate. The idea is to consider an approximating stochastic system in which the chance of one new infection in time Δt is $\beta x(t)s\,\Delta t$, where s is the actual number of infectives and $x(t)$ is the number of susceptibles in the associated deterministic model of Kermack and McKendrick. For the population of

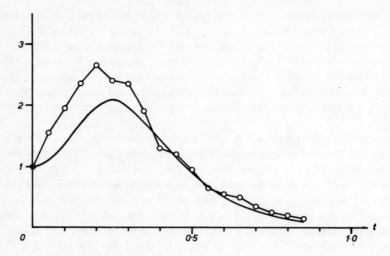

Fig. 6.5   Comparison of mean numbers of infectives, plotted against time, for (i) Kendall's approximating system (continuous curve), and (ii) his Monte Carlo series (linked circles)

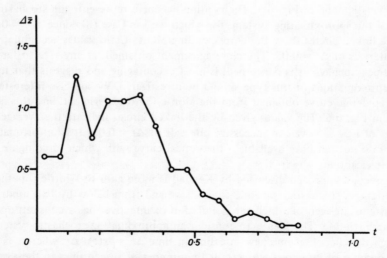

Fig. 6.6   Epidemic curve for Kendall's Monte Carlo experiment given by the average number of new removals in successive intervals of $\Delta t = 0.05$

infectives this amounts to a "generalized" birth-and-death process (Kendall, 1948a) with birth- and death-rates $\beta x(t)$ and γ, respectively. The resulting analysis is rather too complicated to summarize here, but it could lead to some interesting developments.

More recently, Ludwig (1973a) has developed an approximating stochastic system based on rewriting equations (6.28) in terms of the number of infectives and the total number of removed individuals at any given time. Some simple transformations are used, and terms are neglected that involve the variance of the number of removals conditional on the number of infectives. This leads to a set of equations whose number is proportional to n rather than n^2. Numerical computation shows that in general the approximating stochastic system implied by the above procedure shows excellent agreement with the exact results supplied by the original equations.

6.7   Asymptotic approximations

Because of the relative intractability of the general stochastic epidemic model as compared with the simple epidemic, increasing attention has been paid in recent years to the possibility of developing appropriate mathematical approximations (as distinct, for example, from the approximating stochastic systems of Whittle, used in Section 6.5, and of Kendall, described in Section 6.6). So far, the perturbation and diffusion approximations of Bailey, Weiss and McNeil, outlined in Section 5.8, have not been found capable of convenient extensions to the general epidemic. Daniels (1971) has discussed some of the reasons for these difficulties. It is, however, possible that the methods of Daley and Kendall (1965), and the extensions of Barbour (1972), will yield some further results.

The simplest asymptotic result available relates to the distribution of the total size of the epidemic when the relative removal rate is well below the threshold and the chances are that a large epidemic will develop. A very rough heuristic argument runs as follows.

First consider the deterministic model, starting with a trace of infection in a group of n susceptibles. Equation (6.21) shows that the intensity of the epidemic, α say, is given by

$$\alpha = 1 - e^{-n\alpha/\rho}. \tag{6.103}$$

For n/ρ large, a first approximation to the root near to $i = 1$ is evidently

$$\alpha \doteqdot 1 - e^{-n/\rho}.$$

Hence the number of susceptibles escaping infection is approximately

$$m = n(1 - \alpha) \doteqdot n\, e^{-n/\rho}. \tag{6.104}$$

Following the reasoning of Violet Cane (1966), we can argue that there is a large population exposed to infection and a small chance that any given individual will escape infection. If the latter chances are virtually independent, as seems intuitively likely, we should expect to obtain an approximately Poisson distribution, whose parameter, in a large population with n/ρ also large, would be the deterministic value given in (6.104). Cane gives a more detailed heuristic discussion, and shows that the fate of any one individual is practically uncorrelated with that of another. This interesting result for the asymptotic distribution of the number of susceptibles remaining uninfected was, however, first obtained by Daniels (1967) in 1966. He used a fairly intricate analytical procedure to derive asymptotic approximations, both above and below the threshold, starting with Foster's random walk formulation described in Section 6.4. The reader should refer to Daniels' paper for details. and also to Downton (1967a) for a simpler derivation of one of the main formulae.

An interesting asymptotic result for the average duration of the general epidemic was also derived at about the same time by Ridler-Rowe (1967) using some general results for Markov processes due to Reuter (1957, 1961). Ridler-Rowe proved several theorems applicable to an extended model that included the immigration of both susceptibles and infectives (see Section 7.6). This involved a considerable amount of mathematical analysis. The main result of interest here is that if T is the duration-time for an epidemic process starting with a infectives and n susceptibles then the average duration-time is asymptotically given by

$$\bar{T} \sim \gamma^{-1} \log (a + n), \quad n \to \infty. \tag{6.105}$$

It is worth noting that this result requires only that $n \to \infty$ and not that $a \to \infty$.

More recently, Daniels has again used the random walk approach to study the maximum transient size of a closed epidemic, that is, the maximum numbers of circulating infectives ever achieved at any time during the course of the epidemic. This could well be of importance for the planning of health facilities designed to cope with the consequences of epidemics. It should however be noted that, strictly speaking, it is not the infectives as such that need medical care, but those who have been removed and are still receiving care before dying or recovering.

Another type of asymptotic approach has been developed by Nagaev (1970, 1971) and Nagaev and Startsev (1968, 1970). These authors, in a similar way to Daniels (1966), found it more convenient to work with the pair of variables (i, j), where i is the total number of susceptibles who have become infected, and j is the number of removals. Thus

$$i = n - r, \quad j = n - r - s + a. \tag{6.106}$$

The transition probabilities given in (6.58), corresponding to an infection or a removal, respectively, are therefore

$$p_i \equiv \Pr\{(i,j) \to (i+1,j)\} = \frac{n-i}{n+\rho-i}\,,$$

$$q_i \equiv \Pr\{(i,j) \to (i,j+1)\} = \frac{\rho}{n+\rho-i}\,. \tag{6.107}$$

The absorbing boundary for the transformed variables (i,j) is clearly given by the line $j = a + i$.

Now, let X_i, $i = 0, 1, 2, ...$, be independent, geometrically distributed, random variables with probabilities of success given by p_i, and write

$$S_k = \sum_{i=0}^{k} X_i. \tag{6.108}$$

It can then be seen that, if w_n is the final size of the epidemic,

$$\Pr\{w_n > k\} = \Pr\{S_0 < a, S_1 < a+1, ..., S_k < a+k\}. \tag{6.109}$$

The expression in (6.109) is exact, but an explicit formulation is difficult to obtain. Nagaev and Startsev managed to find several tractable approximations valid for n and a both large. Some typical results are illustrated by the following theorems, quoted here without proof. It is assumed that $a \to \infty$, $n \to \infty$, such that $a = o(n)$, and either $c \leqslant \frac{\rho}{n} \leqslant 1 - c$ or $1 + c \leqslant \frac{\rho}{n} = o(a)$, where c is an arbitrarily small fixed positive constant.

Theorem 1

Given the foregoing conditions, the probability of total epidemic size w_n is given asymptotically by

$$\Pr\{w_n > a_n - xb_n\} = \Phi(x)\{1 + o(1)\}, \tag{6.110}$$

where

$$a_n = \frac{a}{\frac{\rho}{n} - 1}, \quad b_n = \left\{ \frac{a\left(\frac{\rho}{n} + \frac{\rho^2}{n^2}\right)}{\left(\frac{\rho}{n} - 1\right)^3} \right\}^{\frac{1}{2}}, \quad \frac{\rho}{n} > 1;$$

$$a_n = \alpha n, \quad b_n = \frac{\left\{\alpha n \left(1 + \frac{(\rho/n)^2}{1 - \alpha}\right)\right\}^{\frac{1}{2}}}{\frac{\rho}{n}(1 - \alpha) - 1}, \quad \frac{\rho}{n} < 1; \tag{6.111}$$

$$\Phi(x) = \frac{1}{\sqrt{2\pi}} \int_{-\infty}^{x} e^{-\frac{1}{2}u^2}\, du,$$

and α is the smallest positive root (as before) of (6.104).

Theorem 2

If we define $\beta = a\left(1 - \dfrac{\rho}{n}\right)$, and if in addition to the previous conditions we
have $|\beta| \to \infty$, $\beta = o(a)$ and $na^{-3} = o(\beta^{-2})$, then

$$\Pr\{w_n \geqslant a_n - xb_n\} = \Phi(x)\{1 + o(1)\}, \tag{6.112}$$

where $a_n = (2an)^{\frac{1}{2}}, \quad b_n = (2n^3a^{-1})^{\frac{1}{4}}. \tag{6.113}$

Theorem 3

Further suppose that $\dfrac{\rho}{an} \geqslant \delta > 0$. Then the probability distribution of w_n
is asymptotically Poisson with parameter an/ρ.

Several other results of a similar nature are also available, covering both total epidemic size and duration time. It is of great interest to see how existing techniques of handling the limiting forms of probability distributions can be applied to the special case of epidemics. At the same time it cannot be denied that the conditions under which the theorems are valid are in most cases highly specialized. Not only does the initial number of susceptibles have to be large, which is perfectly reasonable, but the initial number of infectives has to tend to infinity as well. Moreover, for many of the theorems, these limits have to be approached in a special way. Whether the results are sufficiently robust to provide insight into the behaviour of actual epidemics is a matter for further investigation.

6.8   Estimation of parameters

In the previous sections we have been concerned only with the probability theory of the epidemic process under discussion. We now turn to the problem of estimating the unknown parameters involved, e.g. β and γ or ρ. Since the present model is much more realistic than the simple epidemic described earlier, and since data on the household distribution of cases are often available, it is worth considering the question of estimation in greater detail. When investigating household distributions of cases we are really studying small-scale epidemics occurring in family groups after the disease has been introduced by one, or occasionally more than one, of their members who has contracted the disease elsewhere. The opportunities for cross-infection within such a compact group are usually fairly considerable, and this makes it possible to deal with these intra-household epidemics more or less independently of the course of the epidemic in the community at large. Two main types of analysis arise: the first when we know only the total number of cases occurring in a sufficiently long period of time, and the second when we have the actual dates at which symptoms appear. For reasons given below, we may prefer to use the first type of analysis even when the second is theoretically possible.

6.81   Household distribution of total number of cases

It has already been emphasized above that we do not in practice normally know when a susceptible actually becomes infected (and in the present model infectious as well), and often we do not know when he ceases to be infectious. If the infective is removed from circulation while still clinically infectious, this does not matter, provided removal occurs as specified by the model, but in some diseases symptoms may not occur until after infectiousness has ceased. In this event we can observe none of the transitions from one basic state of the process to another; and in particular we cannot recognize the times of removal in the sense in which "removal" is used in the model. Fortunately, however, we can fall back on the total number of cases, which we shall know with reasonable certainty after the elapse of sufficient time, say a few weeks (but if the time allowed is too long, a new epidemic may be started which will be confused with the first). We can hardly expect to be able to estimate both β and γ from such data since the distribution of ultimate epidemic size depends only on their ratio ρ, and no information is available about the time-scale involved. The results of Section 6.4 are immediately applicable here, and Table 6.2 sets out the probabilities P_w for $a = 1$ and $n = 1, 2, 3, 4$ and 5. This is likely to meet the requirements of most household data arising in practice, though there is a small chance that some groups may have multiple introductions, i.e. a may be greater than unity. Unfortunately, with the negative exponential distribution of incubation periods entailed by the present model, reliable recognition of multiple introductions is very uncertain, and the best course seems to be to neglect the possibility, though one can hardly regard this as an entirely satisfactory expedient. With the peaked distribution of incubation period arising in chain-binomial models and their derivatives (Chapters 14 and 15) this difficulty is much easier to overcome.

Maximum-likelihood estimation

Let us now consider what is specifically involved in the maximum-likelihood estimation of ρ. Suppose the data consist of N households, each containing n susceptibles besides the initial case introducing the disease. Let the number of households with w new cases after the first be a_w, $0 \leqslant w \leqslant n$. Then the maximum-likelihood score for ρ is

$$S(\rho) = \sum_{w=0}^{n} a_w S_w(\rho), \qquad (6.114)$$

where

$$S_w(\rho) = \frac{1}{P_w} \frac{dP_w}{d\rho}. \qquad (6.115)$$

Algebraic expressions for the overall score $S(\rho)$ in terms of ρ and the a_w have been given in Table 6.2. To facilitate rapid calculation, the score coefficients,

$S_w(\rho)$, were computed by EDSAC at Cambridge University Mathematical Lab-
oratory for the ranges $n = 2, 3, 4$ and 5; $\rho = 1\cdot0(0\cdot1)\,10\cdot0$; and these tabulations
are given in the Appendix. When $n = 1$, there is of course no difficulty as an
explicit estimate is immediately available.

The maximum-likelihood equation

$$S(\hat{\rho}) = 0, \tag{6.116}$$

is most easily solved by the usual procedure of calculating $S(\rho)$ at a few trial
values of ρ until we have scores of opposite signs for two sufficiently close
adjacent values ρ_1 and ρ_2. The estimate $\hat{\rho}$ is given by inverse interpolation and
the standard error by $\{I(\rho)\}^{-\frac{1}{2}}$, where the infomation $I(\rho)$ is approximately

$$I(\rho) \doteq \frac{S(\rho_1) - S(\rho_2)}{\rho_2 - \rho_1}. \tag{6.117}$$

After estimation we calculate the P_w from Table 6.2 and the corresponding
expectations NP_w, in order to test the goodness-of-fit.

Illustrative example

As an illustration we can consider the data shown in Table 6.4 given by
Wilson *et al.* (1939) on scarlet fever, which might be expected on general epidemiological grounds to be approximately represented by the present model.

Table 6.4   *Observed and expected numbers for epidemics of scarlet fever
in households of three (n = 2)*

No. of secondary cases (w)	No. of households observed (a_w)	No. of households expected (NP_w)
0	172	169·5
1	42	46·0
2	21	19·5
Total (N)	235	235·0

The score is $S(\rho) = 172S_0(\rho) + 42S_1(\rho) + 21S_2(\rho)$, and if for $n = 2$ we use
the tables in the Appendix, we find $S(5\cdot1) = +0\cdot1917$ and $S(5\cdot2) = -0\cdot0464$.
Hence $I = 2\cdot381$, and the estimate, obtained by inverse interpolation between
the two scores, together with its standard error, is

$$\hat{\rho} = 5\cdot18 \pm 0\cdot66. \tag{6.118}$$

The expected numbers shown in Table 6.4 indicate good agreement with the
observations, and the goodness-of-fit χ^2 is 0·50 on one degree of freedom.
Naturally more extensive investigation would be required before much reliance
could be placed on this result, but it is interesting to note that Wilson *et al.*

obtained a significant departure from expectation when fitting a chain-binomial.

6.82 Household distribution with observed removal times

Let us now suppose that it is legitimate to make use of the observed removal times. Then to exhibit in a simple way the sort of analysis employed, we first consider households of two with $n = a = 1$, and use Foster's representation of the process as a random walk on a lattice. The probability that the first case is removed before infecting the one and only susceptible is $\rho/(1 + \rho)$, and the probability of cross-infection is $1/(1 + \rho)$. Let the observed numbers of households showing these two different patterns be a_0 and a_1, respectively, where $a_0 + a_1 = N$. When cross-infection occurs, there is initially one infective and one susceptible; then two infectives; next, one of these is removed, giving the time of occurrence of the first case observed; finally, the second infective is removed after the elapse of a time-interval t_i in the ith household. The observed case-to-case interval, t_i, is distributed as a negative exponential with frequency function $\gamma e^{-\gamma t_i} dt_i$. It follows that the likelihood of the sample can be written

$$e^L \propto \left(\frac{\rho}{\rho + 1}\right)^{a_0} \left(\frac{1}{\rho + 1}\right)^{a_1} \gamma^{a_1} \exp\left\{-\gamma \sum_{i=1}^{a_1} t_i\right\}. \tag{6.119}$$

Therefore

$$L = \text{const.} + a_1 \log \beta + N \log \gamma - N \log (\beta + \gamma) - \gamma \sum_{i=1}^{a_1} t_i. \tag{6.120}$$

Application of the usual procedure finally gives the following estimates and large-sample variances

$$\hat{\beta} = \frac{a_1^2}{a_0 T}, \quad \hat{\gamma} = \frac{a_1}{T},$$

$$\left. \text{var}(\hat{\beta}) = \frac{\beta(\beta + \gamma)(\beta + 2\gamma)}{N\gamma}, \quad \text{var}(\hat{\gamma}) = \frac{\gamma^2(\beta + \gamma)}{N\beta}, \right\} \tag{6.121}$$

where

$$T = \sum_{i=1}^{a_1} t_i.$$

If we try to apply the same approach to larger households, we run into the difficulty that the joint distribution of the intervals between successive removals is no longer simple in form. However, the distribution between the last two cases is still negative exponential, and we can simplify the treatment by using the information provided by this interval alone, ignoring the others.

As before, we assume there to be a_w households with w cases after the primary one, $0 \leqslant w \leqslant n$, while the probability of exactly w additional cases is P_w. The time-interval between the last two observed removals in the ith family, having w additional cases in all, is taken to be t_{wi}.

Now, the waiting time in the state before the final removal is distributed as a negative exponential with parameter $\beta(n - w) + \gamma$, independently of whether the next transition is an infection or a removal. A similar point occurs in the next section in the specification of equation (6.140), but was overlooked in the present context in the first edition. I am indebted to Mr Kevin Gough for the correction.

The overall likelihood is accordingly

$$e^L \propto P_0^{a_0} \prod_{w=1}^{n} P_w^{a_w} \prod_{i=1}^{a_w} \{\beta(n-w)+\gamma\} \exp\left[-\{\beta(n-w)+\gamma\}t_{wi}\right]. \quad (6.122)$$

Thus
$$L = \text{const.} + \sum_{w=0}^{n} a_w \log P_w + \sum_{w=1}^{n} a_w \log\{\beta(n-w)+\gamma\}$$
$$- \sum_{w=1}^{n}\sum_{i=1}^{a_w} \{\beta(n-w)+\gamma\}t_{wi}. \quad (6.123)$$

In principle, we can proceed by using a suitable optimizing computer program to find the maximum-likelihood estimates of β and γ. Approximate starting values can be obtained as follows.

The quantity P_w is a function of ρ only, so that if we put

$$S(\rho) = \sum_{w=0}^{n} \frac{a_w}{P_w} \frac{dP_w}{d\rho},$$

then $S(\rho)$ is precisely the score already used in Section 6.81 for estimating ρ from the total size of epidemic alone (see equations (6.114) and (6.115)). Differentiating (6.123) with respect to β and γ therefore gives

$$\frac{\partial L}{\partial \beta} = -\frac{\gamma S(\rho)}{\beta^2} + \sum_{w=1}^{n} \frac{(n-w)a_w}{\beta(n-w)+\gamma} - \sum_{w=1}^{n}\sum_{i=1}^{a_w}(n-w)t_{wi},$$
$$\text{and} \quad \frac{\partial L}{\partial \gamma} = -\frac{S(\rho)}{\beta} + \sum_{w=1}^{n} \frac{a_w}{\beta(n-w)+\gamma} - \sum_{w=1}^{n}\sum_{i=1}^{a_w} t_{wi}. \quad \Bigg\} \quad (6.124)$$

Let us suppose that $\hat{\rho}$ is the solution of the equation $S(\hat{\rho})=0$, as appearing in (6.116). Then the second equation of (6.124) gives, after multiplication by β and putting both $\partial L/\partial\gamma$ and $S(\rho)$ equal to zero, the approximate estimate

$$\check{\beta} = \sum_{w=1}^{n} \frac{a_w}{n-w+\rho} \Bigg/ \sum_{w=1}^{n}\sum_{i=1}^{a_w} t_{wi}, \quad (6.125)$$

with
$$\check{\gamma} = \hat{\rho}\check{\beta}. \quad (6.126)$$

Alternatively, one might use (6.124) as the basis for a maximum-likelihood scoring approach, though this would be tedious without computer assistance.

How much information is lost by neglecting all the time-intervals except the last is unknown, and this would certainly be worth a special investigation. We therefore need to develop methods of estimation which will use all, or nearly all, the available data without involving prohibitively heavy arithmetic.

An obvious complication, most easily described for the two-person household, i.e. with $n = a = 1$, is that when there are in fact two removals, a long time might elapse between them. Thus, having observed only a single removal over a reasonably long period of time, we cannot be certain that another will not occur. Conversely, if a second removal is observed a *very* long time, e.g. years, after the first, it seems more likely that the second case is due to a new infection from outside rather than to cross-infection within the family. Sally Ohlsen (1964) proposed to avoid the first difficulty, and to some extent to limit the effect of the second difficulty, by observing what happens in each household for some fixed period of time τ after the first removal. An exact statistical analysis then leads to appropriate estimates of β and γ. This is in many ways an improvement on the previous analysis, but the problem of choosing a suitable value of τ still remains. With a prospective investigation τ could be fixed in advance, but in the analysis of retrospective data it may be very difficult or impossible to assign a value to τ.

Morgan (1965) has investigated this problem further, and gives simple corrections that can be applied to the estimates in (6.121) so as to yield close approximations to Ohlsen's estimates. If τ is large then (6.121) is likely to be reasonably accurate. But if τ is too small much information may be lost and the method of estimation may break down. As Morgan points out, the real reason for choosing a small value of τ is to eliminate the possibility that the second case has been infected from outside. If this seems an appreciable risk, it would be better to include this factor in the analysis from the start by introducing an additional parameter. An expression is given by Morgan for the ensuing likelihood function that could be used in appropriate circumstances for the computerized maximum-likelihood estimation of the three parameters involved.

6.83 Analysis of a single epidemic in a large group

As mentioned above, the difficulty in analysing all the removal data from a large household is that the joint distribution of the successive removal intervals does not have a simple form. The problem presents itself in a specially tantalizing way when we have, say, 20 or 30 cases of disease in a *single* epidemic outbreak. A fair amount of statistical information ought to be available, provided that we can use all the data. Bailey and Thomas (1971) have recently shown how this can be done by providing a rigorous mathematical formulation of the basic probability model, coupled with a computerized algorithm for obtaining maximum-likelihood estimates of the parameters β and γ.

Although, of course, the total size of the epidemic provides information about the relative removal rate ρ, it might be questioned in advance whether data on a succession of inter-removal times would enable β and γ to be estimated separately with any degree of accuracy. A little reflexion shows that this is a reasonable hope. As already shown in Section 6.3, replacing the original time variable t by $\tau = \beta t$ leads to a system of equations involving ρ only. If therefore we replace β and γ by $\lambda\beta$ and $\lambda\gamma$, say, the model in τ-time will be unchanged, but in t-time the process will develop λ times as rapidly. The duration of the whole epidemic or the position of the peak would therefore be expected in principle to supply information about the scaling parameter λ. This implies information about both β and γ, taking into account the estimate of ρ.

Let us first investigate the likelihood of the observed set of inter-removal times, *given* that the epidemic was of total size w. As previously, we suppose that at time t there are r susceptibles and s infectives. In addition, we write u for the total number of removals. If the process starts with one infective and n susceptibles, we have

$$r + s + u = n + 1. \tag{6.127}$$

Since there are $w + 1$ cases in all, there are w observable intervals. Let us write τ_u for the interval between the uth and the $(u + 1)$th removals, $u = 1$, $2,\ldots, w$. The observed data thus consist of the set $(\tau_1, \tau_2,\ldots, \tau_w)$. It is convenient to distinguish the whole past history of the process up to and including the uth removal by the symbol H_u, i.e.

$$H_u \equiv (\tau_1, \tau_2,\ldots, \tau_{u-1}), \quad 2 \leqslant u \leqslant w + 1, \tag{6.128}$$

using the formal symbol H_1, which applies to the first removal, to mean that there are no previously observed data.

Let us indicate the joint likelihood of the whole set of w observed intervals by $f(\tau_1, \tau_2,\ldots, \tau_w) \equiv f(H_{w+1})$. In terms of conditional likelihoods we can thus write

$$\begin{aligned}
f(\tau_1, \tau_2,\ldots, \tau_w) &= f(\tau_1)f(\tau_2 | \tau_1)f(\tau_3 | \tau_1, \tau_2) \ldots f(\tau_w | \tau_1,\ldots, \tau_{w-1}) \\
&= \prod_{u=1}^{w} f(\tau_u | H_u).
\end{aligned} \tag{6.129}$$

The log likelihood L_1 of the observed set of intervals, given w, is thus

$$L_1 = \sum_{u=1}^{w} \log f(\tau_u | H_u). \tag{6.130}$$

It is important for practical purposes to note that we can in general observe only removals but not infections. Now between the uth and $(u + 1)$th removals we have in all $n - u + 1$ susceptibles and infectives. Only one additional variable is therefore required to indicate the state of the process during any given inter-removal interval.

Suppose that there are s circulating infectives immediately following the uth removal. At this moment we have $r = n - s - u + 1$ susceptibles. Let us write $p(s | H_u)$ for the probability of s given the previously observed data, where $1 \leqslant u \leqslant w + 1$. Note that $1 \leqslant s \leqslant w - u + 1$ when $1 \leqslant u \leqslant w$, for if $s = 0$ the process has already terminated. When $u = w + 1$ we simply have $s = 0$, corresponding to the removal of the last infective.

Now let us consider a sub-process starting with m infectives just after the uth removal and continuing with infections only until the $(u + 1)$th removal occurs after an interval τ_u, the number of circulating infectives then being s. We write the probability of this precise sequence of infections and removal, without regard to the time elapsing, but conditional on m and H_u, as $p(s | H_u, m)$. The likelihood of τ_u, given H_u and the observed sequence of infections and removal, can be written as $f(\tau_u | H_u, m, s)$.

The joint likelihood of m, s and τ_u, given H_u, is therefore

$$f(m, s, \tau_u | H_u) = p(m | H_u)p(s | H_u, m)f(\tau_u | H_u, m, s), \tag{6.131}$$

where in general $0 \leqslant s \leqslant n - u$, since all of these points could be reached from the restricted range, given by $1 \leqslant m \leqslant w - u + 1$, that applies just after the uth removal. Also $0 \leqslant \tau_u < \infty$. However, we wish to restrict ourselves to the paths for which $1 \leqslant s \leqslant w - u$, since everything is to be conditional on w. A normalizing factor $C(H_u)$ is thus required, and is given by

$$C^{-1}(H_u) = \sum_{s=1}^{w-u} \sum_{m=1}^{s+1} \int_0^\infty f(m, s, \tau_u | H_u) d\tau_u$$

$$= \sum_{s=1}^{w-u} \sum_{m=1}^{s+1} p(m | H_u) p(s | H_u, m), \qquad (6.132)$$

since

$$\int_0^\infty f(\tau_u | H_u, m, s) d\tau_u = 1. \qquad (6.133)$$

Note that m cannot be greater than $s + 1$ in (6.132) since only one removal can take place between any one removal point and the next.

The normalized likelihood over the admissible range of points is accordingly

$$f(m, s, \tau_u | H_u) = C(H_u) p(m | H_u) p(s | H_u, m) f(\tau_u | H_u, m, s). \qquad (6.134)$$

We can now obtain the conditional likelihood $f(s, \tau_u | H_u)$ by summing (6.134) over m, and $f(\tau_u | H_u)$ by summing over both m and s, i.e.

$$f(s, \tau_u | H_u) = \sum_{m=1}^{s+1} f(m, s, \tau_u | H_u), \qquad (6.135)$$

and

$$f(\tau_u | H_u) = \sum_{s=1}^{w-u} f(s, \tau_u | H_u). \qquad (6.136)$$

An iterative formula connecting $p(s | H_{u+1})$ and $p(s | H_u)$ can now be derived using a simple conditional probability argument. Thus

$$p(s | H_{u+1}) \equiv p(s | H_u, \tau_u)$$

$$= \frac{f(s, \tau_u | H_u)}{f(\tau_u | H_u)}, \qquad 1 \leqslant s \leqslant w - u. \qquad (6.137)$$

It may be noted in passing that $C(H_u)$ cancels when we substitute from (6.134)–(6.136) into (6.137).

Provided that we can calculate $p(s | H_u, m)$ and $f(\tau_u | H_u, m, s)$ in (6.134), equations (6.132)–(6.137) supply a basis for a well-defined sequence of iterations leading directly to the computation of the log likelihood L_1 given in (6.130).

Now $p(s | H_u, m)$ can be calculated immediately from Foster's random walk representation of the progress of an epidemic in terms of the succession of population states indicated by the points (r, s). It follows from (6.58) that in general

$$p(s | H_u, m) = \frac{\rho}{n - s - u + \rho} \prod_{j=n-m-u+1}^{n-s-u+1} \frac{j}{j + \rho}, \qquad m \leqslant s \leqslant n - u. \qquad (6.138)$$

When there are no new infections after the uth removal and before the $(u + 1)$th, we have $s = m - 1$ and

$$p(m - 1 | H_u, m) = \frac{\rho}{n - m - u + 1 + \rho}. \tag{6.139}$$

Next, we must consider the likelihood of any inter-removal time *given* the path pattern actually followed. We have, in fact, a univariate stochastic process starting from the state of m infectives just after the uth removal and proceeding to the state of s infectives just after the $(u + 1)$th removal by means of $s - m + 1$ successive infections followed by a removal. This makes a total of $s - m + 3$ possible states.

Let $p_i \equiv p_i(m, u, \beta, \gamma, t)$ be the probability that this sub-process of $s - m + 3$ states has undergone i transitions by time t. Then p_i is the probability of there being $m + i$ infectives for $0 \leqslant i \leqslant s - m + 1$, while p_{s-m+2} is the probability of having reached the final state of s infectives following the $(u + 1)$th removal. In a manner analogous to the derivation of equations (5.30) for the simple stochastic epidemic in Section 5.3, we can obtain the relevant master equations for the general case of $s \geqslant m$ as

$$\left.\begin{aligned}
\frac{dp_0}{dt} &= -\lambda_0 p_0, \\[2mm]
\frac{dp_i}{dt} &= \lambda_{i-1} p_{i-1} - \lambda_i p_i, \quad 1 \leqslant i \leqslant s - m + 1, \\[2mm]
\frac{dp_{s-m+2}}{dt} &= \lambda_{s-m+1} \, p_{s-m+1},
\end{aligned}\right\} \tag{6.140}$$

where

$$\lambda_i = \beta(m + i)(n - m - i - u + 1) + \gamma(m + i), \quad 0 \leqslant i \leqslant s - m + 1,$$
$$\tag{6.141}$$

the initial conditions being

$$p_0(0) = 1, \quad p_i(0) = 0 \quad \text{if} \quad i \neq 0. \tag{6.142}$$

Care must be taken with the specification of the transition rates λ_i defined in (6.141). As pointed out by Prof. N. G. Becker (personal communication), the term $\gamma(m + i)$ was omitted from equation (16) in the original formulation by Bailey and Thomas (1971). That (6.141) in fact gives the correct form for λ_i can be seen by considering the time waited in the ith state before the relevant transition occurs. Although in general in the sub-process considered we are interested only in new infections, the transition rate for any type of transition is λ_i, and waiting time and type of transition are easily seen to be independent.

Now p_{s-m+2} is the distribution function of the duration time τ_u of the sub-process in question, and dp_{s-m+2}/dt is the frequency function. Hence

$$f(\tau_u | H_u, m, s) = \lambda_{s-m+1} \, p_{s-m+1}(\tau_u), \tag{6.143}$$

using the last equation of (6.140). In principle, $p_{s-m+1}(\tau_u)$ can be found by solving the first $s-m+2$ equations in (6.140) and setting $t = \tau_u$. Mathematically speaking, there is evidently no difficulty about an exact solution. But comparison with the solutions for the simple stochastic epidemic discussed in Section 5.3 suggests that the usual algebraic solutions are likely to be very awkward for numerical computation. Using an electronic computer, Bailey and Thomas found straightforward Runge–Kutta numerical integration to be quite satisfactory. Moreover, computer time could be saved by noticing that the sets of equations in (6.140), for fixed m and variable s, are nested except for the last two equations in each set. For the details of these and other practical computational aspects the reader should consult the paper mentioned.

When $s = m - 1$, there are no new infections and the next transition is simply the $(u + 1)$th removal. The frequency distribution of this interval is evidently

$$f(\tau_u|H_u, m, m-1) = \lambda_0 e^{-\lambda_0 \tau_u}, \tag{6.144}$$

where λ_0 is defined in (6.141).

We also need the initial distribution $p(s|H_1)$ to get the whole sequence of iterations started. From (6.138) it is clear that, with $m = 1$, $u = 0$,

$$p(s|H_1) \propto \frac{\rho}{n-s+\rho} \prod_{j=n}^{n-s+1} \frac{j}{j+\rho}, \quad 1 \leq s \leq w,$$

where normalization over the indicated range is required. Thus, if we write

$$p'(s|H_1) = \frac{\rho}{n-s+\rho} \prod_{j=n}^{n-s+1} \frac{j}{j+\rho}, \tag{6.145}$$

then

$$p(s|H_1) = \frac{p'(s|H_1)}{\sum_{s=1}^{w} p'(s|H_1)}, \quad 1 \leq s \leq w. \tag{6.146}$$

We have thus shown how to compute the ingredients of the right-hand side of (6.134), and can proceed to the evaluation of L_1 for any given β and γ.

Now, statistical information is also available from the total observed epidemic size w. The relevant log likelihood is

$$L_2 = \log P_w, \tag{6.147}$$

where P_w is given by (6.47), and the quantities f_{rs} can be found from (6.49), putting $a = 1$ for the present application. Starting with $f_{n1} = (n + \rho)^{-1}$, all the f_{rs} can be found successively from the recursive relationship

$$f_{rs} = \frac{(r+1)(s-1)f_{r+1,s-1} + \rho(s+1)f_{r,s+1}}{s(r+\rho)}, \tag{6.148}$$

which is obtained by simply rearranging (6.49). Note that for any given w we continue the calculations only to the point where $f_{n-w,1}$ has been found. The latter is then substituted in (6.47) to yield P_w. We could, alternatively, work with the set of equations in (6.52) for the g_{rs}, and then use (6.50) and (6.47). Again, we might make use of Williams' function $f_w(x)$ and base our computations on the formulae in (6.61)–(6.63). It is not clear, however, that there would be any real computational advantages in the two latter approaches.

Since the likelihood of the interval data is calculated conditionally on a given total epidemic size, we can obtain the joint likelihood of the data as a whole simply by multiplying the likelihoods for interval data and total epidemic size. The joint log likelihood is therefore given by

$$L = L_1 + L_2, \tag{6.149}$$

where L_1 and L_2 are given by (6.130) and (6.147), respectively.

To compute maximum-likelihood estimates of β and γ we merely have to maximize L using an appropriate optimizing computer program, such as the CERN program MINROS, in which the function to be maximized is defined by (6.149), and the foregoing mathematics specifies the algorithms to be used in calculating L_1 and L_2. An advantage of MINROS is that it involves an error analysis that supplies standard errors along with the maximum-likelihood estimates.

It will be realized of course that the interval data are not independently distributed, but that the τ_u are intricately correlated with different distributions. Nevertheless, it seems reasonable to make use of the maximum-likelihood approach, provided a degree of caution is exercised. If the likelihood function has a sufficiently marked maximum, the usual optimum properties may well be realized approximately.

In any practical computation it is convenient to have suitable starting values β_0 and γ_0. One method of doing this is to appeal to a deterministic analysis. If w and n are fairly large, the intensity of the epidemic is $i = (w + 1)/n$, so that equation (6.22) in Section 6.2 becomes

$$\frac{n}{\rho} = -\frac{\log(1-i)}{i}.$$

The deterministic estimate of ρ is therefore given by

$$\rho_0 = -\frac{w + 1}{\log\left(1 - \dfrac{w+1}{n}\right)}. \tag{6.150}$$

Again, the theoretical peak height of the epidemic curve is γy_0, where y_0 is given in (6.25). Thus if the observed peak height is h, we can estimate γ_0 as

$$\gamma_0 = \frac{h}{y_0} = \frac{h}{n - \rho_0 - \rho_0 \log(n/\rho_0)}. \tag{6.151}$$

Since we need only an approximate value for h it might easily be determined from visual inspection only. Otherwise, if this is difficult we could assume approximate normality in the observed epidemic curve. If the variance of the histogram for the incidence of new cases is v, the fitted value of h would be

$$h = (w + 1)(2\pi v)^{-\frac{1}{2}}.\tag{6.152}$$

Bailey and Thomas (1971) gave an illustrative example of the use of the above method in analysing data made available by Dr David M. Thompson and Dr William H. Foege on a smallpox outbreak. This involved a total of 30 cases in a population of 120 individuals at risk in a closed community in Abakaliki in south-eastern Nigeria. It was admitted, however, that the model was somewhat oversimplified so far as smallpox was concerned, since no allowance is made in the model for the existence of an appreciable latent period following the receipt of infection. Nevertheless it is useful to demonstrate the feasibility of such statistical analyses of data drawn from field studies. From this point of view the results are quite encouraging.

The data actually consisted of the following 29 inter-removal times (measured in days).

$$13, 7, 2, 3, 0, 0, 1, 4, 5, 3, 2, 0, 2, 0, 5$$

$$3, 1, 4, 0, 1, 1, 1, 2, 0, 1, 5, 0, 5, 5,$$

where the occurrence of zeros corresponds in an obvious way to cases appearing on the same day. Using the foregoing analysis, the following maximum-likelihood estimates are obtained:

$$\hat{\beta} = 0\cdot00088 \pm 0\cdot00025,$$

$$\hat{\gamma} = 0\cdot091 \pm 0\cdot031,\tag{6.153}$$

these figures being rates per day. The covariance matrix of these estimates was computed as

$$\begin{bmatrix} 0\cdot605 \times 10^{-7} & 0\cdot531 \times 10^{-5} \\ 0\cdot531 \times 10^{-5} & 0\cdot942 \times 10^{-3} \end{bmatrix}.\tag{6.154}$$

Now $\hat{\rho} = \hat{\gamma}/\hat{\beta}$, and we can use the easily verified large-sample formula

$$\frac{\text{var}(\hat{\rho})}{\hat{\rho}^2} = \frac{\text{var}(\hat{\beta})}{\hat{\beta}^2} - \frac{2\,\text{cov}(\hat{\beta},\hat{\gamma})}{\hat{\beta}\hat{\gamma}} + \frac{\text{var}(\hat{\gamma})}{\hat{\gamma}^2}$$

to obtain the corresponding standard error. We thus find

$$\hat{\rho} = 103 \pm 37.\tag{6.155}$$

Of course the standard errors in (6.153) and (6.155) are all quite large, as expected. In particular, $\hat{\rho}$ is well below the critical value of 119, as expected from the observed epidemic size, but this result is obviously not significant. Nevertheless, this illustrative example gives an idea of how much information is available from the kind of data presented.

It should, however, be emphasized that the computations involved can be very time-consuming. In fact it needed about $5\frac{1}{2}$ minutes on an IBM System 360 Model 40 computer to calculate a single log likelihood for any given pair of values of β and γ. The whole optimizing process could take several hours. An improvement on this situation was achieved by Bailey and Thomas through the use of a suitable mathematical approximation. It turns out that the cumulants of a function associated with $f(s, \tau_u | H_u)$ can be easily computed, and a gamma-distribution approximation to this function, using the first two cumulants only, can be readily derived. Approximations to $f(\tau_u | H_u)$ and $p(s | H_{u+1})$ then follow. This method was about 18 times as fast as the more accurate procedure already described, the systematic errors all being only a fraction of the corresponding standard errors. It is evident that the search for fast approximations is likely to be of considerable practical importance in the future, when attempts are made to utilize more realistic models than the present one.

Along with parameter estimation one should also consider the problem of goodness-of-fit. This is a difficult matter, especially as the conditional distributions, given H_u, of the τ_u are in general likely to be very skewed and non-normal. The conditional cumulants of any τ_u can be computed fairly easily. Bailey and Thomas (1971) suggest comparing the observed τ_u with their expected conditional distributions, the latter being derived approximately from a few low-order cumulants. Thus if the conditional distributions were all approximately negative exponential we could simply compare τ_u with its conditional mean value $\mu_1'(\tau_u | H_u)$, say. Rescaling the observations as

$$t_u = \frac{\tau_u}{\mu_1'(\tau_u | H_u)}, \tag{6.156}$$

then provides a set of variables all drawn from the negative exponential distribution $f(t) = \mathrm{e}^{-t}$. We could then examine whether the observed distribution function values $F_u = 1 - \mathrm{e}^{-t_u}$ could reasonably have come from a $(0, 1)$ rectangular distribution. Further sophisticated discussion seems unnecessary at present, especially for small-sample data like the smallpox material looked at above. At the same time there is here an important area of statistical research which should receive further investigation in the future.

6.9 Modifications and extensions

So far in this chapter we have essentially confined ourselves to a single form of the underlying model for a general epidemic (whether deterministic or stochastic), and in particular have assumed the existence of homogeneous mixing. As with the simple epidemic models of Chapter 5, a variety of modifications and extensions can be envisaged. Major extensions, involving substantially new features, will be introduced in later chapters. But it is convenient to review here a range of smaller developments, any one of which might of course assume much greater importance in the future.

Several interrelated groups

First of all, there is the possibility of allowing for non-homogeneous mixing by recognizing the existence of two or more distinct groups of individuals. A few deterministic results for the case of only two groups were first given many years ago by Wilson and Worcester (1945f). It is convenient to assume homogeneous mixing within each group, plus a measure of cross-infection between different groups. It was mentioned in Section 5.10 how Becker (1968) had extended to several groups Haskey's (1957) results for a simple stochastic epidemic with two groups, on the assumption that all inter- and intra-cross-infection rates were equal. Using the same simplifying assumptions, Becker also showed how results might be obtained for a general stochastic epidemic involving several groups.

Recently, Watson (1972) has studied a more general model for many groups, in which the members of any group mix homogeneously amongst themselves, but to a lesser extent with individuals of other groups. Specifically, we envisage a population of size N divided into m distinct groups C_r $(1 \leqslant r \leqslant m)$. We define β_{ij} as the infection-rate in C_i due to infectives in C_j $(1 \leqslant i,j \leqslant m)$, and γ_i as the removal-rate in C_i. The β_{ij} are then expressed in more readily interpretable parameters by means of the relationship

$$\beta_{ij} = \frac{\beta_i p_{ij} N_i}{N_j},\qquad(6.157)$$

where β_i is the infection-rate in C_i and p_{ij} is the rate of mixing between C_i and C_j. With this definition of p_{ij} there are certain constraints involved, e.g.

$$p_{ij} = p_{ji}, \quad p_{ii} = 1, \quad 0 \leqslant p_{ij} \leqslant 1.\qquad(6.158)$$

In particular, if all $p_{ij} = 1$, we have universal homogeneous mixing, while if $p_{ij} = 0$ $(i \neq j)$ there are m completely separate populations. There is also an interesting special case of "equivalent" classes, defined by

$$N_i = N_0, \quad \gamma_i = \gamma, \quad \beta_{ij} = \begin{cases} \beta, & i=j, \\ q\beta, & i \neq j, \end{cases}\qquad(6.159)$$

where $0 \leqslant q \leqslant 1$.

Noting the apparent intractability of the general stochastic version, Watson examined the deterministic approximation and showed how the intensities of the sub-epidemics in the several groups could be computed by the iterative solution of a set of simultaneous nonlinear equations.

In the special case of equivalent groups, a multidimensional linear birth-and-death process can be used as an upper boundary process approximating the numbers of infectives in the several groups during the early stages. This approach is an extension of that already described for a single population in Section 6.5. For large q there is a threshold, which when exceeded leads to a major outbreak affecting a majority of classes. But when q is small, there are three distinguishable possibilities: (1) a localized outbreak only, having a minor character in the initially affected group; (2) a restricted outbreak, giving rise to major outbreaks in a small number of groups; and (3) a generalized outbreak, involving major epidemics in most groups. Since, in principle, many public health interventions involve changes in the model parameters, it seems probable that qualitative theorems of this type could provide useful practical insights.

Generalized infection and removal rates

Another modification of the original homogeneous mixing assumption is provided by ideas of Severo (1969a) already introduced in the context of the simple epidemic in Section 5.10. We there saw that the probability of one new infection in time Δt might be expressed as $\beta r^{1-b} s^a \Delta t$ instead of $\beta r s \Delta t$, where r and s were the numbers of susceptibles and infectives, respectively. The parameters a and b were called the "infection power" and the "safety-in-numbers" power, respectively, and were susceptible of a certain broad physical interpretation. For a general epidemic, with removal as well, Severo suggested introducing a *removal power* c such that the chance of a removal in Δt was $\gamma s^{1+c} \Delta t$. The parameter c is intended to reflect in some measure the characteristics of a specific disease or environmental circumstances. Use of the recursive techniques of Severo (1967a), already mentioned in Sections 5.9, 5.10 and 6.3, leads to an algorithm for computing the relevant probabilities. In discussion, Severo (1969a) pointed out how this approach could in principle be employed to estimate the five parameters β, γ, a, b and c, from data on a series of independent households. These data would have to specify the state of each household, with regard to the numbers of both infectives and susceptibles, at each of a number of arbitrary times. Unfortunately, as emphasized in Section 6.8, real data rarely tell us anything about the numbers of infectives or uninfected susceptibles, at any time. We can usually determine, at most, the instants of removal of infectives from circulation, or, alternatively, the total number of removals that have occurred up to any given time. To deal with such situations would seem to require a rather intricate extension of Severo's methods. (If this could be done, however, it would also apply to the simpler problem involving β and γ only, investigated by Bailey and Thomas (1971) and described in Section 6.8.)

Cooke's deterministic model

Mention should also be made of the extended deterministic model of Cooke (1967), further developed by Hoppensteadt and Waltman (1970). This model has certain features not present in the model of Section 6.2. For instance, the infected individuals fall into two classes: (1) those who are infected but not yet infectious; and (2) those who are both infected and infectious to others. It is further assumed that individuals in class (1) have to reach a certain threshold of accumulated dosage of infection before being able to infect others.

Again, if an individual becomes infectious at time t, he recovers at time $t + \sigma$, where σ is some fixed constant. The effect of the threshold is to lead to functional equations rather than ordinary differential equations. Hoppensteadt and Waltman pay special attention to establishing the existence, uniqueness, and continuous dependence of solutions on the equations of the model. A number of numerical results are also presented in graphical form. In a subsequent paper Hoppensteadt and Waltman (1971) extend the model to cover the possibility of removed individuals losing their immunity and returning to an infectious state. See also Hethcote (1970), Wilson (1972), Cooke and Yorke (1973), and later work by Waltman.

It is of course most valuable to have such results established with a high degree of mathematical rigour. At the same time there are still many unanswered questions as to how far the model is epidemiologically appropriate, and whether the additional complexities introduced are capable of providing an improved understanding of real data. The possibility of investigating the implications of a stochastic analogue should also be considered.

Small epidemics in large populations

Another source of model modification stems from the discussion by Bailey (1964b) of the obvious fact that so many epidemic outbreaks are of relatively small extent. In some cases, following the notion in Section 5.1 about an effective number of independent groups within a population, we might think that a small total epidemic was really due to a large epidemic in a small sub-population. However, obvious sociological considerations suggest that the contacts occurring in a modern city are likely to be fairly extensive. If this is so, the idea of a large epidemic in a small sub-group may often be untenable. Now small outbreaks tend to be the rule when the relative removal rate ρ is greater than the initial number of susceptibles n (see, e.g., Section 6.5). Moreover, since the change in the total number of susceptibles is then relatively small, we can approximate the behaviour of the group of infectives by a suitably defined linear birth-and-death process.

Bailey pointed out that in such a case the general stochastic epidemic model of Section 6.3 leads to an epidemic curve given by

$$w = \gamma a\, e^{(\beta n - \gamma)t}. \tag{6.160}$$

For $\rho = \gamma/\beta > n$, this curve falls continuously from the initial value of $w(0) = \gamma a$. Thus we do *not* have an epidemic curve of typical unimodal shape.

Now the general stochastic epidemic entails an infectious period with a negative-exponential distribution (i.e. proportional to a χ_2^2 variable). It is easy to modify the model by supposing the infectives to pass through *two* negative-exponential stages, giving an infectious period distribution proportional to a χ_4^2 variable. The whole multidimensional stochastic process is still Markov in character. For small epidemics the process is linear, as before, and the partial differential equation for the moment-generating function is easily written down. Tractable ordinary differential equations for the stochastic means can be derived in the usual way by picking out coefficients of the terms that are linear in the relevant dummy variables. These equations are, as expected, identical with the corresponding deterministic equations. It is easy to show that the resultant epidemic curve is now in *unimodal* form.

A similar result can be obtained by keeping the infectious period negative exponential, but introducing a latent period which has a negative-exponential distribution instead of being identically zero. It is obvious that introducing many stages for both latent and infectious periods must lead to a fairly flexible general model.

It follows that there is a *prima facie* case for considering that the multi-dimensional birth-and-death type of process could be quite useful in describing small epidemics in large populations. There are, however, some serious difficulties in the modified models described above, as pointed out by Morgan (1964). Using computer calculations, he showed that the epidemic curves, though indeed unimodal, were extremely skew and would not in general represent typical data at all adequately. Moreover, the stochastic means themselves could be unsatisfactory since an appreciable proportion of epidemics would have very few cases indeed and would probably not be classified as epidemics at all. Morgan therefore recommended modifying the model so as to include only those realizations that survived beyond a predetermined time-interval τ. This leads to some improvement in the shape of the epidemic curve. Amongst other results, Morgan demonstrated that the model involving a χ_4^2 distribution of the infectious period could yield a nearly symmetrical epidemic curve if a suitable selection of realizations were chosen, ignoring those that were "too small" or "too large".

These ingenious modifications seem very promising, but it is evident that further work is required to take into account the way in which actual epidemics are sampled. Many of those examined do in fact show approximately symmetrical epidemic curves, but others have ragged tails. To what extent do we really neglect small isolated outbreaks in practice? And in what way is it justified in a theoretical assessment to neglect outbreaks that are too large or last too long, on the grounds that the birth-and-death model is then no longer valid?

The cost of epidemics

Another aspect of epidemics that has received some attention in recent years is the question of the economic cost of an epidemic. This problem was initially raised by Becker (1970a) and further developed in the context of the simple stochastic epidemic by Jerwood (1970). Subsequent applications to the more realistic general stochastic epidemic have been made by Jerwood (1971), Gani (1973), Gani and Jerwood (1972), and Downton (1972a, b). The general idea is to specify the cost of any given epidemic outbreak as a random variable

C, defined in terms of a linear function of the duration time T and the stochastic integral W under the infective path $Y(t)$. Thus

$$C = aW + bT, \tag{6.161}$$

where a and b are appropriate constants, and

$$W = \int_0^T Y(t)dt. \tag{6.162}$$

The investigation of C as defined in (6.161) leads to a good deal of interesting mathematics, but it is perhaps too early to say what the practical implications are likely to be. There is a basic difficulty in the formulation (6.161), since any costs related to the general stochastic epidemic as normally interpreted would arise from the treatment of removals rather than from the numbers of infectives circulating at various times during the epidemic. The subsequent fate of the removals in terms of disposal and treatment is in fact independent of the precise patterns of circulating infectives. One might well argue that the cost of an epidemic is more directly related to the total size of epidemic, since this is the total number of actual cases to be dealt with. The pattern of removal might also be important, especially if the facilities available for handling patients are limited in extent and thus liable to overload. (Incidentally, it is worth pointing out that Downton (1972b) finally shows that the mean area under the infectives trajectory is equal to the mean epidemic size divided by the relative removal rate.) Obviously, further study of these problems is needed, especially in relation to the practical issues of medical treatment and public health control.

Branching process models

Mention should also be made of explorations into age-dependent branching process formulations using, for example, the theoretical approach described by Harris (1963). In the applications described by Bharucha-Reid (1956, 1958) a latent period is easily introduced having a general distribution of length, but the infectious period is contracted to a point. Bharucha-Reid confines his detailed discussion to the case of latent periods with negative exponential distribution, and also supposes that each infective gives rise to no more than two further infections.

The disadvantage of the approach so far is that it involves a one-dimensional branching process describing only the number of infectives, and not taking into account the changing number of susceptibles. As it stands, therefore, the theory might be used to model the initial stages of an epidemic or describe the behaviour of small epidemics, but it cannot supply theorems of more general validity. If, however, the approach could be further developed to include models of somewhat greater realism covering, for example, both latent periods and non-zero infectious periods as well as accounting for the susceptible population, . then considerable strides forward might be made.

Direct removal of susceptibles

In many diseases, e.g. poliomyelitis, a certain proportion of infected individuals never show sufficiently marked symptoms to be recognized as actual cases of disease. Nevertheless, such individuals may well be infectious and so contribute to the spread of the epidemic. This is the problem of so-called "carriers", which will be discussed explicitly in Chapter 10. In the meantime we note here an extension to the general stochastic epidemic by Sakino and Hayashi (1959) and Sakino (1962b) which envisages the possibility that certain susceptibles pass directly to the state of immune removal without going through the intermediate stage of being infectious. The extent to which this notion is biologically realistic seems uncertain. It could well be true of disease where some susceptibles acquire permanent immunity as the result of a series of small immunizing doses of infection, but would not apply where circulating infectives were simply not recognized at removal because of the complete absence of overt symptoms. However, so far as the theory goes, both deterministic and stochastic discussions are available. Typical results include extensions of investigations previously described in Sections 6.2 and 6.4.

7

Recurrent epidemics and endemicity

7.1 Introduction

In the detailed theory discussed in the previous two chapters we have been thinking in terms of epidemic processes in communities of susceptibles, ranging from small households to large populations, which tend to exhibit certain characteristic forms of transient behaviour, such as minor outbreaks dying rapidly away or true epidemics building up to a peak of activity before slowly declining. At all events, after the elapse of a sufficiently long period of time a final stable state is reached, so that we can talk of the total size of epidemic and discuss its magnitude, probability distribution, and the chain of events by which it is attained. Over comparatively short periods of time, say a few months, such a picture may be quite suitable for epidemics in small groups of individuals like households or school classrooms, but it is clearly untenable if we consider the behaviour of the commoner infectious diseases in larger communities. When a disease is rare, like plague or smallpox in Britain, any outbreak that occurs can be regarded as an isolated phenomenon: it is *epidemic* in the strict sense. Even though, with diseases like measles, poliomyelitis, diphtheria, influenza, the common cold, etc., there may be periodic outbreaks of an epidemic nature, the infection is kept alive all the time by a constant low-level spread to new susceptibles. The stock of susceptibles is constantly replenished by new recruits to the population, and also in some cases by the loss of immunity in those previously attacked. It is also possible that some diseases are constantly introduced *de novo* by the genetic mutation of normally harmless and widely distributed organisms to more virulent forms.

Broadly speaking, therefore, these commoner infectious diseases, of which measles and the common cold may be regarded as fairly typical, are really *endemic*. They are constantly with us, though often presenting considerable fluctuation in prevalence. The general level may tend to be oscillatory, and measles, for example, has both an approximately two-year cycle and shorter seasonal variations as well. In such a situation we often speak of *recurrent epidemics*, and the elucidation of the relevant large-scale phenomena is clearly of considerable importance. Quantitative investigations of this kind present great difficulty, but when sufficiently advanced they may be expected to describe the behaviour of epidemic processes in large populations in terms not automatically derivable from the equally important complementary studies of small-scale data, where we seek to fit appropriate biological models in detail.

The early deterministic work of Soper (1929) on the periodicity of recurrent outbreaks of measles met with difficulties in providing a satisfactory description of actual events since it entailed *damped* epidemic waves. Further investigations along similar lines were made later by Wilson and Worcester in a series of papers (1941a to 1945f). Subsequently, the problem was reconsidered by Bartlett (1953 to 1960c). He made several major advances by formulating a more realistic stochastic model. This showed how an *undamped* series of epidemic outbreaks could arise, and led to the concept of a critical community size above which oscillations would tend to be maintained, as well as explaining other observable phenomena. Bartlett's work quoted above is primarily related to measles so far as practical interpretations are concerned. However, some attention (Bartlett, 1960a, c; 1964, 1966) has also been given to chickenpox, but this involves additional complications because of its connection with shingles (herpes zoster).

In Section 7.2 we introduce the basic deterministic model which under appropriate conditions yields a steady state, about which natural periodic oscillations are possible. Unfortunately, as mentioned above, the latter are damped, in contradiction with observed epidemiological phenomena. This finding persists even when modifications are made, as in Section 7.3, to allow for an incubation period or seasonal variations in infection-rate (the forced seasonal component remains, but the longer natural periodic waves disappear). Two special cases of undamped waves are noted in Section 7.3, one depending on a rather specialized model with constant parameters, the other involving a certain pattern of public health intervention tending to regulate the epidemic swings.

To investigate the possible causes of undamped waves and the phenomenon of the fade-out of infection, a stochastic analogue of the basic deterministic model is described in Section 7.4. The analysis shows that an undamped series of epidemic outbreaks is possible if new cases of disease are permitted to enter the community. A modified stochastic model is then developed in Section 7.5, involving the introduction of new infectives explicitly. An inverse correlation between the average renewal time for successive epidemic outbreaks and community size is established. This is shown to be in approximate agreement with observed data.

In Section 7.6 certain asymptotic approximations are pursued, valid for large numbers of susceptibles and infectives. Analysis of the basic stochastic model without reintroduction of infection shows that, in the absence of extinction or fade-out of infection, stochastic fluctuations will persist indefinitely. Further, a more detailed analysis indicates that the passage-time to extinction is very sensitive to community size. The existence of a critical level is suggested, above which the disease tends to maintain itself and below which fade-out occurs. Again, this is in conformity with observed data on measles in the UK, the USA, and elsewhere.

Finally, some simulation studies are discussed in Section 7.7. These provide additional confirmation of the theoretical analyses, which often rely on extensive approximations, by showing broad qualitative agreement with observed epidemiological phenomena.

7.2 Basic deterministic model

Let us now return to the simple deterministic set-up described in Section 6.2, where we envisaged a community of n individuals comprising, at time t, x susceptibles, y infectives in circulation, and z individuals who were isolated, dead, or recovered and immune. We further postulated infection- and removal-rates β and γ, so that there were $\beta xy \, \Delta t$ new infections and $\gamma y \, \Delta t$ removals in time Δt. An additional assumption to be made here is that the stock of susceptibles is continually replenished. The simplest way to do this is to introduce a birth-parameter μ, so as to give $\mu \, \Delta t$ new susceptibles in time Δt. If the population is to remain stable the arrival of new susceptibles must be balanced by an appropriately defined death-rate. The simplest model that can be constructed avoids explicit reference to a death-rate by concentrating on the groups of susceptibles and infectives, the former at any rate being supposed not subject to death. This is equivalent to assuming that, on average, the deaths of removed individuals are just balanced by the births of new susceptibles. The basic differential equations are accordingly

$$\left.\begin{aligned} \frac{dx}{dt} &= -\beta xy + \mu, \\ \frac{dy}{dt} &= \beta xy - \gamma y. \end{aligned}\right\} \tag{7.1}$$

Equilibrium values x_0 and y_0 are given by equating the differential coefficients to zero. Thus

$$x_0 = \gamma/\beta, \quad y_0 = \mu/\gamma. \tag{7.2}$$

The equations for small departures from these equilibrium values are obtained by writing

$$x = x_0(1 + u), \quad y = y_0(1 + v), \tag{7.3}$$

and substituting (7.3) in (7.1). This yields

$$\left.\begin{array}{r}
\sigma \dfrac{du}{dt} = -(u + v + uv), \\[3mm]
\tau \dfrac{dv}{dt} = u(1 + v),
\end{array}\right\} \qquad (7.4)$$

where $\sigma = \gamma/\beta\mu, \quad \tau = 1/\gamma.$

If we now neglect the product uv and eliminate u from the two equations in (7.4), we obtain the second-order differential equation in v

$$\frac{d^2v}{dt} + \frac{1}{\sigma}\frac{dv}{dt} + \frac{1}{\sigma\tau} v = 0, \qquad (7.5)$$

which has the solution

$$\left.\begin{array}{r}
v_1 = v_0 e^{-t/2\sigma} \cos \xi t, \\[3mm]
\xi = \left(\dfrac{1}{\sigma\tau} - \dfrac{1}{4\sigma^2}\right)^{\frac{1}{2}},
\end{array}\right\} \qquad (7.6)$$

where

for a suitably chosen origin of time. We then obtain the solution for u given by

$$\left.\begin{array}{r}
u_1 = v_0(\tau/\sigma)^{\frac{1}{2}} e^{-t/2\sigma} \cos (\xi t + \psi), \\[3mm]
\cos \psi = -\tfrac{1}{2}(\tau/\sigma)^{\frac{1}{2}}, \quad 0 \leqslant \psi \leqslant \pi.
\end{array}\right\} \qquad (7.7)$$

where

The solutions u_1 and v_1, which are linearized or first-order components only, clearly involve damped harmonic trains of waves with period $2\pi/\xi$. In his application to measles, Soper took τ equal to two weeks, the approximate incubation period, and from the data available to him he estimated σ in London to be roughly $68 \cdot 2$ weeks. Equations (7.6) then give the period $2\pi/\xi = 73 \cdot 7$ weeks, with a peak-to-peak damping factor of $\exp(-\pi/\sigma\xi) = 0 \cdot 58$.

For somewhat larger oscillations we ought to take into account the non-linear character of the equations (7.4). For this purpose it is convenient to write

$$\left.\begin{array}{r}
u = u_1 + a_{11}u_1^2 + a_{12}u_1v_1 + a_{22}v_1^2 + ..., \\[3mm]
v = v_1 + b_{11}u_1^2 + b_{12}u_1v_1 + b_{22}v_1^2 + ...,
\end{array}\right\} \qquad (7.8)$$

where the coefficients, a_{ij} and b_{ij}, can be found in terms of τ/σ by straightforward substitution in (7.4). If τ/σ is small, so that $\psi \sim \tfrac{1}{2}\pi$, we have approximately

$$\left.\begin{array}{r}
u = u_1'(1 + \tfrac{1}{3}v_1), \\[3mm]
v = v_1 + \tfrac{1}{3}v_0^2 e^{-t/\sigma} \cos 2\xi t,
\end{array}\right\} \qquad (7.9)$$

where $u_1' = -v_0(\tau/\sigma)^{\frac{1}{2}} e^{-t/2\sigma} \sin \xi t.$

It will be noticed that the damping coefficient has relatively little influence on the period $2\pi/\xi$, which, for small τ/σ, is roughly $2\pi(\sigma\tau)^{\frac{1}{2}} = 2\pi(\beta\mu)^{-\frac{1}{2}}$, and so largely depends on the birth-rate for new susceptibles and the infection-rate. As an alternative to the foregoing approximate discussion we can always investigate special cases by step-by-step numerical solution of (7.1), though care is needed to ensure sufficient accuracy and to avoid mistaken conclusions about the effect of damping.

Another way of representing the oscillatory behaviour of the process is to plot the path traced by the point (x, y). This also allows a convenient method of comparing the deterministic solution with paths followed by actual realizations of the stochastic analogue. It can be shown that the deterministic curve found in this way has the form of a spiral converging on the equilibrium point (x_0, y_0), and that this occurs in spite of the non-linear form of (7.1). An elegant argument due to G. E. H. Reuter (Bartlett, 1956) is as follows. Consider the function

$$f(u, v) = \{(1 + u) - \log(1 + u)\} + (\tau/\sigma)\{(1 + v) - \log(1 + v)\}. \quad (7.10)$$

Differentiating with respect to t and using (7.4) gives

$$\frac{df}{dt} = -\frac{u^2}{\sigma(1 + u)} \leqslant 0. \quad (7.11)$$

Thus f continually decreases along any path for which t increases. Since $f \geqslant 1 + \tau/\sigma$, it follows that f tends to a finite limit $f_0 \geqslant 1 + \tau/\sigma$, as t tends to infinity. Now the curves $f = c$ are closed, surround the point (x_0, y_0), and shrink down as c tends to $1 + \tau/\sigma$. By considering the second differential coefficient d^2f/dt^2 we can show that $f_0 = 1 + \tau/\sigma$, so that the point (x, y) must actually tend to (x_0, y_0).

An important consequence of the above discussion is that, while the additional assumption of a constant influx of fresh susceptibles is sufficient to account for epidemic waves with a period of about the right order of magnitude, the damping down to a steady endemic state entailed by the calculations is at variance with observed epidemiological facts. Before passing on to stochastic models we must first look at the effect of certain modifications to the present process, especially as the introduction of an incubation period, for example, was once wrongly thought to counteract the damping.

7.3 Modified deterministic models

7.31 Seasonal variations in infection-rate

As mentioned in Section 7.1, not only do records of measles notifications tend to show an approximately biennial cycle, but there are appreciable seasonal variations as well. The precise reasons for the latter do not immediately concern us here, but it may be noted in passing that relevant factors may be the assembling and dispersion of schoolchildren at beginning and end of term, possible seasonal changes in the virulence or viability of the infecting organism, meteorological conditions which at times may facilitate the spread of infection, and so on.

The simplest modification is to try replacing the infection-rate β by $\beta' = \beta + \beta_1 \cos \omega t$, where $2\pi/\omega = 52$ weeks. We suppose the relative amplitude of these forced oscillations, $\rho = \beta_1/\beta$, to be small. Substituting the new value of β in (7.1), and using (7.3), gives equations corresponding to (7.4). These can now be dealt with as before by eliminating u to yield the modified form of (7.5), namely

$$\frac{d^2v}{dt^2} + \frac{1}{\sigma}\frac{dv}{dt} + \frac{1}{\sigma\tau}v = -\frac{\rho\omega}{\tau}\sin \omega t. \tag{7.12}$$

The particular integral of (7.12) representing the forced oscillation term is, by a standard result, of type $V = A \cos(\omega t + \epsilon)$, where the amplitude is

$$A = \frac{\rho\omega}{\tau}\left\{\left(\frac{1}{\sigma\tau} - \omega^2\right)^2 + \left(\frac{\omega}{\sigma}\right)^2\right\}^{-\frac{1}{2}}. \tag{7.13}$$

Since the rate at which new notifications actually occur is given by γy, we have

$$\gamma y = \mu(1 + v)$$
$$\doteqdot \mu(1 + v_1 + V), \tag{7.14}$$

where v_1 is the first-order solution in (7.6). If we take $\tau = 2$, $\sigma = 68\cdot2$, as before, and $\omega = \pi/26$, then substituting in (7.13) gives A as approximately $8\cdot1\rho$. This shows that a 10 percent variation in β', as envisaged by Soper, would lead to seasonal variations of about 80 percent in the rate of notifications. Studies made by L. Linnert (unpublished University of Manchester report) revealed a value of approximately 60 percent in Manchester for the years 1917–1951.

Again, the order of magnitude of predicted variation is correct, but while the forced seasonal waves persist, the longer natural period will still theoretically disappear. The above treatment is slightly different from Bartlett (1956) in that he considered variation in the incidence of new infections, whereas we have looked at changes in the rate of removal, which correspond more directly to notifications. There is, of course, little difference in the general implications.

7.32 Allowance for incubation period

Another possible source of error in the use of the simple continuous-infection model is that it makes no allowance for the effect of a fairly well-defined incubation period, such as is clearly recognizable in measles. Soper believed, wrongly as it happened because of an inaccurate numerical method, that the introduction of an incubation period into the model would offset the damping effect.

However, as first pointed out by Wilson and Worcester (1945e), the appropriate coefficient in Soper's model is really only halved.

If we suppose that there is a latent period of length a after infection, at the end of which the infected individual becomes infectious, the processes of infection and removal then proceeding as before, the deterministic equations will be

$$\left.\begin{array}{l}\dfrac{dx(t)}{dt} = -\beta x(t)y(t-a) + \mu, \\[2mm] \dfrac{dy(t)}{dt} = \beta x(t)y(t-a) - \gamma y(t).\end{array}\right\} \tag{7.15}$$

The equilibrium values are exactly the same as for (7.1). If we now put $D \equiv d/dt$, the equations for u and v are found to be

$$\left.\begin{array}{l}\left(D + \dfrac{1}{\sigma}\right)u + \dfrac{1}{\sigma}e^{-aD}v = 0, \\[2mm] -\dfrac{1}{\tau}u + \left(D + \dfrac{1}{\tau} - \dfrac{1}{\tau}e^{-aD}\right)v = 0.\end{array}\right\} \tag{7.16}$$

A short heuristic treatment of (7.16), using an operational method, is as follows If we assume that the infectious period is short, both β and γ are large and τ tends to zero. In this case the differential equation for v reduces to

$$\left\{\left(D + \dfrac{1}{\sigma}\right)e^{aD} - D\right\}v = 0. \tag{7.17}$$

The form of the solution depends on the roots of

$$(D + 1/\sigma)e^{aD} - D = 0.$$

If we write this as

$$aD = -\log\{1 + 1/(\sigma D)\},$$

and expand the logarithm in negative powers of D, we obtain the series

$$aD = -\dfrac{1}{\sigma D} + \dfrac{1}{2\sigma^2 D^2} - \dots . \tag{7.18}$$

The first approximation to (7.18) is given by $D = (-a\sigma)^{-\frac{1}{2}}$, and the second by

$$aD = -\dfrac{1}{\sigma D} - \dfrac{a}{2\sigma},$$

which is equivalent to the equation

$$\dfrac{d^2w}{dt^2} + \dfrac{1}{2\sigma}\dfrac{dw}{dt} + \dfrac{1}{\sigma a}w = 0. \tag{7.19}$$

Comparing this with (7.5) shows that the approximate solution here is similar to the previous one, except that we now have a instead of τ, and the damping coefficient is halved.

7.33   Two interacting groups of individuals

We now consider the type of deterministic model treated in Section 7.2, but involving two groups instead of only one. Moreover, we suppose there to be interaction between the two groups, which might be actual migration of susceptibles or infectives from one group to the other, or might merely be visits involving ultimate return to the original group. To allow for the first contingency we introduce emigration rates, θ and ϕ, for susceptibles and infectives, respectively. Similarly, we need additional parameters to allow for susceptibles of one group to be infected by infectives of the other group. A suitable extension of the previous equations (7.1) is

$$\left.\begin{aligned}
\frac{dx_1}{dt} &= -(\beta_1 y_1 + \beta_2 y_2)x_1 + \mu + \theta(x_2 - x_1), \\[2mm]
\frac{dy_1}{dt} &= (\beta_1 y_1 + \beta_2 y_2)x_2 - \gamma y_1 + \phi(y_2 - y_1),
\end{aligned}\right\} \qquad (7.20)$$

with two similar equations for the second group. The equilibrium values of x_1 and x_2 are $\gamma/(\beta_1 + \beta_2)$, and of y_1 and y_2 are μ/γ. To obtain the equations for small departures from equilibrium, let us now write

$$x_j = \frac{\gamma}{\beta_1 + \beta_2}(1 + u_j), \quad y_j = \frac{\mu}{\gamma}(1 + v_j), \quad j = 1, 2. \qquad (7.21)$$

Substituting (7.21) in (7.20) and the two similar equations for the second group, gives, with $d/dt \equiv D$,

$$\left.\begin{aligned}
\left(D + \frac{1}{\sigma'} + \theta\right)u_1 + \frac{\alpha}{\sigma'}v_1 - \theta u_2 + \frac{1-\alpha}{\sigma'}v_2 &= 0, \\[2mm]
-\gamma u_1 + \{D + \gamma(1 - \alpha) + \phi\}v_1 - \{\gamma(1 - \alpha) + \phi\}v_2 &= 0,
\end{aligned}\right\} \qquad (7.22)$$

and two similar equations with suffixes 1 and 2 interchanged, where we have put

$$\alpha = \frac{\beta_1}{\beta_1 + \beta_2}, \quad \sigma' = \frac{\gamma}{\mu(\beta_1 + \beta_2)}. \qquad (7.23)$$

It is interesting to observe that if we add each equation in (7.22) to the corresponding one with interchanged suffixes, we obtain

$$\left.\begin{aligned}
\left(D + \frac{1}{\sigma'}\right)U + \frac{V}{\sigma'} &= 0, \\[2mm]
DV - \gamma U &= 0,
\end{aligned}\right\} \qquad (7.24)$$

where
$$U = u_1 + u_2, \quad V = v_1 + v_2.$$

Now these two equations in U and V are exactly the same as equations (7.4) in u and v, neglecting uv and writing σ' for σ. Similar solutions therefore apply. In particular, the damping term has coefficient $1/\sigma'$. On the other hand, if we subtract corresponding pairs of equations, the result is

$$\left.\begin{array}{c} \left(D + \dfrac{1}{\sigma'} + 2\theta\right) U' - \dfrac{1 - 2\alpha}{\sigma'} V' = 0, \\[2ex] -\gamma U' + \{D + 2\gamma(1 - \alpha) + 2\phi\}V' = 0, \\[2ex] U' = u_1 - u_2, \quad V' = v_1 - v_2. \end{array}\right\} \qquad (7.25)$$

where

Eliminating U' and V' from (7.25) gives a quadratic in D whose roots determine the solutions required. It is sufficient to remark here that the coefficient of D is $(\sigma')^{-1} + 2\gamma(1 - \alpha) + 2(\theta + \phi)$, which contains only positive terms, showing that the damping of U' and V' is greater than that of U and V.

Presumably, analogous results could be obtained for several interacting groups. In the case of a very large number of very small groups having a geographical spread, we could consider the limiting form of a spatially continuous distribution of population. This problem will be taken up in Section 9.2.

7.34 Models with undamped waves

All the recurrent epidemic models discussed so far in this chapter are capable of explaining the existence of epidemic waves in terms of oscillations about a steady state. Unfortunately, the harmonic trains of waves are always damped, and this has led to a virtual abandonment of the deterministic theory in favour of the stochastic approach of the next section, where an undamped series of outbreaks is possible.

Nevertheless, it is well known in biophysics (e.g. Rashevsky, 1964) that sustained, undamped oscillations are possible in certain multi-compartment systems (sometimes with as few as three compartments) subject to appropriate interactions and feedbacks. It would be interesting to know if this kind of explanation could be invoked in an epidemic context. The possibility of undamped waves arising from a deterministic model is established by considering the following two special cases.

First, suppose we have a disease which is lethal to all those contracting it. Thus all removals are in fact deaths, and make no further contribution to the life of the community. Let us also suppose that the disease is sufficiently virulent to suppress any live births amongst circulating infectives. New susceptible births therefore arise solely from the susceptible group itself. If μ is the birth-rate per individual, equation (7.1) is replaced by

$$\left.\begin{array}{l} \dfrac{dx}{dt} = -\beta xy + \mu x, \\[2mm] \dfrac{dy}{dt} = \beta xy - \gamma y, \end{array}\right\} \qquad (7.26)$$

for which the steady-state solution is

$$x_0 = \gamma/\beta, \quad y_0 = \mu/\beta. \qquad (7.27)$$

Use of (7.3) then quickly leads to

$$\frac{du}{dt} = -\mu v, \quad \frac{dv}{dt} = \gamma u, \qquad (7.28)$$

to first order in the small quantities u and v. Eliminating u, say, from (7.28) yields the familiar equation

$$\frac{d^2v}{dt^2} + \gamma\mu v = 0, \qquad (7.29)$$

which has an undamped solution

$$v = v_0 \sin(\gamma\mu)^{\frac{1}{2}}t. \qquad (7.30)$$

Secondly, consider a relatively small series of outbreaks in a population sufficiently large for the number of susceptibles to remain effectively constant and equal to n. We are therefore concerned with a single equation

$$\frac{dy}{dt} = n\beta y - \gamma y = my, \qquad (7.31)$$

where

$$m = n\beta - \gamma. \qquad (7.32)$$

We thus have a simple deterministic population model for the group of infectives, with solution

$$y = y_0 e^{mt}. \qquad (7.33)$$

If $m > 0$ the epidemic curve given by $w = \gamma y$ is rising, and if $m < 0$ the curve is falling.

Suppose now that when the epidemic curve is rising exponentially with *positive* $m = m_1$ it continues to do so until it reaches the value $w = a$. At this point, the public health authorities take action. As a result of a special campaign, people not only move around less, thus reducing β, but they stay home more readily at the first signs of illness, thus increasing γ. If these parameter changes are sufficiently large, m will take the *negative* value $m = m_2$. The epidemic curve now falls exponentially until it reaches the level $w = b$, when public health action ceases. The parameter m then reverts to m_1 and the process is repeated, the epidemic curve undergoing an undamped series of oscillations between the levels a and b.

Of course, those examples are greatly oversimplified, but they show that regulatory mechanisms leading to undamped waves are quite possible even in deterministic models. The possible extension of these ideas to more realistic configurations is a matter worthy of further investigation.

7.4 Basic stochastic model

It is clear from the foregoing discussion that the deterministic model originally proposed by Soper has had some success, especially in predicting epidemic waves from assumptions not explicitly involving such fluctuations. Nevertheless, the waves are in general subject to appreciable damping, leading to a stable epidemic state. This is true when allowance is made for such modifications as seasonal variation in infection-rate or the introduction of an incubation period. It was, however, shown at the end of the previous section that undamped waves could occur either in a rather specialized model involving a certain balance between birth, death and infection, or in a model where the infection and removal rates were to some extent controllable by public health policy.

In practice epidemiological records do not reveal damped oscillations converging to a steady endemic level. As demonstrated by Bartlett (1957), using extensive measles data from the UK, oscillations tend to persist when community size is apparently above a certain critical level. Below this level there is a strong tendency to "fade-out", suggestive of the extinction of a stochastic process. Bartlett observed a continuous pattern of epidemic peaks and troughs with no fade-out in two towns of more than 650 000 inhabitants; occasional fade-out in three towns having 180 000–415 000 inhabitants; and invariable fade-out in 14 towns with populations of 113 000 or less. It was also observed that the mean period between epidemics tended to be negatively correlated with community size. Detailed analysis suggested a critical level of about 250 000 total population for measles. A similar figure was later obtained by Bartlett (1960c) in his analysis of United States measles data. Black (1966) has further refined and confirmed Bartlett's results in a detailed study of measles endemicity in 19 island communities, where the reintroduction of disease was minimal and the effects of population dispersion could be observed.

The net result of these conclusions is that a stochastic investigation appears to be essential if the absence of damping in large communities and the occurrence of fade-out in small ones is to receive a reasonably realistic explanation. It is interesting to note that we are proposing to appeal to stochastic formulations in situations where the gross population sizes are relatively large (although the susceptible populations would in general be much smaller).

We shall first consider the appropriate stochastic version of the simplest non-spatial deterministic model developed in Section 7.2. Thus all we require is the extension of the model described in Section 6.3 to the case where the renewal of susceptibles is permitted. We write $p_{rs}(t)$ for the probability that there are r susceptibles and s infectives at time t. There are now three types of transition in time Δt to be taken into account, and these are represented by

$$
\left.
\begin{array}{lll}
\text{(i)} & \Pr\{(r,s) \to (r-1, s+1)\} = \beta rs\,\Delta t, \\[2mm]
\text{(ii)} & \Pr\{(r,s) \to (r, s-1)\} \quad\; = \gamma s\,\Delta t, \\[2mm]
\text{(iii)} & \Pr\{(r,s) \to (r+1, s)\} \quad\; = \mu\,\Delta t.
\end{array}
\right\}
\tag{7.34}
$$

The general method of procedure, also referred to in Section 6.3, leads to the partial differential equation

$$
\frac{\partial \Pi}{\partial t} = \beta(w^2 - zw)\frac{\partial^2 \Pi}{\partial z\,\partial w} + \gamma(1-w)\frac{\partial \Pi}{\partial w} + \mu(z-1)\Pi,
\tag{7.35}
$$

where

$$
\Pi(z, w, t) = \sum_{r,s} p_{rs}(t) z^r w^s
\tag{7.36}
$$

is the probability-generating function. We shall not attempt here the complete solution of either (7.35) or of the equivalent set of differential-difference equations in the probabilities. Nevertheless, several important features of the solution can be deduced by the following arguments based on approximations to the model.

In discussing the epidemic situation in Section 6.5, where there was no renewal of susceptibles, it was seen that the critical threshold behaviour of the process could be predicted in general terms by supposing that initially the number of susceptibles was actually constant, instead of slowly diminishing. This meant that we could regard the population of infectives as subject to an ordinary birth-and-death process with birth- and death-rates βn and γ, respectively, where n was the initial number of susceptibles. A similar argument can be applied in the present context a little more generally: although we shall ignore the depletion of the stock of·susceptibles by infection, we shall to some extent take account of the accession of fresh susceptibles by supposing these to increase deterministically at rate μ. The approximate birth- and death-rates for the population of infectives are therefore $\beta(n + \mu t)$ and γ.

Now it has been shown by D. G. Kendall (1948) that the chance, P, of extinction for a birth-and-death process with time-dependent birth- and death-rates $\lambda(t)$ and $\nu(t)$, is given by

$$
P = \left\{\frac{J}{1+J}\right\}^a,
\tag{7.37}
$$

where

$$
J = \int_0^\infty \nu(t) \exp\left[\int_0^t \{\nu(\tau) - \lambda(\tau)\}d\tau\right]dt,
\tag{7.38}
$$

and a is the initial population size. In the present context we have $\lambda(t) = \beta(n + \mu t)$ and $\nu(t) = \gamma$. Substitution in (7.38) yields therefore

$$
\left.
\begin{aligned}
J &= \int_0^\infty \gamma \exp\left\{(\gamma - \beta n)t - \tfrac{1}{2}\beta\mu t^2\right\}dt \\
&= \zeta \exp\left\{\tfrac{1}{2}\zeta^2(f-1)^2\right\} \int_{\zeta(f-1)}^\infty \exp\left(-\tfrac{1}{2}u^2\right)du,
\end{aligned}
\right\}
\tag{7.39}
$$

where $\qquad \zeta = \dfrac{\gamma}{(\beta\mu)^{\frac{1}{2}}}, \quad f = \dfrac{n\beta}{\gamma} = \dfrac{n}{\rho}.$

The quantity ρ here is the relative removal-rate of Chapter 6.

It is instructive to compare these results with those for the corresponding situation in which no fresh susceptibles are added, i.e. $\mu = 0$. In the latter case the chance of extinction, P, is given by (cf. Section 6.5)

$$
\left.
\begin{aligned}
P_{\mu=0} &= (\rho/n)^a, \quad \rho < n, \\
&= 1, \qquad\quad \rho \geqslant n.
\end{aligned}
\right\}
\tag{7.40}
$$

Now when $\mu \neq 0$, there is no sharp cut-off at $\rho = n$. The chance of extinction varies continuously, having the value $\left\{1 + \left(\dfrac{2}{\pi\zeta^2}\right)^{\frac{1}{2}}\right\}^{-a}$ at $\rho = n$, and the asymptotic form

$$
\left.
\begin{aligned}
P_{\mu\neq0} &\sim \left(\frac{\rho}{n}\right)^a \left\{1 - \frac{a\rho^2}{n(n-\rho)\zeta^2}\right\}, \\
\end{aligned}
\right\}
\tag{7.41}
$$

when $\qquad\qquad \rho \ll n.$

If however, ρ is much larger than n, so that $f \to 0$, then $P \to 1$ provided J is large. This will require ζ to be large. The rough value suggested by the deterministic treatment of Section 7.2 is $\zeta = \gamma/(\beta\mu)^{\frac{1}{2}} = (\sigma/\tau)^{\frac{1}{2}} = 5 \cdot 84$, which is quite sufficient to make $1 - P$ negligibly small.

The essential difference between the full stochastic model and the corresponding deterministic one can easily be seen from the foregoing approximations. It is the phenomenon of extinction that gives the stochastic process an entirely different character, at any rate in a comparatively small isolated community. For in this case after a major outbreak the numbers of susceptibles and infectives will both be fairly low. If we consider the progress of the process from this point, the appropriate value of ρ/n is likely to be quite large and extinction is very probable. If new cases of the disease are permitted to enter the community a fresh outbreak will occur as soon as the population of susceptibles has increased sufficiently. Moreover, this recurrence of outbreaks will involve no damping, as with the deterministic version.

7.5 Modified stochastic model

Following up the remarks at the end of the last section, we see that in a community which is not completely isolated a series of major outbreaks will occur, each of which is triggered off by the arrival of new cases from outside, whenever the density of susceptibles has grown large enough.

We can examine the consequences of this a little more closely by means of the following approximate argument. Let us assume new infectives to arrive randomly at an average rate ϵ, so that the chance of one new arrival in time Δt is $\epsilon \Delta t$. Suppose that at $t = 0$, the number of susceptibles is negligible, but that it increases deterministically at a rate μ, which is much greater than ϵ. Suppose further that we neglect, as before, the ultimate reduction in the number of susceptibles when infection actually does spread. Then it is easily seen that the effects of each freshly introduced infective are independent of each other. The probability of no epidemic occurring up to time t is, therefore, approximately given by

$$\prod_{0<u<t} \{1 - \epsilon\, du + \epsilon\, du\, P(u)\} \sim \exp\left[-\epsilon \int_0^t \{1 - P(u)\}du\right], \quad (7.42)$$

where $P(u)$ is the chance of extinction with one new infective at time u, when the number of susceptibles is taken to be μu. We now use the approximation to $P(u)$ given by (7.40), i.e.

$$P(u) = \sigma/u, \quad u > \sigma, \\ = 1, \quad u \leqslant \sigma, \qquad\qquad (7.43)$$

where $\sigma = \gamma/\beta\mu$, as previously defined in equation (7.4). It follows that the required probability is

$$\exp\left\{-\epsilon \int_0^t (1 - \sigma/u)du\right\} = \left(\frac{t}{\sigma}\right)^{\epsilon\sigma} e^{-\epsilon(t-\sigma)}, \quad t > \sigma. \quad (7.44)$$

The lower limit to the integral is now σ, since all factors on the left of (7.42) are unity in the interval $0 < u < \sigma$. If $F(t)$ is the distribution function of the time elapsing before the occurrence of a major epidemic, then the expression in (7.44) is just $1 - F(t)$. Differentiation gives the corresponding frequency distribution, which in terms of a variable $T = t/\sigma$, is

$$dF = k(T-1)T^{k-1}e^{-k(T-1)}dT, \quad T > 1, \\ \text{where} \quad k = \epsilon\sigma = \epsilon\gamma/\beta\mu. \qquad (7.45)$$

This distribution has a mode at $T_m = 1 + k^{-\frac{1}{2}}$. We could assume that the mean $\overline{T}$ was roughly of the same form. Bartlett's (1956) calculations showed that, as expected, $\overline{T}$ is relatively insensitive to variations in k, unless k is less than about 2, when $\overline{T}$ increases rapidly. Put another way, we may say that the average renewal time $\bar{t}$ is directly proportional to σ, but is relatively uninfluenced by ϵ provided the latter is not too small. The proportionality of $\bar{t}$ to σ may be contrasted with the proportionality of the analogous deterministic period to $(\sigma\tau)^{\frac{1}{2}}$.

It can now be seen in general terms just how the present stochastic model leads to a permanent and undamped succession of outbreaks, which although not following a strict cycle will exhibit a pattern of behaviour determined by the distribution of epidemic renewal time. Comparison with the deterministic process can also be made by considering the path of the point (r, s). The corresponding deterministic path traced by (x, y), as described in Section 7.2, was in general a converging spiral. Although the whole line $y = 0$ was a possible path, it was never reached from any point within the positive quadrant. In the stochastic model, however, the path is very likely to drop to the x-axis whenever the number of susceptibles falls below the threshold value, after which it will follow the x-axis until a new infective arrives.

From the point of view of interpreting actual data, we could assume that the immigration rate ϵ of new infectives was approximately proportional to the total community size n. Thus we could write $\bar{T} \doteq 1 + an^{-\frac{1}{2}}$, and $\bar{t} \doteq \sigma + bn^{-\frac{1}{2}}$. In Bartlett's (1957) detailed discussion of the UK material, observed pairs of values of $\bar{t}$ and $100\,n^{-\frac{1}{2}}$ were plotted graphically. An approximately linear relation was in fact evident, and it is interesting to record that the ordinate corresponding to $n = \infty$, namely $\bar{t} = \sigma$, was not inconsistent with the value $\sigma = 68\cdot2$ used by Soper in analysing his London data (Section 7.2).

Thus certain well-marked features of the epidemiological records of measles are explicable in a broad qualitative way by means of the stochastic model described, whereas so far no satisfactory deterministic model has been found.

7.6   Asymptotic approximations

7.61   Basic stochastic model

Let us first look at the large-sample behaviour of the basic stochastic model described in Section 7.4. If the numbers of susceptibles and infectives are large enough, we can assume as a first approximation that the chance of extinction is negligible and that an equilibrium point (x_0, y_0) exists, corresponding to the solution of the deterministic equations (7.1). This allows us to carry through an orthodox time-series type of analysis.

We now write $X(t)$ and $Y(t)$ for the random variables describing the numbers of susceptibles and infectives at time t, taking the specific values r and s, respectively, as indicated near the beginning of Section 7.4. The transition probabilities given in (7.34) imply that we can represent the stochastic changes ΔX and ΔY over Δt as follows. First, we consider ΔX as compounded of a loss due to infection, having a Poisson distribution with mean $\beta XY\,\Delta t$, and a gain arising from the arrival of new susceptibles, having a Poisson distribution with mean $\mu\,\Delta t$. Secondly, we conceive ΔY as made up of a Poisson gain due to infection, having parameter $\beta XY\,\Delta t$, and a loss from removals defined by a Poisson distribution with parameter $\gamma Y\,\Delta t$.

It is convenient in the subsequent work to replace the foregoing Poisson variables with similar variables having the means adjusted to zero. Thus we can specify the following large-sample stochastic analogue of the deterministic equations (7.1):

$$\left.\begin{array}{l}\Delta X = -\beta XY\,\Delta t + \mu\,\Delta t - \Delta Z_1 + \Delta Z_2, \\ \Delta Y = \beta XY\,\Delta t - \gamma Y\,\Delta t + \Delta Z_1 - \Delta Z_3,\end{array}\right\} \quad (7.46)$$

where the independent random variables ΔZ_1, ΔZ_2 and ΔZ_3 are adjusted Poisson variables having zero means and variances $\beta XY\,\Delta t$, $\mu\,\Delta t$ and $\gamma Y\,\Delta t$, respectively.

The deterministic equilibrium position is

$$x_0 = \gamma/\beta, \quad y_0 = \mu/\gamma, \quad (7.47)$$

as previously given in (7.2). For small stochastic departures from this position, we put

$$X = x_0(1+U), \quad Y = y_0(1+V), \quad (7.48)$$

where $U \equiv U(t)$ and $V \equiv V(t)$ are small random variables, corresponding to the deterministic expressions in (7.3).

Equations (7.46) are of course strictly non-linear stochastic equations. But they can be conveniently linearized by substituting (7.48) in (7.46), using (7.47), and retaining only first-order terms in U and V. We thus obtain

$$\left.\begin{array}{l}x_0\,\Delta U = -\mu(U+V)\Delta t - \Delta Z_1 + \Delta Z_2, \\ y_0\,\Delta V = \mu U\,\Delta t + \Delta Z_1 - \Delta Z_3,\end{array}\right\} \quad (7.49)$$

where, to first order in U and V, the variances of ΔZ_1, ΔZ_2 and ΔZ_3 are $\mu(1+U+V)\Delta t$, $\mu\,\Delta t$ and $\mu(1+V)\Delta t$, respectively.

Substituting $\Delta U = U(t+\Delta t) - U(t)$ and $\Delta V = V(t+\Delta t) - V(t)$ on the left-hand side of (7.49) leads to

$$\left.\begin{array}{l}x_0 U(t+\Delta t) = (x_0 - \mu\,\Delta t)U(t) - \mu V(t)\,\Delta t - \Delta Z_1 + \Delta Z_2, \\ y_0 V(t+\Delta t) = y_0 V(t) + \mu U(t)\,\Delta t + \Delta Z_1 - \Delta Z_3.\end{array}\right\} \quad (7.50)$$

We next express the variances and covariances of the equilibrium distribution of U and V as σ_U^2, σ_V^2 and σ_{UV}^2, respectively. Since we have arranged for U and V to be small, it follows that

$$\left.\begin{array}{l}\sigma_U^2 \doteq E\{U(t)\}^2 = E\{U(t+\Delta t)\}^2, \\ \sigma_V^2 \doteq E\{V(t)\}^2 = E\{V(t+\Delta t)\}^2, \\ \sigma_{UV}^2 \doteq E\{U(t)V(t)\} = E\{U(t+\Delta t)V(t+\Delta t)\}.\end{array}\right\} \quad (7.51)$$

The two equations in (7.50) can now be squared and cross-multiplied, after which we take expectations. Retaining only terms of order Δt leads, after a little reduction, to the equations

$$\left.\begin{aligned} x_0(\sigma_U^2 + \sigma_{UV}^2) &= 1, \\ y_0\sigma_{UV} &= -1, \\ x_0\sigma_U^2 - y_0(\sigma_{UV} + \sigma_V^2) &= 1, \end{aligned}\right\} \qquad (7.52)$$

which easily solve to yield

$$\sigma_U^2 = \frac{1}{x_0} + \frac{1}{y_0}, \quad \sigma_{UV} = -\frac{1}{y_0}, \quad \sigma_V^2 = \frac{1}{y_0} + \frac{x_0}{y_0^2}. \qquad (7.53)$$

These results are valid for sufficiently small stochastic fluctuations about the equilibrium position, and demonstrate that in the absence of fade-out the oscillations will be indefinitely maintained. This is in sharp contrast to the damped waves predicted by the deterministic model of Section 7.2.

7.62 Modified stochastic model

Secondly, we shall look more closely at the modified stochastic model discussed in Section 7.5, where it is assumed in addition that new infectives are introduced randomly at rate ϵ. In the notation of Section 6.3, we write $p_{rs}(t)$ for the probability of there being exactly r susceptibles and s infectives at time t, and define the probability-generating function

$$P(z, w, t) = \sum_{r,s} p_{rs}(t)z^r w^s \qquad (7.54)$$

(corresponding to the function in (6.30), but now referred to t-time). The relevant partial differential equation for $P(z, w, t)$ can be written down more or less immediately using a standard method (Bailey, 1964a, Sec. 7.4). In fact, we require the analogue of (6.31), putting $\tau = \beta t$, and allowing for the random Poisson introduction of susceptibles and infectives, at rates μ and ϵ, respectively We evidently have

$$\frac{\partial P}{\partial t} = \beta(w^2 - zw)\frac{\partial^2 P}{\partial z\,\partial w} + \gamma(1 - w)\frac{\partial P}{\partial w} + \mu(z - 1)P + \epsilon(w - 1)P. \qquad (7.55)$$

We are specially interested in the stable distribution reached in the limit $t \to \infty$, particularly the distribution of Y which will allow us to gauge the chance of an extreme value falling to zero. We evidently have $\partial P/\partial t = 0$. If we write

$$Q(z, w) = P(z, w, \infty), \qquad (7.56)$$

equation (7.55) becomes

$$\beta(w^2 - zw)\frac{\partial^2 Q}{\partial z\,\partial w} + \gamma(1 - w)\frac{\partial Q}{\partial w} + \mu(z - 1)Q + \epsilon(w - 1)Q = 0. \quad (7.57)$$

Further, let

$$q_{rs} = p_{rs}(\infty), \qquad (7.58)$$

so that

$$Q(z, w) = \sum_{r,s} q_{rs} z^r w^s. \qquad (7.59)$$

Now the limiting distribution of Y, the number of infectives, is given by $Q(1, w)$. So we put $z = 1$ in (7.57), and divide through by $w - 1$. This yields

$$\beta w \left[\frac{\partial^2 Q}{\partial z\,\partial w}\right]_{z=1} - \gamma \left[\frac{\partial Q}{\partial w}\right]_{z=1} + \epsilon [Q]_{z=1} = 0. \qquad (7.60)$$

We next substitute from (7.59) to obtain

$$\beta \sum_{r,s} rsq_{rs} w^s - \gamma \sum_{r,s} sq_{rs} w^{s-1} + \epsilon \sum_{r,s} q_{rs} w^s = 0. \qquad (7.61)$$

Picking out the coefficient of w^s gives in general

$$\beta s \sum_r rq_{rs} - \gamma(s + 1) \sum_r q_{r,s+1} + \epsilon \sum_r q_{rs} = 0, \quad s > 0, \qquad (7.62)$$

and

$$-\gamma \sum_r q_{r1} + \epsilon \sum_r q_{r0} = 0, \quad s = 0. \qquad (7.63)$$

Let us now write

$$q_s = \sum_r q_{rs}, \quad \bar{r}_s q_s = \sum_r rq_{rs}, \qquad (7.64)$$

so that $\bar{r}_s$ is the mean number of susceptibles, given s infectives. Equation (7.62) now takes the form

$$\beta s q_s \bar{r}_s - \gamma(s + 1)q_{s+1} + \epsilon q_s = 0, \quad s > 0, \qquad (7.65)$$

and (7.63) becomes

$$\epsilon q_0 = \gamma q_1. \qquad (7.66)$$

In equation (7.65) we shall assume that ϵ is small enough to be neglected and shall write for convenience

$$G_s = sq_s, \qquad (7.67)$$

thus obtaining

$$G_{s+1} \sim \frac{\beta \bar{r}_s}{\gamma} G_s = \frac{\bar{r}_s}{x_0} G_s \qquad (7.68)$$

Unfortunately, this relationship still contains the unknown quantity $\bar{r}_s$, but some useful approximations are possible. To begin with, in the absence of the introduction of new infections, i.e. $\epsilon = 0$, it follows from (7.48) and (7.53) that var $(X) \sim (x_0/y_0)$ var (Y). Thus C.V. $(X) \sim (y_0/x_0)^{\frac{1}{2}}$ C.V. (Y). Hence the coefficient of variation of X is much less than the coefficient of variation of Y if $y_0 \ll x_0$. In these circumstances X is more stable than Y, and we can use a large-sample approximation for $\bar{r}_s$ based on the assumption that $\epsilon = 0$.

Taking expectations of the exact stochastic equations in (7.46) shows that

$$\mu = \beta E(XY) = \gamma E(Y). \tag{7.69}$$

Therefore

$$E(Y) = \mu/\gamma = y_0, \tag{7.70}$$

the precise deterministic value. On the other hand, we have from (7.69)

$$\mu/\beta = E(XY) \equiv \text{cov}(X, Y) + E(X) E(Y)$$
$$= x_0 y_0 \sigma_{UV} + y_0 E(X), \tag{7.71}$$

using (7.48) and (7.70). Substituting from (7.47) and (7.53) into (7.71) now gives

$$E(X) \sim x_0 + \frac{x_0}{y_0}, \tag{7.72}$$

thus providing a better approximation than $E(X) \sim x_0$.

In a large population we can assume that the regression is approximately linear, at least to the order of accuracy envisaged. Hence

$$\bar{r}_s \sim x_0 + \frac{x_0}{y_0} + \frac{\text{cov}(X, Y)}{\text{var}(Y)} (s - y_0)$$

$$= x_0 + \frac{x_0}{y_0} - \frac{x_0(s - y_0)}{x_0 + y_0}. \tag{7.73}$$

We can now substitute (7.73) in (7.68) to give

$$G_{s+1} \sim \left(1 + \frac{1}{y_0} - \frac{s - y_0}{x_0 + y_0}\right) G_s.$$

Since the left-hand side of this relationship is approximately equal to $G_s + \partial G_s/\partial s$, it follows that

$$\frac{\partial \log G_s}{\partial s} \sim \frac{1}{y_0} - \frac{s - y_0}{x_0 + y_0}. \tag{7.74}$$

Integrating with respect to s, taking exponentials and substituting into (7.67), quickly leads to

$$q_s \sim \frac{C}{s} \exp\left[-\frac{\{s-y_0-(x_0+y_0)/y_0\}^2}{2(x_0+y_0)}\right]. \tag{7.75}$$

The constant C can be obtained by integration since $\int_{-\infty}^{\infty} q_s ds = 1$. As the exponential term on the right of (7.75) may be expected to provide its main contribution in the neighbourhood of $s = y_0$, we can set the factor C/s equal to C/y_0 as a first approximation. Integration is then immediate, and gives

$$C \sim y_0\{2\pi(x_0+y_0)\}^{-\frac{1}{2}}. \tag{7.76}$$

Therefore

$$q_s \sim \frac{y_0}{s\{2\pi(x_0+y_0)\}^{\frac{1}{2}}} \exp\left[-\frac{\{s-y_0-(x_0+y_0)/y_0\}^2}{2(x_0+y_0)}\right]. \tag{7.77}$$

Now the mean recurrence time to zero infectives, $\bar{R}$ say, for the kind of population process being considered is (Bartlett, 1960a, Sec. 3.4)

$$\bar{R} = \frac{1-q_0}{\epsilon q_0} \sim \frac{1}{\gamma q_1} \tag{7.78}$$

for small q_0, using (7.66). Substituting from (7.77) into (7.78) therefore gives

$$\bar{R} \sim \frac{\{2\pi(x_0+y_0)\}^{\frac{1}{2}}}{\gamma y_0} \exp\left\{\frac{(y_0+x_0/y_0)^2}{2(x_0+y_0)}\right\} \tag{7.79}$$

as the average recurrence-time from, say, $Y = y_0$ to $Y = 0$.

For y_0 large, as we have assumed, the mean recurrence-time will also be large, and this will give the order of magnitude of the passage-time to zero, even in the case when $\epsilon = 0$, which is the situation in which we are specially interested. To gain some idea of the implications of (7.79), we can express $\bar{R}$ in terms of y_0 and the ratio x_0/y_0. Let us suppose that the latter remains approximately constant for communities of different sizes, and use the value already proposed in Section 7.2 for measles in London, namely $x_0/y_0 = 34\cdot1$ together with $\gamma = \frac{1}{2}$ week. We now have $\bar{R}$ as a function of y_0. Some values given by Bartlett (1960a, b) are shown in Table 7.1.

Table 7.1   *Mean recurrence-time $\bar{R}$ in terms of y_0*

y_0	50	100	150	200	250	300	400
$\bar{R}$ (years)	0·6	0·8	1·2	2·1	3·9	7	24

The figures in Table 7.1 should perhaps be regarded as no more than indicative, especially for the smaller y_0. Nevertheless, they clearly imply a rapid rise in the theoretical extinction-time when y_0 rises above about 200, that is, when the removal-rate γy_0 rises above about 100 cases per week. This suggests the existence of a critical community size, above which measles would appear to maintain itself, while in smaller communities the disease would tend to fade out and have to be re-introduced from outside before another epidemic could be triggered off. These results are in quite good agreement with the UK and American data already referred to at the beginning of Section 7.4.

For a detailed discussion the reader should refer to Bartlett (1957, 1960c), where various complicating factors inevitable in real data, such as under-reporting of cases, are investigated and allowed for. The ability of the stochastic modelling to explain several essential features of real epidemic processes, already noted in previous sections, is quite remarkable.

Finally, mention should be made of some theorems of Ridler-Rowe (1967). These have already been referred to in Section 6.7 in the context of the general stochastic epidemic without any immigration of infectives or susceptibles. For the extended model involving immigration of both infectives and susceptibles, Ridler-Rowe used some general results for Markov processes due to Reuter (1957, 1961) to prove the following asymptotic theorems.

The expected duration-time $\overline{T}$ from the start of the process, with a infectives and n susceptibles, to the point at which the infectives first become extinct is given by

$$\overline{T} \sim \gamma^{-1} \log(a + n), \quad n \to \infty. \tag{7.80}$$

This result may be compared with that of Bartlett in (7.79). The difference of form is presumably due to the fact that Bartlett is concerned with appropriate passage-times to zero starting near to the equilibrium point, whereas Ridler-Rowe considers starting from a point for which the number of susceptibles (though not necessarily the number of infectives) is very large and a long way from the equilibrium point.

It was also shown that the process is "non-dissipative". The sum of all the individual probabilities in the limiting distribution is unity, so that the process tends to infinity, as $t \to \infty$, only with probability zero.

Another result is that as the susceptible immigration-rate tends to zero, then the number of infectives is asymptotically distributed like a Poisson variable with parameter ϵ/γ.

7.7 Simulation studies

It will be seen from the foregoing sections that detailed investigation of fully stochastic models for recurrent epidemics presents very considerable difficulties. Nevertheless, by the use of various approximate arguments the broad features of large-scale processes can be discerned, although some of these are necessarily confined to the initial stages. For these reasons it is desirable to supplement the theoretical work with simulation studies on artificially constructed series of observations, involving the application of Monte Carlo methods.

We can then obtain further information on the long-term behaviour of an epidemic series without recourse to approximate and heuristic probability arguments, although of course a different kind of uncertainty is introduced.

Methods of constructing such artificial realizations of stochastic processes have been described by several writers, e.g. Kendall (1950) and, in the present context, Bartlett (1953). Details need not be given here, but it may be mentioned that the basic idea is to use a source of random numbers to obtain a series of quantities which represents a succession of independent observations derived from some appropriate frequency distribution. In this way we can produce artificial realizations of epidemic processes in which the random elements of infection, removal, etc., are properly introduced in accordance with the theoretical model adopted.

Bartlett (1953), for example, studied such a series chosen to mimic the behaviour of a boarding-school subject to recurrent epidemics of measles. This is fairly close to an idealized community in which epidemics tend to be sustained by the influx of susceptibles, e.g. new entrants at the beginning of each term, and the introduction of new infection, e.g. occasional boys catching measles during the holidays but not developing symptoms until after the beginning of term. With constants chosen *a priori* to be in reasonable conformity with known facts, a series was generated corresponding to 13 years' experience at such a school. During this time six major outbreaks occurred, having an average period of 125 weeks between them. The expected type of stochastic stability was observed, later epidemics being quite comparable in size with the earlier ones. There were also four minor epidemics not leading to a big build-up of cases. No precise statistical fitting to real data was possible, but the behaviour of the artificial series was in broad agreement both with the predictions already derived from stochastic models (in contrast with the implications of deterministic versions) and also with the general character of actual epidemiological data, e.g. Cheeseman (1950).

In the artificial series just described recurrence of epidemics was ensured by repeated introduction of small numbers of new cases from outside the group. On the other hand, the arguments of Section 7.4 point to the existence of a critical size of community. Below this critical value extinction will be the normal fate of any epidemic that happens to occur, a series of outbreaks being maintained only by the re-entry of infection. Above the critical size the chance of extinction will become progressively smaller. An artificial process was constructed by Bartlett (1956) which mimicked in many respects the behaviour of ectromelia in mice, as studied experimentally by Greenwood *et al.* (1936). Owing to the labour involved in computing with a continuous-infection model, a chain-binomial representation was used instead. Although this is quite a different process (see Chapters 8 and 14) so far as fine structure is concerned, it is unlikely to show substantial large-scale differences. The artificial series in question (using an incubation period of 4 days) ran for the equivalent of nearly three years, or about thirty cycles, before extinction occurred. Again, we have the right type of qualitative agreement with mathematical theory and empirical fact.

A more ambitious study specifically related to the spread of measles is that reported by Bartlett (1957, 1960a, 1961), in which a computer was used to build up artificial processes extended in space as well as time (see also Section 9.5). This provided further support in a general way of previous ideas. It also suggested that for appropriate values of the basic constants, the critical size for relatively isolated towns should be somewhere in the neighbourhood of 200 000 individuals, provided that the initial swing of susceptibles is sufficiently like the quasi-equilibrium values expected to occur later. Smaller critical sizes would apply to non-isolated districts because of the immigration of new infectives.

As mentioned at the beginning of Section 7.4, a detailed analysis of actual data, both in the UK and the USA, suggested a critical level round about the 250 000 mark. The simulation studies are in broad qualitative agreement with this observed figure, and thus provide additional confirmation of the correctness of the underlying models, whose mathematical properties have been investigated in Section 7.4, 7.5 and 7.6.

8
Discrete-time models

8.1 Introduction

So far we have been considering, almost exclusively, processes that occur in continuous time, although some of the simulations referred to in Section 7.7 (e.g. Bartlett, 1960a, 1961) in fact used discrete-time analogues when these were more convenient. For theoretical purposes the continuous-time models have been found more tractable, though they are certainly not without difficulties.

Simple discrete-time models, essentially using a fixed latent period with infectiousness confined to a single point of time, were first used around 1928 for teaching purposes by Lowell J. Reed and Wade Hampton Frost in the United States (see Wilson and Burke, 1942; Abbey, 1952; Maia, 1952). Independent developments, with specific statistical applications to measles data, were made in the United Kingdom by Greenwood (1931 and later). Most subsequent work has been of an applied statistical nature, and it will be more appropriate to describe this *in extenso* in Chapter 14 of Part 3, which deals with applications as opposed to general theory.

Very little general theory appears to exist. Firescu and Tăutu (1967) have used a Markov chain model to describe the passage of an individual between a variety of states, such as "uninfected susceptible", "uninfected immune", "healthy carrier", "typical case", etc. The transition probabilities p_{ij}, of passing from state i to state j, are regarded as fixed. So far as endogenous factors affecting the individual are concerned, this model certainly entails a fair degree of realism. Unfortunately, it also makes the probability of infection totally independent of the number of infectives in the population.

Another approach has been adopted by Bartoszyński (1967, 1969) utilizing a discrete-time Galton–Watson process (see Harris, 1963). This admits variable latent and infectious periods but, as with Bharucha-Reid's (1956, 1958) application of an age-dependent branching process to the continuous-time situation (see end of Section 6.9), it confines attention to a one-dimensional process describing the number of infectives and neglects the changing number of

156

susceptibles. Bartoszyński also discussed an extension of this model to cover
the possibility of several sub-habitats with migration between them, and a
further development (Bartoszyński, 1972) deals with the problem of a population consisting of a large number (conceptually infinite in the model) of
different families.

The principal theory capable of taking into account both infectives and susceptibles, especially their interaction, is that of Gani (1969) and Gani and
Jerwood (1971). This work uses a Markov chain approach and forms the basis
of the main presentation in the current chapter in Sections 8.2–8.5. Some
asymptotic results, analogous to the continuous-time theory of Section 7.6 for
reucrrent epidemics, are given in Section 8.6.

8.2   Basic models

Let us first describe a little more explicitly the model alluded to in the
foregoing introductory section. We assume that, following the receipt of
infection by any susceptible, there ensues a latent period of fixed length. The
subsequent infectious period is considered to be contracted to a single point
of time. In the chain-binomial models of Reed, Frost and Greenwood the
infective is then effectively "removed" from circulation. If he recovers and
returns to the population, he is assumed to remain immune to further infection. At the moment of infectiousness of any given infective, the chance of
contact with any specified susceptible, sufficient or adequate to transmit the
infection, is indicated by $p = 1 - q$. It is evident that new cases will occur in
distinct groups or generations, the generation time being equal to the fixed
latent period. We can take the latter as the discrete unit of time for the evolution of the whole process. At each generation the actual number of new cases
will have a binomial distribution depending on the parameter p. The precise
form of the distribution varies according to our choice of certain additional
biological assumptions.

Let us write S_t for the random variable indicating the number of infected
persons just prior to time t who become infectious at time t, and R_t for the
random variable indicating the number of susceptibles remaining uninfected at
time t. It is evident that

$$R_t = S_{t+1} + R_{t+1}. \tag{8.1}$$

In the Greenwood specification it is supposed that a susceptible's chance of
being infected depends only on the presence of *some* infectives, and not on
their actual number. Suppose that the random variables R_t and S_t take the
specific values at time t given by r_t and s_t, respectively. If $s_t = 0$, the epidemic
realization in question terminates immediately, since there are no further infectives. If, on the other hand, $s_t \geqslant 1$, we can write for the Greenwood model

$$\Pr\{S_{t+1} = s_{t+1} | R_t = r_t, S_t = s_t\} = \frac{r_t!}{r_{t+1}! \, s_{t+1}!} p^{s_{t+1}} q^{r_{t+1}}, \quad s_t \geqslant 1. \tag{8.2}$$

In the Reed–Frost version, however, it is assumed that the chance of infection *does* depend on the number of infectives present. Thus the chance of any given susceptibles escaping infection from any of the s_t infectives present is q^{s_t}. The chance of acquiring infection at this stage is therefore $1 - q^{s_t}$. The probability, in the Reed–Frost model, of s_{t+1} infectives occurring at time $t + 1$ is thus

$$\Pr\{S_{t+1} = s_{t+1}|R_t = r_t, S_t = s_t\} = \frac{r_t!}{r_{t+1}!\, s_{t+1}!}\,(1 - q^{s_t})^{s_{t+1}}\, q^{s_t r_{t+1}}, \left.\begin{array}{c} \\ \\ s_t \geqslant 0. \end{array}\right\} \quad (8.3)$$

The binomial character of the distributions in (8.2) and (8.3), and the fact that the discrete stochastic processes involve chains of related distributions, have led to the use of the term *chain-binomial models*. These distributions are used extensively in Chapter 14 as a basis for the maximum-likelihood estimation of the basic parameter p (and also other modifying parameters that may need to be introduced). But these practical statistical applications tend to obscure the fact that the processes involved have certain basic Markov chain aspects that are of importance in a general theoretical analysis.

Thus if we re-write (8.2) in the form

$$\Pr\{R_{t+1} = r_{t+1}|R_t = r_t\} = \frac{r_t!}{r_{t+1}!\,(r_t - r_{t+1})!}\, p^{r_t - r_{t+1}}\, q^{r_{t+1}}, \quad (8.4)$$

it is clear that in the Greenwood model we have a univariate Markov chain for the random variable R_t.

Similarly, we can reformulate (8.3) as

$$\Pr\{R_{t+1} = r_t - s_{t+1}, S_{t+1} = s_{t+1}|R_t = r_t, S_t = s_t\}$$

$$= \frac{r_t!}{s_{t+1}!\,(r_t - s_{t+1})!}\,(1 - q^{s_t})^{s_{t+1}}\, q^{s_t(r_t - s_{t+1})}, \quad (8.5)$$

which shows that the Reed–Frost model can be described in terms of a bivariate Markov chain for the pair of variables R_t and S_t.

In order to develop further the implications of this Markov chain format we first need some preliminary mathematical results which are derived in the following section.

8.3   Preliminary theory

It is convenient to discuss a Markov chain $\{X_t\}$ having a finite space state, with transition matrix

$$\mathbf{M} = \{m_{ij}\}, \quad \begin{array}{l} 0 \leqslant m_{ij} \leqslant 1 \quad \text{for } i \neq j, \\ 0 < m_{jj} \leqslant 1, \\ i, j = 0, 1, 2, ..., k. \end{array} \left.\right\} \quad (8.6)$$

Because of our interest in epidemic chain-binomial processes we are concerned with chains that terminate at time $T = t$ when $X_t = X_{t-1}$, interpreting X_t as the variable number of susceptibles.

We now define the diagonal matrix of probabilities

$$\mathbf{Q} = \text{diag}\{m_{ij}\} = \{m_{ij}\,\delta_{ij}\}, \tag{8.7}$$

where δ_{ij} is the Kronecker delta, and all $m_{jj} > 0$. It is also convenient to define

$$\mathbf{P} = \mathbf{M} - \mathbf{Q}, \tag{8.8}$$

which is the matrix of transition probabilities with all diagonal elements set equal to zero.

If we wish to obtain the probability that the process terminates at $T = t$, given that the process commences at $t = 0$ with $X_0 = i$, we first write the chance of terminating in state j at time t, starting in state i at time zero, as

$$\Pr\{T = t, X_t = X_{t-1} = j \,|\, X_0 = i\} = \{\mathbf{P}^{t-1}\}_{ij}\, m_{jj}. \tag{8.9}$$

We can now sum (8.9) over $0 \leqslant j \leqslant k$ to give

$$\Pr\{T = t \,|\, X_0 = i\} = \sum_{j=0}^{k} \Pr\{T = t, X_t = X_{t-1} = j \,|\, X_0 = i\}$$

$$= \sum_{j=0}^{k} \{\mathbf{P}^{t-1}\}_{ij}\, m_{jj}, \quad \text{using (8.9)},$$

$$= \mathbf{A}_i'\, \mathbf{P}^{t-1}\, \mathbf{Q}\mathbf{E}, \quad 1 \leqslant t \leqslant \infty, \tag{8.10}$$

where $\mathbf{A}_i'$ is a row vector representing the initial probability distribution, and containing $k + 1$ elements, all zero except for the $(i + 1)$th which is unity, and $\mathbf{E}$ is a column vector of $k + 1$ unit elements, i.e.

$$\left.\begin{aligned} \mathbf{A}_i' &= [0, 0, ..., 0, 1, 0, ..., 0], \\ \mathbf{E}' &= [1, 1, ..., 1, ..., 1]. \end{aligned}\right\} \tag{8.11}$$

and

The matrix representation on the right of (8.10) is easily verified by multiplying through the factors indicated.

The probability-generating function $\Pi_i(\theta)$ of the time to termination T is thus given by

$$\Pi_i(\theta) = \sum_{t=1}^{\infty} \theta^t \Pr\{T = t \,|\, X_0 = i\}$$

$$= \sum_{t=1}^{\infty} \mathbf{A}_i'\, \theta^{t-1}\, \mathbf{P}^{t-1}\, \theta\mathbf{Q}\mathbf{E}, \quad \text{using (8.10)},$$

$$= \mathbf{A}_i'(\mathbf{I} - \theta\mathbf{P})^{-1}\theta\, \mathbf{Q}\mathbf{E}, \quad 0 \leqslant \theta \leqslant 1, \tag{8.12}$$

where $\mathbf{I}$ is an identity matrix of $k + 1$ rows and columns. Note that the inverse in (8.12) always exists since $|\theta\mathbf{P}| < 1$.

The distribution in (8.10) has been called a Markov geometric distribution because it is somewhat analogous in structure to the ordinary geometric distribution given by $f(x) = p^{x-1}q$ for $1 \leqslant x < \infty$ and $0 < p = 1 - q < 1$. Moreover, the probability-generating function is $(1 - \theta p)^{-1}\theta q$ which corresponds to (8.12).

We can check that (8.10) represents a proper distribution by putting $\theta = 1$ in (8.12). Thus, let

$$c_i \equiv \Pi_i(1) = \mathbf{A}_i' (\mathbf{I} - \mathbf{P})^{-1} \mathbf{Q} \mathbf{E}. \tag{8.13}$$

It follows from (8.13) that

$$(\mathbf{I} - \mathbf{P})^{-1} \mathbf{Q} \mathbf{E} = \mathbf{C}, \tag{8.14}$$

where $\mathbf{C}$ is a column vector of the elements $\{c_i\}$. If we multiply (8.14) through by $\mathbf{I} - \mathbf{P}$, we obtain the set of equations

$$\mathbf{Q} \mathbf{E} = (\mathbf{I} - \mathbf{P}) \mathbf{C}. \tag{8.15}$$

From the definitions of $\mathbf{E}$, $\mathbf{P}$ and $\mathbf{Q}$ above we can easily verify that the solution $\mathbf{C}$ of (8.15) is in fact a column vector of unit elements. Thus every $c_i = 1$.

In order to keep track of the final state X_T at which the process terminates, we can work with the joint probability-generating function $\Pi_i(\theta, \phi)$ for the pair of variables (T, X_T). It follows from (8.9) that

$$\Pi_i(\theta, \phi) = \sum_{t=1}^{\infty} \sum_{j=0}^{k} \theta^t \phi^j \{\mathbf{P}^{t-1}\}_{ij} \, m_{jj}. \tag{8.16}$$

Let us now define $\mathbf{\Phi}$ as the diagonal matrix for which the jth diagonal element is ϕ^j, all other elements being zero, i.e.

$$\mathbf{\Phi} = \{\delta_{ij}\phi^j\}. \tag{8.17}$$

Then it is easy to see that we can write

$$\sum_{j=0}^{k} \{\mathbf{P}^{t-1}\}_{ij} \, \phi^j m_{jj} \equiv \mathbf{A}_i' \, \mathbf{P}^{t-1} \mathbf{\Phi} \mathbf{Q} \mathbf{E}, \tag{8.18}$$

using an argument more or less identical with that which led to the matrix product form in (8.10). Substituting (8.18) into (8.16) gives

$$\Pi_i(\theta, \phi) = \sum_{t=1}^{\infty} \theta^t \mathbf{A}_i' \, \mathbf{P}^{t-1} \mathbf{\Phi} \, \mathbf{Q} \mathbf{E}$$

$$= \mathbf{A}_i' \, (\mathbf{I} - \theta\mathbf{P})^{-1} \, \mathbf{\Phi} \, \theta \, \mathbf{Q} \mathbf{E}, \tag{8.19}$$

which reduces to (8.12) when $\theta = 1$. Gani and Jerwood (1971) give the result (8.19) in the form

$$\Pi_i(\theta, \phi) = \mathbf{A}_i'(\phi) (\mathbf{I} - \theta \mathbf{P}(\phi))^{-1} \theta \, \mathbf{Q} \mathbf{E}, \tag{8.20}$$

where
$$\mathbf{A}_i'(\phi) = [0, 0, ..., \phi^i, ..., 0],$$
and
$$\mathbf{P}(\phi) = \{m_{ij}\phi^{j-i}(1-\delta_{ij})\}. \tag{8.21}$$

The two forms are identical, since

$$
\begin{aligned}
\mathbf{A}_i'(\phi)\,(\mathbf{I}-\theta\mathbf{P}(\phi))^{-1} &= \mathbf{A}_i'\,\boldsymbol{\Phi}\cdot(\mathbf{I}-\theta\boldsymbol{\Phi}^{-1}\mathbf{P}\boldsymbol{\Phi})^{-1}\\
&= \mathbf{A}_i'\,\boldsymbol{\Phi}\cdot\{\boldsymbol{\Phi}^{-1}(\mathbf{I}-\theta\mathbf{P})\boldsymbol{\Phi}\}^{-1}\\
&= \mathbf{A}_i'\,\boldsymbol{\Phi}\cdot\boldsymbol{\Phi}^{-1}(\mathbf{I}-\theta\mathbf{P})^{-1}\,\boldsymbol{\Phi}\\
&= \mathbf{A}_i'(\mathbf{I}-\theta\mathbf{P})^{-1}\boldsymbol{\Phi}\,. \tag{8.22}
\end{aligned}
$$

From (8.12) the mean termination time $\mu = E(T)$ is quickly found by picking out the coefficient of θ, i.e.

$$\mu = \mathbf{A}_i'(\mathbf{I}-\mathbf{P})^{-2}\,\mathbf{Q}\mathbf{E} = \mathbf{A}_i'(\mathbf{I}-\mathbf{P})^{-1}\,\mathbf{E}, \tag{8.23}$$

since, as noted above after equation (8.15), $\mathbf{Q}\mathbf{E} = (\mathbf{I}-\mathbf{P})\mathbf{E}$. Similarly, we can derive the variance $\sigma^2 = \mathrm{var}\,(T)$ as

$$
\begin{aligned}
\sigma^2 &= 2\mathbf{A}_i'\mathbf{P}(\mathbf{I}-\mathbf{P})^{-3}\,\mathbf{Q}\mathbf{E} + \mathbf{A}_i'(\mathbf{I}-\mathbf{P})^{-2}\,\mathbf{Q}\mathbf{E} - \{\mathbf{A}_i'(\mathbf{I}-\mathbf{P})^{-1}\,\mathbf{E}\}^2\\
&= \mathbf{A}_i'\{2\mathbf{P}(\mathbf{I}-\mathbf{P})^{-2}\,\mathbf{E} + (\mathbf{I}-\mathbf{P})^{-1}\,\mathbf{E}\} - \{\mathbf{A}_i'(\mathbf{I}-\mathbf{P})^{-1}\,\mathbf{E}\}^2. \tag{8.24}
\end{aligned}
$$

The mean and variance of the final state, $E(X_T)$ and $\mathrm{var}\,(X_T)$, can also be found in the same way, as can the covariance of T and X_t, and any other higher moments of interest.

8.4   Chain-binomial applications

The results derived in Section 8.3 for the Markov geometric distribution can now be applied, with certain modifications and adaptations, to the Greenwood and Reed–Frost chain-binomials introduced in Section 8.2. The starting point in each case is to identify the appropriate transition matrix $\mathbf{M}$ defined in (8.6).

8.41   Greenwood model

As indicated by (8.4), the sequence of random variables $\{R_t\}$ for the numbers of susceptibles at each stage constitutes, in the Greenwood version, a univariate Markov chain. The epidemic comes to an end at time $T = t$ if $R_t = R_{t-1}$ or if $R_t = 0$. It follows from (8.4) that the elements of $\mathbf{M} = \{m_{ij}\}$, for an initial number of susceptibles $r_0 = k$, are given by

$$
\begin{aligned}
m_{ij} &= \binom{i}{j}p^{i-j}q^j, \quad 0 \leqslant j \leqslant i,\\
&= 0, \qquad\qquad\quad i < j \leqslant k. \tag{8.25}
\end{aligned}
$$

The matrix $\mathbf{M}$ thus has the lower triangular form

$$\mathbf{M} = \begin{bmatrix} 1 & 0 & 0 & \cdots & 0 \\ p & q & 0 & \cdots & 0 \\ p^2 & 2pq & q^2 & \cdots & 0 \\ \vdots & & & & \\ p^k & kp^{k-1}q & \binom{k}{2}p^{k-2}q^2 & \cdots & q^k \end{bmatrix} \qquad (8.26)$$

The vector of initial probabilities is now $\mathbf{A}'_k$, where

$$\mathbf{A}'_k = [0; 0, ..., 0, 0, 1], \qquad (8.27)$$

and $\mathbf{P}$ and $\mathbf{QE}$ are given by

$$\mathbf{P} = \begin{bmatrix} 0 & 0 & 0 & \cdots & 0 \\ p & 0 & 0 & \cdots & 0 \\ p^2 & 2pq & 0 & \cdots & 0 \\ \vdots & & & & \\ p^k & kp^{k-1}q & \binom{k}{2}p^{k-2}q^2 & \cdots & 0 \end{bmatrix}, \qquad (8.28)$$

and $\quad (\mathbf{QE})' = [1, q, q^2, ..., q^k]. \qquad (8.29)$

It follows that the joint probability-generating function for the pair of variables (T, R_T), i.e. the duration time T and the number of susceptibles present at time T, is given by (8.19) or (8.20) with $i = k$, e.g. by

$$\Pi_k(\theta, \phi) = \mathbf{A}'_k(\mathbf{I} - \theta\mathbf{P})^{-1}\mathbf{\Phi}\,\theta\mathbf{QE}, \qquad (8.30)$$

where the relevant $\mathbf{A}'_k$, $\mathbf{P}$, $\mathbf{QE}$ and $\mathbf{\Phi}$ are given by (8.27), (8.28), (8.29) and (8.17).

If we want to work, as is more usual, with the epidemic size $W_T = k - R_T$, i.e. the total number of cases over and above the initial number of infectives, instead of R_T, then we require the modified joint probability-generating function

$$\Pi'_k(\theta, \phi) = \phi^k \Pi_k(\theta, \phi^{-1}). \qquad (8.31)$$

8.42   Reed–Frost model

This time, as shown by (8.5), it is the pair of variables (R_t, S_t) that exhibits the Markov chain property. We can still use the Markov geometric distribution, provided an appropriate modification is made.

We shall assume, as for the Greenwood model, that $r_0 = k_j$ and also, for convenience, that $s_0 = 1, 2, ..., k$, though s_0 could in fact have finite values greater than k. Now, for any given value of t, there are $(k + 1)^2$ possible states, since each of the random variables in the pair (R_t, S_t) may take any of the values indicated by $r_t, s_t = 0, 1, ..., k$. These $(k + 1)^2$ states can be numbered in terms of submatrices of a complete matrix $\mathbf{M}$. When this is done in an appropriate way the previous theory applies.

In general, $\mathbf{M}$ is built up from $(k + 1)^2$ submatrices $\mathbf{M}_{ij}$; $i, j = 0, 1, ..., k$, whose elements are defined by

$$\{\mathbf{M}_{ij}\}_{rs} = \binom{s+j}{j}(1 - q^i)^j (q^i)^s, \quad \text{if } r = s + j, \\ = 0, \qquad\qquad\qquad\qquad\quad r \neq s + j, \tag{8.32}$$

and each submatrix consists of a single diagonal or subdiagonal set of non-null elements. An example of $\mathbf{M}$ for $k = 3$ is shown in full detail in Table 8.1.

We also need extended definitions of $\mathbf{Q}$ and $\mathbf{P}$. It is sufficient, in following the spread of infection, to use the $k(k + 1) \times (k + 1)$ and $k(k + 1) \times k(k + 1)$ matrices given, respectively, by

$$\mathbf{Q} = \begin{bmatrix} \mathbf{M}_{10} \\ \mathbf{M}_{20} \\ \vdots \\ \mathbf{M}_{k0} \end{bmatrix}, \qquad \mathbf{P} = \begin{bmatrix} \mathbf{M}_{11} & \mathbf{M}_{12} & ... & \mathbf{M}_{1k} \\ \mathbf{M}_{21} & \mathbf{M}_{22} & ... & \mathbf{M}_{2k} \\ \vdots & & & \vdots \\ \mathbf{M}_{k1} & \mathbf{M}_{k2} & ... & \mathbf{M}_{kk} \end{bmatrix} \tag{8.33}$$

The joint distribution of (T, R_T) can now be expressed in terms of a bivariate probability-generating function analogous to (8.30). The matrix $\mathbf{E}$ can be defined as before, but $\mathbf{\Phi}$ must be extended to a partitioned matrix $\mathbf{\Psi}$ of k^2 submatrices, such that the submatrices on the leading diagonal are all $\mathbf{\Phi}$, the rest being null. Further, the vector of initial probabilities must now be $\mathbf{A}'_{s_0 k}$, where

$$\mathbf{A}'_{s_0 k} = [0, 0, ..., 0, 1, 0, ..., 0], \tag{8.34}$$

the single unit element being in the $(s_0 k)$th place of the $k(k + 1)$ elements.

With these modified definitions, we can write the joint probability distribution of (T, R_T) as

$$\Pi_k(\theta, \phi) = \mathbf{A}'_{s_0 k}(\mathbf{I} - \theta\mathbf{P})^{-1}\mathbf{\Psi}\,\theta\,\mathbf{QE}, \tag{8.35}$$

using the relationship in (8.31) to obtain the joint probability-generating function of (T, W_T).

8.43 General comments

Although much remains to be done in developing the above approach to

Table 8.1 *Chain-binomial model: transition matrix M for k = 3*

s_t	r_t	$r_{t+1}=0$				$r_{t+1}=1$				$r_{t+1}=2$				$r_{t+1}=3$			
	$s_{t+1}=$	0	1	2	3	0	1	2	3	0	1	2	3	0	1	2	3
0	0	1	·	·	·	·	·	·	·	·	·	·	·	·	·	·	·
	1	1	·	·	·	·	·	·	·	·	·	·	·	·	·	·	·
	2	1	·	·	·	·	·	·	·	·	·	·	·	·	·	·	·
	3	1	·	·	·	·	·	·	·	·	·	·	·	·	·	·	·
1	0	·	1	·	·	·	·	·	·	·	·	·	·	·	·	·	·
	1	·	q	·	·	p	·	·	·	·	·	·	·	·	·	·	·
	2	·	q^2	·	·	$1-q^2$	·	·	·	·	·	·	·	·	·	·	·
	3	·	q^3	·	·	$1-q^3$	·	·	·	·	·	·	·	·	·	·	·
2	0	·	·	1	·	·	·	·	·	·	·	·	·	·	·	·	·
	1	·	·	q^2	·	·	$2pq$	·	·	p^2	·	·	·	·	·	·	·
	2	·	·	q^4	·	·	$2(1-q^2)q^2$	·	·	$(1-q^2)^2$	·	·	·	·	·	·	·
	3	·	·	q^6	·	·	$2(1-q^3)q^3$	·	·	$(1-q^3)^2$	·	·	·	·	·	·	·
3	0	·	·	·	1	·	·	·	·	·	·	·	·	·	·	·	·
	1	·	·	·	q^3	·	·	$3pq^2$	·	·	$3p^2q$	·	·	p^3	·	·	·
	2	·	·	·	q^6	·	·	$3(1-q^2)q^4$	·	·	$3(1-q^2)^2q^2$	·	·	$(1-q^2)^3$	·	·	·
	3	·	·	·	q^9	·	·	$3(1-q^3)q^6$	·	·	$3(1-q^3)^2q^3$	·	·	$(1-q^3)^3$	·	·	·

provide the degree of theory already existing for the simple and general stochastic epidemics in continuous time, it does provide a more general basis for further discussion than is available from the simple statistical applications of Chapter 14. The latter rely heavily on the enumeration of individual chains, which is feasible for relatively small family groups but awkward for groups with large numbers of initial susceptibles. The Gani and Jerwood approach not only provides convenient computational algorithms for calculating the probabilities of duration times and total epidemic size, but also relates chain-binomial models to the general theory of stochastic processes.

8.5 Modifications and extensions

A number of extensions and modifications to the foregoing theory are worth considering. For example, changes could be made in the probabilities m_{ij} in (8.25) or $(\mathbf{M}_{ij})_{rs}$ in (8.32) without affecting the Markovian structure of the processes or changing the methods of obtaining the distributions of duration times and total epidemic sizes.

Thus Gani and Jerwood (1971) gave an example of investigating the effects of inoculation, in which, after the initial outbreak of infection, all remaining susceptibles are inoculated. Let us suppose that the effect of inoculation is to increase the probability q of no contact with infection from the initial value of q_0 at $t = 0$ to some maximum value $q_1 > q_0$ after one latent period, after which q gradually declines to $q_\infty = q_0$ again. While the structure of the Greenwood and Reed—Frost models remains unchanged over any single discrete time-interval, the whole Markov process now becomes nonhomogeneous in time with probability q_t of no contact in $(t, t + 1)$. For the Greenwood model the matrices $\mathbf{P}$ and $\mathbf{QE}$, defined in (8.28) and (8.29) respectively, are simply adjusted to $\mathbf{P}_t$ and $\mathbf{Q}_t\mathbf{E}$ obtained by substituting p_t and q_t for p and q on the right hand sides. The probability of, for example, an epidemic of duration t is then

$$\Pr\{T = t \,|\, X_0 = k\} = \mathbf{A}'_k \mathbf{P}_0 \mathbf{P}_1 \dots \mathbf{P}_{t-2} \mathbf{Q}_{t-1} \mathbf{E}, \qquad (8.36)$$

which may be compared with the time-homogeneous result previously given in (8.10) for $X_0 = i$. Gani and Jerwood give a numerical illustration of the computation of mean duration-time and mean epidemic size in relation to inoculation compared with no-inoculation. It would be interesting to pursue such an investigation in the context of specific diseases and intervention policies (see also Chapter 20).

Gani and Jerwood also point out that, for the Greenwood model, the Markov chain with transition matrix (8.26) can be regarded as embedded at fixed time-intervals in a pure death process in continuous time. If, following Bailey (1964, Section 8.5), we write $X(t)$ for the number of survivors at time

t in a death process having parameter μ, then

$$\Pr\{X(t+\tau) = j \mid X(t) = i\} = \binom{i}{j} e^{-j\mu\tau}(1 - e^{-\mu\tau})^{i-j}$$

$$= \binom{i}{j} q^j p^{i-j}, \tag{8.37}$$

if we write
$$p = 1 - e^{-\mu\tau}. \tag{8.38}$$

Since (8.37) corresponds exactly with the transition probabilities given in (8.25), it follows that the transition probability matrix $\mathbf{M}$ in (8.26) characterizes the Markov chain $\{R_t\}$ embedded at times $j\tau$ in the pure death process $\{X(t)\}$, subject to the interpretation (8.38).

We might hope to find that the Reed–Frost model could be embedded in the simple stochastic epidemic. This apparently is not the case, though there is some analogy over a *single* discrete time-interval.

More recently, however, Ludwig has shown that certain connections can be established between Reed–Frost models and more general models, provided that attention is restricted to the final size of epidemic. Thus, suppose we extend the Reed–Frost model by incorporating an infectious period which is of non-zero duration. This certainly increases realism, but means that the "age-structure" of the infected population must be dealt with explicitly in describing the progress of the epidemic in time. At time t we may suppose that there are r susceptibles and s infectives, the ages of the latter since infection being u_j, $1 \leqslant j \leqslant s$.

We may however argue as follows. Let the contact-rate for any given infective be $\beta(u)$, where u is the time that has elapsed since he was infected. Write $Q(u)$ for the probability of no contact, during the time-interval $(0, u)$, between a given susceptible and an infective of age u. Then it follows in the usual way that

$$\frac{dQ(u)}{du} = -\beta(u)\, Q(u). \tag{8.39}$$

Therefore,

$$Q(u) = \exp\left\{ -\int_0^u \beta(v)\, dv \right\}. \tag{8.40}$$

The chance that there will never be any contact adequate to infect the susceptible is $Q(\infty) \equiv Q$, say.

If there are a infectives initially, we define Q_0 as

$$Q_0 = Q^a, \tag{8.41}$$

so that Q_0 is the probability that a given susceptible never has any adequate contact with any of the initial infectives.

Now let us write $p(w|n)$ for the probability that w individuals are eventually infected out of an initial group of n susceptibles, i.e. a final epidemic size w. We can regard the initial group of n susceptibles as consisting of w "losers" and $n - w$ "winners". There are of course $\binom{n}{w}$ ways of making this decomposition. The probability of all the w "losers" becoming infected is $p(w|w)$, by definition. And the probability that each of the $n - w$ "winners" escapes contact, both with the initial a infectives and with the w "losers", is $Q_0^{n-w} Q^{w(n-w)}$. The probability of an epidemic of size w is therefore given by

$$p(w|n) = \binom{n}{w} p(w|w) \, Q_0^{n-w} \, Q^{w(n-w)}. \tag{8.42}$$

Further, since every epidemic that starts with n susceptibles must have a final size w for which $0 \leqslant w \leqslant n$, we also have

$$\sum_{w=0}^{n} p(w|n) = 1. \tag{8.43}$$

By induction on n we can use (8.42) and (8.43) to calculate $p(w|n)$. We start with $p(0|0) = 1$; $p(0|1) = Q_0$, $p(1|1) = 1 - Q_0$; $p(0|2) = Q_0^2$, etc., etc.

It is thus evident that the final epidemic size has a probability distribution $p(w|n)$ that depends solely on a, n and Q. The complications introduced by an extended infectious period disappear if we restrict attention to the distribution of epidemic size. So far as the latter is concerned, all models of the type considered with homogeneous mixing and single types of infectives and susceptibles are equivalent to a Reed–Frost formulation.

Ludwig also considers extensions to models involving several types of infectives or susceptibles. The epidemic size-distributions can now be computed in terms of appropriately defined Markov chains. These ideas have some importance for the interference models of Elveback $et\ al.$ (1971) discussed in Chapter 18.

8.6 Asymptotic approximations

So far, very few asymptotic approximations to discrete-time models are available. One would certainly expect that the explicit Gani–Jerwood theory of Sections 8.3–8.5 would be susceptible of such a development, but this still remains to be done. As things stand, however, there are only a few results in discrete endemic theory analogous to some of the continuous-time results in Section 7.6.

Let us use the notation of Section 8.2 and write S_t for the random variable indicating the number of infected persons just prior to time t who become infectious at time t, and R_t for the random variable indicating the number of susceptibles remaining uninfected at time t. Following Bartlett (1960a, c), but with a change of notation, we may define an extended chain-binomial model as follows.

The R_t susceptibles at time t give rise to the next generation of infectives S_{t+1}, and are subsequently augmented by an influx of μ new susceptibles. Thus

$$R_{t+1} = R_t - S_{t+1} + \mu, \tag{8.44}$$

which is the appropriate extension of equation (8.1). We shall suppose μ to be constant, corresponding to a regular input of fresh susceptibles. It may be shown that the alternative formulation of a random influx will have little effect on the amplitude of oscillations, provided μp is small.

Now S_{t+1} is a random variable having a binomial distribution with parameter $1 - q^{S_t}$, the number of "trials" being R_t, as in equations (8.3) or (8.5). We can therefore write the large-sample discrete stochastic equation, analogous to the continuous-time formulation in the second line of (7.46), as

$$S_{t+1} = R_t(1 - q^{S_t}) + Z_t, \tag{8.45}$$

where Z_t is an adjusted binomial variable with zero mean and variance $R_t q^{S_t}(1 - q^{S_t})$.

In a deterministic formulation, equation (8.44) would imply that the equilibrium value of S_t was μ. If the equilibrium value of R_t is taken to be ν, equation (8.45) leads to the relation

$$\mu = \nu(1 - q^\mu). \tag{8.46}$$

In a large-sample analysis of the approximate amplitude of small stochastic fluctuations some care is necessary, the theoretical difficulties being greater than those encountered previously in the continuous-time discussion of Section 7.6. We first observe that equation (8.44) shows that, exactly,

$$E(S_t) = \mu. \tag{8.47}$$

For small stochastic departures from the deterministic equilibrium, we can write

$$R_t = \nu(1 + U_t), \quad S_t = \mu(1 + V_t), \tag{8.48}$$

where U_t and V_t are small random variables, corresponding to the continuous-time definitions in (7.48). Substitution in equation (8.45) yields

$$\mu(1 + V_{t+1}) = \nu(1 + U_t)\{1 - q^\mu \exp(\mu V_t \log q)\} + Z_t. \tag{8.49}$$

Neglecting small quantities, we therefore have, approximately,

$$\mu \sim \nu(1 - q^\mu), \tag{8.50}$$

which may be compared with the exact relationship in (8.46) based on deterministic assumptions.

We now linearize the basic stochastic equations of the process given in

(8.44) and (8.45), by substituting from (8.48) and using (8.50). This quickly leads to

$$U_{t+1} + \frac{\mu}{\nu} V_{t+1} = U_t, \\ V_{t+1} \sim U_t + CV_t + Z_t/\mu, \quad \Biggr\} \tag{8.51}$$

where

$$C = -\nu q^\mu \log q. \tag{8.52}$$

Next we express the variances and covariances of the equilibrium distribution of U_t and V_t, represented by U and V, as σ_U^2, σ_V^2 and σ_{UV}^2, respectively. Now, from (8.47) and (8.48) we see that $E(V_t) = 0$, and can assume, at least approximately, that $E(U_t) = 0$. Thus

$$\sigma_U^2 = E(U_t^2) = E(U_{t+1}^2), \\ \sigma_V^2 = E(V_t^2) = E(V_{t+1}^2), \\ \sigma_{UV} = E(U_t V_t) = E(U_{t+1} V_{t+1}), \quad \Biggr\} \tag{8.53}$$

corresponding to (7.51). So far as the variable Z_t is concerned, it is by definition independent of the other variables, and has zero mean, and variance

$$\begin{aligned} \text{var}(Z_t) &= R_t q^{S_t}(1 - q^{S_t}) \\ &\sim \nu q^\mu (1 - q^\mu) \\ &\sim \mu q^\mu, \end{aligned} \tag{8.54}$$

where, for the equilibrium situation, we have replaced R_t and S_t by their approximate means and have used (8.50). Proceeding as before in Section 7.6, we square and cross-multiply the two relationships in (8.51), after which we take expectations. We obtain almost immediately

$$2\sigma_{UV} + \frac{\mu}{\nu} \sigma_V^2 = 0, \\ \sigma_V^2 \sim \sigma_U^2 + C^2 \sigma_V^2 + 2C\sigma_{UV} + \mu^{-1} q^\mu, \\ \sigma_{UV} + \frac{\mu}{\nu} \sigma_V^2 \sim \sigma_U^2 + C\sigma_{UV}, \quad \Biggr\} \tag{8.55}$$

corresponding to (7.52).

It should be noticed that the first relationship in (8.55) is exact for larger fluctuations as well, and shows, using (8.48), that

$$\text{cov}(R, S) = -\tfrac{1}{2} \text{var } S. \tag{8.56}$$

For small fluctuations we can solve (8.55) to give, after a little reduction

$$\sigma_V^2 \sim \frac{q^\mu}{\mu(1-C)\left(1+C-\frac{\mu}{2\nu}\right)},$$ (8.57)

and

$$\sigma_U^2 = \frac{\mu(1+C)}{2\nu}\sigma_V^2.$$ (8.58)

Formula (8.57) differs slightly from that given by Bartlett (1960a, c) in that the term $\mu/2\nu$ appears in a factor of the denominator instead of μ/ν. From (8.50), we can write

$$q^\mu \sim 1 - \frac{\mu}{\nu}.$$ (8.59)

If μ/ν is small (as it is with measles, for example), it follows that

$$\log q \sim -\frac{1}{\nu}, \quad C \sim 1 - \frac{\mu}{\nu}, \quad \mu \ll \nu.$$ (8.60)

Substituting (8.60) in (8.57) and (8.58) then leads to

$$\sigma_U^2 \sim \frac{1}{2\mu}, \quad \sigma_V^2 \sim \frac{\nu}{2\mu^2}, \quad \mu \ll \nu \quad \text{(discrete-time)}.$$ (8.61)

These results also include a factor of $\frac{1}{2}$ not shown in Bartlett's formulae.

These discrete-time variances in (8.61) may be compared with the corresponding continuous-time values appearing in (7.53). To obtain a valid analogy we should equate the corresponding steady-state values. Thus in (7.53) we must put $x_0 = \nu$ and $y_0 = \mu$. Hence if $\mu \ll \nu$, the continuous-time variances are approximately

$$\sigma_U^2 \sim \frac{1}{\mu}, \quad \sigma_V^2 \sim \frac{\nu}{\mu^2}, \quad \mu \ll \nu \quad \text{(continuous-time)}.$$ (8.62)

It is interesting to observe that the discrete-time values are just one-half the continuous-time values, although we can still consider that the general orders of magnitude are the same.

When a discrete-time model is used for convenience in simulation studies (see reference to Bartlett's work in Section 9.5 below), we might expect the smaller variance, compared with the continuous-time model, to lead to an increased time to extinction, a phenomenon actually observed by Bartlett (1960a, Sec. 7.2; 1960c, Sec. 4) in his computer simulations.

9

Spatial models

9.1 Introduction

A major aspect of the spread of infectious disease which we have not so far considered is the problem of the geographical distribution of cases. This is in general a very difficult matter, especially in view of the complications that readily arise, as we have seen in Chapters 5—8, even when the spatial aspect is ignored. We have of course already considered some departures from pure homogeneous mixing in Sections 5.10 and 6.9, either in terms of several interacting groups of individuals, or in terms of a modification of the transition rates or probabilities. But these extensions do not involve a direct appeal to a two-dimensional distribution of susceptibles, infectives, and removed individuals.

However, there is an obvious tendency in many communities for susceptibles who are situated a long way from infected persons, to have a smaller chance of infection than those who are in closer contact with the disease.

In Section 9.2 we consider a deterministic model in which the population is supposed to be spread out continuously, and in which infection is assumed in the limit to be both local and isotropic. A somewhat less specialized model is described in Section 9.3, and this permits the derivation of two interesting theorems for epidemic outbreaks. Stochastic formulations are discussed in Section 9.4, including the possibility of using a percolation-theoretic approach. The final section deals with various simulation studies and their implications.

9.2 A deterministic model

In Section 7.3 on modified deterministic models of recurrent epidemics or endemics we considered the extension of a single-group model to the case of two interacting groups of individuals. The basic equations are given in (7.20), where parameters are included to cover the possible introduction of new susceptibles as well as the migration of susceptibles and infectives. We now see what happens when these notions are further extended to the case of a very large number of very small groups, which in the limit leads to a spatially

171

continuous distribution of population, with x and y representing spatial *densities* of susceptibles and infectives.

An appropriate analogue of (7.20) is easily seen to be

$$\left.\begin{array}{l}\dfrac{\partial x}{\partial t} = -\beta x(y + \alpha\nabla^2 y) + \mu + \theta\nabla^2 x, \\[2mm] \dfrac{\partial y}{\partial t} = \beta x(y + \alpha\nabla^2 y) - \gamma y + \phi\nabla^2 y, \end{array}\right\} \tag{9.1}$$

where $\qquad x \equiv x(\xi, \eta, t) \quad y \equiv y(\xi, \eta, t),$

and $\qquad \nabla^2 \equiv \dfrac{\partial^2}{\partial\xi^2} + \dfrac{\partial^2}{\partial\eta^2},$

ξ and η being chosen to designate the spatial coordinates. Although we have used the same symbols here as previously, it will be realized that their interpretations must be somewhat different. An important element of these equations is the introduction of the operator ∇^2, which emerges from the assumption that infection and migration are both local and isotropic. The first-order equations for small fluctuations, corresponding to (7.22), are

$$\left.\begin{array}{l}\left(D + \dfrac{1}{\sigma} - \theta\nabla^2\right) u + \dfrac{1}{\sigma}(1 + \alpha\nabla^2)v = 0, \\[2mm] -\gamma u + \{D - (\phi + \alpha\gamma)\nabla^2\}v = 0. \end{array}\right\} \tag{9.2}$$

Although such equations, studied by Turing (1952) in connection with models for biological growth, may in general have solutions which are undamped in space and time, this is not the case here. For consider a component of the general solution of (9.2) having the form $\exp\{at + i(b\xi + c\eta)\}$, where b and c, but not necessarily a, are real. Substitution in (9.2) leads to

$$\left\{a + \dfrac{1}{\sigma} + \theta(b^2 + c^2)\right\} \{a + (\phi + \alpha\gamma)(b^2 + c^2)\} + \dfrac{\gamma}{\sigma}\{1 - \alpha(b^2 + c^2)\} = 0. \tag{9.3}$$

If we substitute $a = a_1 + ia_2$ in (9.3), and pick out the imaginary part, we obtain

$$a_2\left\{\dfrac{1}{\sigma} + \theta(b^2 + c^2) + (\phi + \alpha\gamma)(b^2 + c^2)\right\} + 2a_1 a_2 = 0. \tag{9.4}$$

Using the inequality $b^2 + c^2 \geqslant 0$, and assuming $a_2 \neq 0$, then gives

$$a_1 \leqslant -\dfrac{1}{2\sigma}. \tag{9.5}$$

It therefore follows that the damping in time is at least as large as that which occurs in the corresponding non-spatial model of Section 7.2.

An interesting application of this theory is to the way in which a disease spreads from a focus of infection freshly introduced into a susceptible area. The second equation of (9.1) can be written as

$$\left.\begin{array}{c} \dfrac{\partial y}{\partial t} = Ay + B\nabla^2 y, \\[2mm] \end{array}\right\} \tag{9.6}$$

where $\qquad\qquad A = (\beta x - \gamma), \quad B = \phi + \alpha\beta x.$

Initially, when x can be taken as approximately constant, (9.6) is a standard diffusion equation. Solution by means of the Fourier transform for spatial coordinates, namely

$$M = \int\int \{\exp(ip\xi + iq\eta)\} y\, d\xi\, d\eta, \tag{9.7}$$

is fairly straightforward. Multiplying (9.6) by $\exp(ip\xi + iq\eta)$ and integrating with respect to ξ and η, gives

$$M = C\exp\{At - B(p^2 + q^2)t\}, \tag{9.8}$$

where C is an arbitrary constant. Inversion yields

$$\begin{aligned} y &= \frac{1}{2\pi}\int\int \exp\{(-ip\xi - iq\eta)\} M\, dp\, dq \\[2mm] &= \frac{C}{2Bt}\exp\left\{At - \frac{\xi^2 + \eta^2}{4Bt}\right\}, \end{aligned} \tag{9.9}$$

where C can be determined by the initial conditions $y = y_0$, $t = t_0$. Now if y_R is the total amount of infection outside a circle of radius R, we have

$$\begin{aligned} y_R &= \int_{\xi^2 + \eta^2 \geqslant R^2} y\, d\xi\, d\eta \\[2mm] &= 2\pi C\exp\left\{At - \frac{R^2}{4Bt}\right\}. \end{aligned} \tag{9.10}$$

From (9.10) it follows that

$$R = 2(AB)^{\frac{1}{2}}t\left\{1 - \frac{\log(y_R/2\pi C)}{At}\right\}^{\frac{1}{2}}. \tag{9.11}$$

Hence $R \to 2(AB)^{\frac{1}{2}}t$ as $t \to \infty$. The circle of radius R corresponding to any given value y_R grows at a rate R/t, and this *velocity of propagation* therefore has the limiting value

$$2(AB)^{\frac{1}{2}} = 2\{(\beta x - \gamma)(\phi + \alpha\beta x)\}^{\frac{1}{2}}.$$

It was suggested by Dr Halliday in the discussion on Soper's paper (1929) that a measles epidemic starting in September took about 24 weeks to spread over the whole of Glasgow. If, for the purposes of rough calculation, we regarded the latter as a circle with a radius of two miles, then the approximate velocity of propagation would be $\frac{1}{12}$ mile per week.

How far such approximate calculations may have practical value is an open question. Nevertheless, the examination of these deterministic processes is an important stage in the development of more realistic models. It also provides useful standards of comparison as well as suggestions to be further investigated in the stochastic analogues to be considered in Section 9.4.

9.3 Spatial threshold theorems

The deterministic model discussed in Section 9.2 involves spatially continuous densities of susceptibles and infectives, and also assumes that infection and migration are both local and isotropic. In the present section we shall adopt the somewhat different formulation introduced by D. G. Kendall (in discussion on Bartlett, 1957). The specification of this model, which ignores the effects both of migration and of the accession of fresh susceptibles, is as follows.

Consider an infinite uniform two-dimensional population for which there are σ individuals per unit area. Let the numbers of individuals in an area dS surrounding a point P who are susceptible, infective or removed be $\sigma x \, dS$, $\sigma y \, dS$ and $\sigma z \, dS$, respectively, where x, y and z are functions of both time and position, and satisfy $x + y + z = 1$. (This definition of x, y and z as proportions should be contrasted with the slightly different usage of Section 6.2.) An argument similar to that previously used in Section 6.2 leads to the basic differential equations, analogous to (6.1), given by

$$\left. \begin{array}{l} \dfrac{\partial x}{\partial t} = -\beta\sigma x \bar{y}, \\[2mm] \dfrac{\partial y}{\partial t} = \beta\sigma x \bar{y} - \gamma y, \\[2mm] \dfrac{\partial z}{\partial t} = \gamma y, \end{array} \right\} \qquad (9.12)$$

where $\bar{y}$ is the spatially weighted average of y indicated by

$$\bar{y}(P, t) = \iint \lambda(PQ)\, y(Q, t)\, dS. \qquad (9.13)$$

In (9.12) the parameters β and γ are constants, and the explicit factor σ in the term $\beta\sigma x \bar{y}$ is used to keep the infection-rate independent of density. It is supposed in (9.13) that dS is an areal element situated at Q, and that $\lambda(PQ)$ is a suitably chosen non-negative weighting coefficient. If y is constant over the plane we shall still want the integral in (9.13) to converge, and can arrange that

$$\int\int \lambda(PQ)dS = 1. \tag{9.14}$$

We now multiply the third equation in (9.12) by $\lambda(PQ)$ and integrate to give

$$\frac{\partial \bar{z}}{\partial t} = \gamma \bar{y}, \tag{9.15}$$

where $\bar{z}$ is defined in a manner similar to $\bar{y}$. Dividing (9.15) into the first equation of (9.12) now gives, *for a fixed point P*,

$$\frac{dx}{d\bar{z}} = -\frac{\sigma x}{\rho}, \tag{9.16}$$

writing $\rho = \gamma/\beta$, as before. Let the initial conditions be

$$x(P, 0) = 1 - \epsilon(P), \quad y(P, 0) = \epsilon(P), \quad z(P, 0) = 0. \tag{9.17}$$

Integrating (9.16) therefore gives

$$x(P, t) = \{1 - \epsilon(P)\}\exp\{- \sigma\bar{z}(P, t)/\rho\}. \tag{9.18}$$

We can now eliminate x from (9.18) and the third equation in (9.12), using $x + y + z = 1$, to obtain

$$\frac{1}{\gamma}\frac{\partial z}{\partial t} = \epsilon + (1 - \epsilon)(1 - e^{-\sigma\bar{z}/\rho}) - z, \tag{9.19}$$

which, with the condition $z(P, 0) = 0$, is sufficient to determine z for all P and t. The value of x can then be derived from (9.18), and that of y by subtraction of x and z from unity.

Let us suppose that initially we have the infection uniformly spread over a circle, centred on the origin O and having radius a, so that

$$\begin{aligned}\epsilon(P) &= \alpha, \quad OP < a, \\ &= 0, \quad OP > a.\end{aligned} \right\} \tag{9.20}$$

The treatment of (9.19) is still difficult without some further restrictions and we shall suppose that $\lambda(PQ)$ vanishes if PQ is greater than some constant b, i.e.

$$\begin{aligned}\lambda(PQ) &> 0, \quad 0 < PQ \leqslant b, \\ &= 0, \quad PQ > b.\end{aligned} \right\} \tag{9.21}$$

Now it follows from (9.12) that, as $t \to \infty$, x decreases and z increases. Since they are bounded they must tend to limits X and Z, respectively. Further, it can be seen that the limit Y of y must be zero, so $X = 1 - Z$, and we need only find $Z(P)$ to investigate the ultimate behaviour of the epidemic. From (9.19) we find

$$\left.\begin{aligned} Z &= \alpha + (1-\alpha)(1 - e^{-\sigma \tilde{Z}/\rho}), && OP < a, \\ &= 1 - e^{-\sigma \tilde{Z}/\rho}, && OP > a. \end{aligned}\right\} \qquad (9.22)$$

It is obvious that $Z(P) > 0$ if $OP < a$, and we can show that the inequality also holds if $OP > a$. For if A is a point such that $Z(A) = 0$, it follows from the second equation of (9.22) that $\tilde{Z}(A) = 0$. The conditions in (9.21) then imply that $Z(P) = 0$ almost everywhere inside a circle with centre at A and of radius b. If this argument is continued in the direction AO we arrive at a contradiction in a finite number of steps. It therefore follows that $Z(P) > 0$ everywhere. This yields the important result that the effects of the epidemic ultimately extend over the whole plane.

Another valuable result involving a new threshold theorem depends on the conjecture (which requires further investigation) that $Z(P)$ decreases steadily as $OP \to \infty$, at least for P sufficiently distant from the origin. In this event it can be seen that $Z(P)$ and $\tilde{Z}(P)$ must both tend to the same limit, ζ say. Equation (9.22) then gives

$$\zeta = 1 - e^{-\sigma \zeta/\rho}. \qquad (9.23)$$

Now (9.23) always has a zero root; but there is a (unique) positive root if and only if $\sigma > \rho$. When this condition holds, it can be shown by a suitable *reductio ad absurdum* argument that $Z(P)$ converges to the positive root, i.e. $\zeta > 0$. We then have a *pandemic,* in which the proportion of individuals contracting the disease is ultimately at least as great as ζ, however far we go away from the initial focus of infection. The quantity ζ may be called the *severity* of the pandemic. Accepting the conjecture mentioned above, we therefore have Kendall's Pandemic Threshold Theorem:

(i) There will be a pandemic if and only if the population density σ *exceeds* the threshold density $\rho = \gamma/\beta$;

(ii) if there is a pandemic then its severity ζ is given by the unique positive root of equation (9.23).

It will be realized that there is a close resemblance between this result and the non-spatial threshold theorem of Kermack and McKendrick for closed populations. Indeed, equation (9.23) is equivalent to equation (6.22) if in the latter we replace N and i by σ and ζ, respectively. Numerical values of corresponding densities and severities can therefore be determined by reference to Table 6.1. Thus if $\sigma = 1.05\rho$ we have a severity of about 9 percent.

Later, Kendall (1965) examined in more detail the behaviour of a one-dimensional version of the above model. Equations (9.12) and (9.13), suitably reinterpreted, still stand. The population is now seen as distributed along a line, $\sigma x(s, t)$ and $\sigma y(s, t)$ being the local densities of susceptibles and infectives, respectively, at distance s from the origin and at time t. It is convenient to replace $\bar{y}$, the spatially weighted average of y, by $y + k\partial^2 y/\partial s^2$, where k is some positive constant.

Instead of trying to find the most general solution of the modified equations, we look for travelling waves by putting

$$x(s, t) = x(s - ct), \quad y(s, t) = y(s - ct), \qquad (9.24)$$

where c (> 0) is the velocity of the waves. Investigation of the possible forms of solution then shows that there are no waves unless the population density σ exceeds the threshold value ρ. This constitutes a Threshold Theorem for waves.

Moreover, when $\sigma > \rho$ no waves can have a smaller velocity than $2\{k(\sigma - \rho)/\sigma\}^{\frac{1}{2}}$, but all waves are possible with velocities greater than or equal to this minimum. It seems likely, however, that an initial local concentration of infectives would generate waves travelling in opposite directions, with asymptotic velocities equal to the minimum. Although this one-dimensional model is somewhat over-simplified, it could have some relevance to the spreading edge of a pandemic, such as occurs from time to time with influenza. For more recent and detailed discussions of these problems see Mollison (1970; 1972a, b).

A two-dimensional investigation would naturally be much more complicated, and certain aspects have already been studied by Mollison (1970).

9.4 Stochastic models

Although the extension of deterministic theory to cover the important features of a spatial distribution of disease, described in Section 9.2, was not without certain difficulties, the analogous generalization in the stochastic case is considerably more complex. Even the basic equation corresponding to (9.1) above appears rather formidable at first sight. Instead of merely using the probability-generating function $\Pi(z, w, t)$, containing the two auxiliary variables z and w, we replace the latter by two *functions*, $z(\mathbf{a})$ and $w(\mathbf{a})$, where the vector $\mathbf{a} \equiv (\xi, \eta)$. We now investigate the appropriate "point" stochastic process (Bartlett, 1954, 1955) by means of the probability-generating *functional* $\Pi\{z(\mathbf{a}), w(\mathbf{a}), t\}$. The required expression for $\partial\Pi/\partial t$ can be written down formally by much the same procedure as that referred to previously. This is most easily done by inspecting the relevant scheme of possible transitions and corresponding operators (e.g. Bartlett, 1956), namely

Type of transition	Rate	Operator
$w(\mathbf{a}) \rightarrow 1$	γ	$\dfrac{\partial}{\partial w(\mathbf{a}) d\mathbf{a}}$
$1 \rightarrow z(\mathbf{a})$	$\mu \, d\mathbf{a}$	1
$z(\mathbf{a})w(\mathbf{b}) \rightarrow w(\mathbf{a})w(\mathbf{b})$	β	$\dfrac{\partial^2}{\partial z(\mathbf{a})\partial w(\mathbf{b}) d\mathbf{a} d\mathbf{b}}$
$w(\mathbf{a}) \rightarrow w(\mathbf{b})$	$\phi \, d\mathbf{a}$	$\dfrac{\partial}{\partial w(\mathbf{a}) d\mathbf{a}}$
$z(\mathbf{a}) \rightarrow z(\mathbf{b})$	$\theta \, d\mathbf{a}$	$\dfrac{\partial}{\partial z(\mathbf{a}) d\mathbf{a}}$

Alternatively, an extension of Bailey (1964, Sec. 7.4) may be used.

It will be noticed that we are here using the special notation for functional derivatives (e.g. Hopf, 1952), in contrast with the ordinary partial differential operators appearing before. If the process envisaged is spatially and temporally homogeneous, then γ and μ are constants, but β, θ and ϕ are all functions of the vector displacement $\mathbf{a} - \mathbf{b}$. If, in addition, the process is assumed to be isotropic, then only the modulus $|\mathbf{a} - \mathbf{b}|$ is involved. The equation for $\partial\Pi/\partial t$ is therefore

$$\frac{\partial\Pi}{\partial t} = \int \gamma\{1 - w(\mathbf{a})\}\frac{\partial\Pi}{\partial w(\mathbf{a})d\mathbf{a}}d\mathbf{a} + \int \mu\{z(\mathbf{a}) - 1\}\Pi d\mathbf{a}$$

$$+ \iint \beta(\mathbf{a} - \mathbf{b})w(\mathbf{b})\{w(\mathbf{a}) - z(\mathbf{a})\}\frac{\partial^2\Pi}{\partial z(\mathbf{a})\partial w(\mathbf{b})d\mathbf{a}d\mathbf{b}}d\mathbf{a}d\mathbf{b}$$

$$+ \iint \phi(\mathbf{a} - \mathbf{b})\{w(\mathbf{b}) - w(\mathbf{a})\}\frac{\partial\Pi}{\partial w(\mathbf{a})d\mathbf{a}}d\mathbf{a}d\mathbf{b}$$

$$+ \iint \theta(\mathbf{a} - \mathbf{b})\{z(\mathbf{b}) - z(\mathbf{a})\}\frac{\partial\Pi}{\partial z(\mathbf{a})d\mathbf{a}}d\mathbf{a}d\mathbf{b}. \tag{9.25}$$

Some simplification results if we can treat the numbers of susceptibles as approximately constant, as in the initial stages of an epidemic. We should then have Π as a functional of $w(\mathbf{a})$ only. Representing the actual number of susceptibles by the constant approximating density $n(\mathbf{a}) = n$, we obtain

$$\frac{\partial\Pi}{\partial t} = \int \gamma\{1 - w(\mathbf{a})\}\frac{\partial\Pi}{\partial w(\mathbf{a})d\mathbf{a}}d\mathbf{a}$$

$$+ n\iint \beta(\mathbf{a} - \mathbf{b})w(\mathbf{b})\{w(\mathbf{a}) - 1\}\frac{\partial\Pi}{\partial w(\mathbf{b})d\mathbf{b}}d\mathbf{a}d\mathbf{b}$$

$$+ \iint \phi(\mathbf{a} - \mathbf{b})\{w(\mathbf{b}) - w(\mathbf{a})\}\frac{\partial\Pi}{\partial w(\mathbf{a})d\mathbf{a}}d\mathbf{a}d\mathbf{b}. \tag{9.26}$$

The process defined by (9.26) is of "multiplicative" type, for which the "backward" equation is simpler than the above "forward" one. Suppose, for example, that we wish to study the consequences of introducing a single case of infection into a population of susceptibles. Let $\Pi(\mathbf{v})$ be the appropriate probability-generating functional. Then it can be shown that $\Pi(\mathbf{v})$ satisfies

$$\frac{\partial\Pi(\mathbf{v})}{\partial t} = \gamma\{1 - \Pi(\mathbf{v})\} + n\int \beta(\mathbf{u} - \mathbf{v})\Pi(\mathbf{v})\{\Pi(\mathbf{u}) - 1\}d\mathbf{u}$$

$$+ \int \phi(\mathbf{v} - \mathbf{u})\{\Pi(\mathbf{u}) - \Pi(\mathbf{v})\}d\mathbf{u}. \tag{9.27}$$

We can obtain the chance of extinction $p_t(\mathbf{v})$ at time t, by putting $w(\mathbf{a}) \equiv 0$.

This yields

$$\frac{\partial p_t(\mathbf{v})}{\partial t} = \gamma\{1 - p_t(\mathbf{v})\} + n \int \beta(\mathbf{u} - \mathbf{v}) p_t(\mathbf{v})\{p_t(\mathbf{u}) - 1\} d\mathbf{u}$$

$$+ \int \phi(\mathbf{v} - \mathbf{u})\{p_t(\mathbf{u}) - p_t(\mathbf{v})\} d\mathbf{u}. \tag{9.28}$$

If we make the further homogeneity assumption that

$$p_t(\mathbf{v}) = p_t(\mathbf{u}) = p_t,$$

then (9.28) reduces to

$$\left.\begin{array}{c} \dfrac{\partial p_t}{\partial t} = \gamma(1 - p_t) + n p_t(p_t - 1)B, \\[2mm] \text{where} \qquad B = \int \beta(\mathbf{u}) d\mathbf{u}. \end{array}\right\} \tag{9.29}$$

This is actually identical with the equation for the chance of extinction of a simple birth-and-death process with birth- and death-rates γ and nB, having as solution

$$p_t = \frac{\gamma\{e^{(nB-\gamma)t} - 1\}}{nB e^{(nB-\gamma)t} - \gamma}. \tag{9.30}$$

Of course, it will be realized that this applies only to the beginning of the process. There appear to be considerable difficulties in developing a satisfactory discussion of the long-term stability of such a spatial process. The rough arguments previously used for non-spatial models in Sections 7.4 and 7.5 do not readily generalize, since a process extended in the plane is likely to show heterogeneity of phase at different points.

We can also obtain equations for moment densities. An equation for the mean density of infectives given by

$$m(\mathbf{a}, t)da \equiv E\{ds(\mathbf{a}, t)\}, \tag{9.31}$$

where $ds(\mathbf{a}, t)$ is the stochastic number of infectives at time t in da, can be derived directly from (9.27), namely,

$$\frac{\partial m(\mathbf{a})}{\partial t} = -\gamma m(\mathbf{a}) + n \int \beta(\mathbf{a} - \mathbf{b}) m(\mathbf{b}) d\mathbf{b}$$

$$- m(\mathbf{a}) \int \phi(\mathbf{a} - \mathbf{b}) d\mathbf{b} + \int \phi(\mathbf{b} - \mathbf{a}) m(\mathbf{b}) d\mathbf{b}. \tag{9.32}$$

Let us now use the bivariate Fourier transform for $m(\mathbf{a})$ given by

$$M(\mathbf{p}) = \int\int \{\exp i(p\xi + q\eta)\} m(\mathbf{a}) d\xi d\eta, \tag{9.33}$$

where $\mathbf{a} \equiv (\xi, \eta)$ and $\mathbf{p} \equiv (p, q)$. Let the corresponding transforms of β and ϕ be $B(\mathbf{p})$ and $\Phi(\mathbf{p})$, respectively. The transform of equation (9.32) is then

$$\frac{\partial M(\mathbf{p})}{\partial t} = \{-\gamma + nB(\mathbf{p}) - \Phi(0) + \Phi(-\mathbf{p})\}M(\mathbf{p}), \qquad (9.34)$$

where $B(0) \equiv B$, appearing in (9.29) above. The solution of (9.34) is therefore

$$M(\mathbf{p}) = \exp\left[\{nB(\mathbf{p}) - \gamma - \Phi(0) + \Phi(-\mathbf{p})\}t\right]. \qquad (9.35)$$

In the special case when infection and diffusion are purely local and isotropic the solution (9.35) corresponds to the solution of the deterministic process represented by (9.6).

Equations for higher-order product densities, which arise in connection with the present type of process, are more easily obtained from the "forward" equations corresponding to (9.27). For a more detailed discussion of the theory briefly indicated in this section, the works by Bartlett (1954, 1955, 1956, 1960a) should be consulted. Extensions of Bartlett's approach to the initial geographical spread of host-vector and carrier-borne epidemics have recently been made by Radcliffe (1973).

Further work was done by Neyman and Scott (1964) for a spatial model incorporating some specific realistic features that had not previously been incorporated, and using a position-dependent branching process model with discrete-time parameter corresponding to the incubation period. Thus the number of susceptibles infected by an infective is made to depend on the position of the latter. Again, an individual who becomes infected at any point is permitted to move away and become infectious at some other place. However, it is a dominant feature of epidemic processes that the stock of susceptibles at risk is diminished by each new infection. This characteristic is not incorporated in Neyman and Scott's model. The latter would therefore be approximately valid at the start of the process but would become progressively less so as the epidemic built up. (See also Section 20.4 on vaccination models.)

How serious the limitation is for the conclusions arrived at is difficult to gauge. In particular it appears that, under fairly broad conditions, the probability of an epidemic building up in a small community is the same as the probability of an explosive outbreak over a major larger area (compare for example the deterministic pandemic threshold theorem in Section 9.3). Moreover, this is very similar to the practical view of public health authorities who usually believe that a focus of infection due to insanitary conditions in any one part of a country may be a source of danger for the whole community. Further discussion of Neyman and Scott's model has been given by Bartoszyński (1969) and Bartoszyński, Łoś and Wycech-Łoś (1965).

A rigorous general theoretical treatment is not yet available for any two-dimensional stochastic epidemic process, though Morgan and Welsh (1965) obtained some interesting theorems for a rather special kind of stochastic infection process taking place amongst susceptibles distributed over all points of a square lattice. The latter is represented by the points (x, y), where x and y are non-negative integers. The process starts with one infective at $(0, 0)$, and the infection spreads in a random Poisson way to neighbouring susceptibles, but *only* in the direction of increasing x and y. This approach was subsequently generalized by Hammersley (1966), using first-passage percolation theory.

The possibility of couching certain two-dimensional infection problems in percolation-theoretic terms is worth noting. There is a basic contrast between the classical diffusion type of models and percolation models. In the simplest example of a one-dimensional Pólya walk, a moving particle moves in steps of unit length along a line starting from the origin. After any number of steps, the particle moves with probability $\frac{1}{2}$ to either right or left. The stochastic mechanism resides, in a sense, in the particle itself.

In the percolation analogue we still have a moving particle, but now the stochastic mechanism lies in the intrinsic properties of the space rather than in the particle. The analogy to the Pólya walk above is that each point of the line has equal probabilities (each one-half) of being "right-sense" or "left-sense". The process starts from the origin, with the particle moving at each step in whatever direction is attached to the point from which the step starts. Thus the motion of the particle is determined by the properties of the space or medium. Movement continues in one direction until the particle meets successive points of opposite sense. It then oscillates between them.

Extensions of a more realistic kind can obviously be made to two or three dimensions. Hammersley and Welsh (1965) give an infectious disease example that might be treated via a percolation model. Thus, consider the trees to be planted in a large orchard at the vertices of a square lattice. It is supposed, for simplicity, that the distances between trees are such that only nearest neighbours can be infected. Let the probability of an infected tree infecting a susceptible tree be p. In ordinary percolation theory we can determine the probability $P_N(p)$ that under these conditions the disease will spread from a given tree to more than N other trees. To introduce a time element, we can assume that the time elapsing between a tree becoming infected and its infecting a neighbouring tree has some statistical distribution, e.g. negative exponential. We can now adopt the approach of first-passage percolation theory and consider the time at which the infection first passes beyond some given region.

Relatively little seems to have been done in developing these approaches in an epidemic context. One difficulty is that making the stochastic mechanism a property of the space often, but not always, seems at variance with the usual epidemiological picture of disease transmission. Another difficulty is that the extensive mathematical work carried out so far on percolation processes, although derived from concrete physical problems, appears to have a highly specialized and abstract character, whose relevance to concrete epidemiological phenomena is by no means clear. Further research in this area would however be well worth undertaking.

9.5 Simulation studies

We have already referred in Section 7.7 to the simulation studies of Bartlett (1957, 1960a, 1961) to examine various problems connected with recurrent epidemics, and we mentioned that the artificial processes built up were extended in space as well as time. This provided a greater degree of realism, especially in the context of real data on large towns and cities in the UK. In fact a 6 × 6 spatial grid of cells was used in the computer simulations. Each cell was treated individually in a non-spatial way as a sub-population, the spatial element being introduced by having a certain degree of migration of infectives between cells having a common boundary. For smaller total populations the usual continuous-time model was used, but for community sizes of the order of 100 000 a discrete-time analogue was used (see Section 8.6) to avoid complications and save time. Bartlett (1960a, Section 7.1; 1960ç, Section 4; 1961) later concluded that the spatial aspect in this type of model was less important than previously supposed. Not only could it be shown, theoretically, that to a first approximation the critical size should be uninfluenced by spatial factors unless there was a diffusion of individuals in the population, but simulation results obtained for the model having a 6 × 6 grid of cells did not differ substantially from results for a corresponding model without the spatial element.

However, the introduction of a spatial element into Bartlett's simulations appears to have been more for the purpose of achieving greater realism and relevance to actual available data than for studying spatial phenomena *per se*. A simulation investigation for the latter purpose was carried out by Bailey (1967a). He considered a population of susceptibles located at the points of a square lattice bounded by the lines $x = \pm k$, $y = \pm k$, the total population thus being of size $n = (2k + 1)^2$. The majority of calculations used $k = 5$, with $n = 121$, but a few more were carried out for $k = 10$, with $n = 441$. It was supposed that an epidemic was started by the single susceptible at the origin becoming infected, the disease subsequently spreading to nearest neighbours in the kind of discrete-time manner already described in Chapter 8. Two versions were possible, the simple epidemic without removal and the general epidemic with removal.

In the simple epidemic it was assumed that there was a fixed latent period following the receipt of infection followed by a very short infectious period, ideally contracted to a point. At this moment the chance of any exposed susceptible becoming infected was p. If a given susceptible was exposed to r infectives the chance of contracting the disease was $1 - (1 - p)^r$. Since in the simple epidemic there is no recovery, it was assumed that each infective became infectious again at an infinite series of time-instants all separated by intervals equal to the latent period.

In the general epidemic, on the other hand, an infective became non-infectious and immune after the first infectious point, just as in ordinary chain-binomial theory.

Bailey chose to assume that the *eight* nearest neighbours to any infective were at risk. This choice was determined partly by the feeling that the use of the usual four nearest neighbours was unduly restricting, and partly by considerations of the limited core storage available on the small computer actually employed. Thus when $p = 1$ the infection spreads deterministically and, with eight nearest neighbours being at risk (unless already infected), has covered by the gth generation a complete square whose sides are given by $x = \pm g = y$. All the susceptibles on the boundary of this square become infected at the next generation. When $g = k$ the disease has spread through the whole population and has reached the boundary. The edge-effects are thus very simple. With values of p smaller than unity, the situation is more complicated, but we can still expect some degree of symmetry *vis-à-vis* the boundaries.

With these ideas in mind, it is reasonable to run off a set of simulated epidemics for any given value of p (the values 0·2, 0·4, 0·6 and 0·8 were actually investigated), and summarize the results by showing (a) the average epidemic curve for the sub-population of individuals located along the boundary of any given square centred on the origin, e.g. $x = \pm l = y$, $(1 \leqslant l \leqslant k)$, and (b) the average epidemic curve for the average individual in the sub-population just mentioned. It is also of interest to consider (c) the epidemic curve for the whole population, ignoring the spatial aspects.

Fig. 9.1 and 9.2 show the results obtained with the simple epidemic for $p = 0·2$ and 0·8, respectively, using sets of 25 simulations. They also exhibit at (d) the completion time distribution. Since the areas under the (b) graphs must all be unity, they can be regarded as frequency distributions. They are thus directly comparable with one another and represent one method of characterizing the advancing epidemic wave. It appears from the (b) graphs in Fig. 9.1 and 9.2 that the wave advances at a more or less steady rate. When p is small, e.g. 0·2 in Fig. 9.1 (b), the wave is more spread out the further one moves from the initial focus. But with p larger, e.g. 0·8 in Fig. 9.2 (b), the waves travel out to the boundary almost unchanged in form.

This more or less linear spread is also implied by the (c) curves for the whole population, at least to the point at which edge-effects begin to be felt. This phenomenon was confirmed in a large population of 441 individuals, i.e. $k = 10$, with $p = 0·6$, for which an almost constant increase of 7·5 new cases per generation was observed for the first ten generations, after which a sharp fall occurred, as expected.

Corresponding results for the general epidemic, in which individuals remain immune and non-infectious after the first, and only, point of infectiousness, are shown in Fig. 9.3 and 9.4. Comparison of Fig. 9.1 and 9.3 (for which a different scaling was necessary) shows that we now have a very different phenomenon. The outbreak of the general epidemic for $p = 0·2$ is very much a localized affair, remaining largely near to the origin and having less and less influence as we move further away. On the other hand, when $p = 0·8$, as in

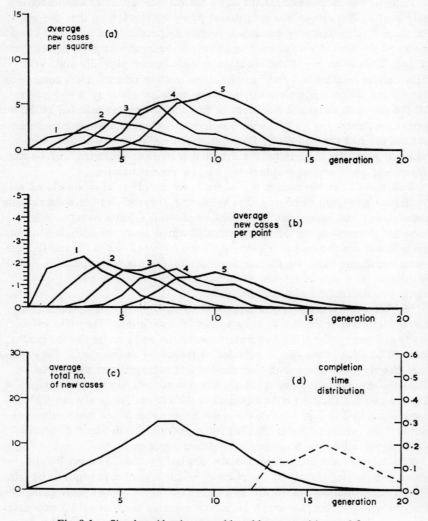

Fig. 9.1   Simple epidemic on an 11 × 11 square with $p = 0.2$

Fig. 9.4, the results are hardly distinguishable from the simple epidemic of Fig. 9.2.

There is obviously a threshold effect here, as we should expect. Table 9.1 shows the distribution of total epidemic size over the range of values $p = 0.20$ (0.04) 0.36. Although the sample sizes are quite small, with only 25 simulations in each set, there is a very marked change in form from a J-shaped

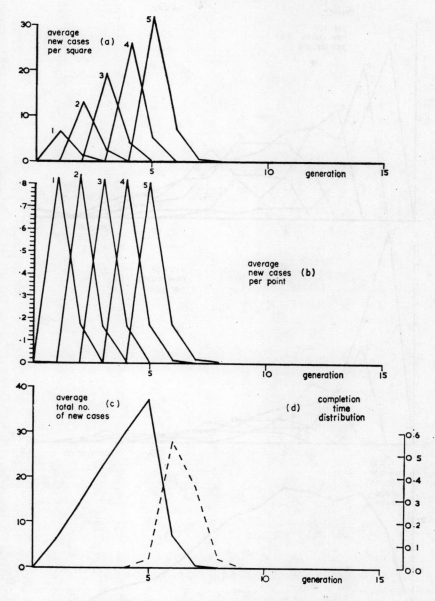

Fig. 9.2   Simple epidemic on an 11×11 square with $p = 0.8$

distribution with maximum ordinate at the lower end when $p = 0.24$ to a
J-shaped distribution with the maximum at the opposite end when $p = 0.32$.

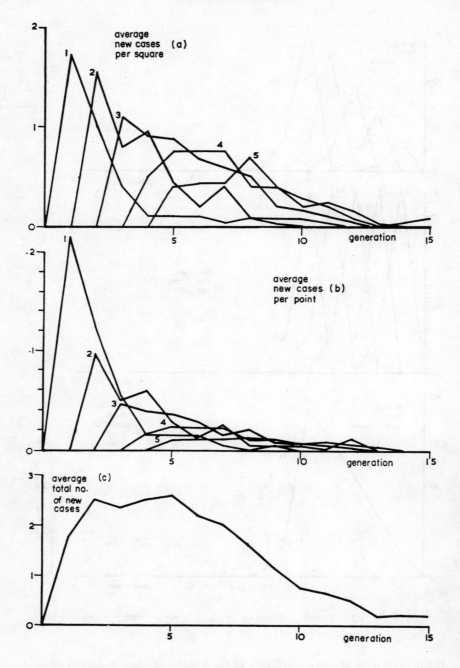

Fig. 9.3   General epidemic on an 11×11 square with $p = 0\cdot2$

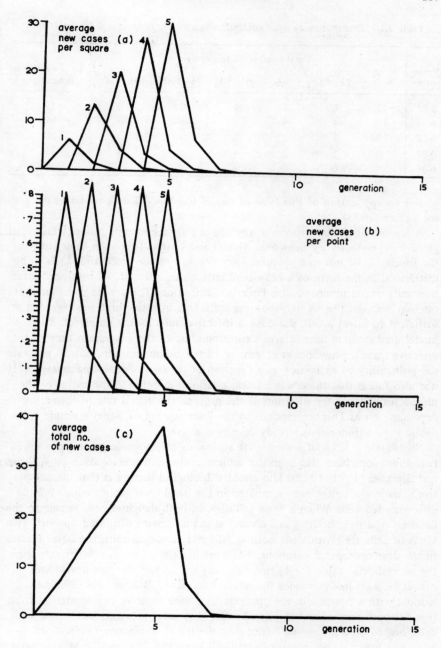

Fig. 9.4   General epidemic on an 11 × 11 square with $p = 0.8$

Table 9.1   *Distribution of total epidemic size over the range p = 0·20 (0·04) 0·36*

Value of p	Total number of new cases						Total number of simulations
	0−20	21−40	41−60	61−80	81−100	101−200	
0·20	13	6	5	1	0	0	25
0·24	10	4	6	2	3	0	25
0·28	8	1	3	8	5	0	25
0·32	2	1	2	4	8	8	25
0·36	0	0	0	1	3	21	25

For an application of this type of model to observed data on ferret distemper see Kelker (1973).

A somewhat similar process to the above simple epidemic model was investigated independently by Schwöbel, Geidel and Lorenz (1966) in their study of the formation of infected plaques. They considered the susceptible cells to be distributed in the form of a hexagonal lattice. An infected cell produced infective units whose number had a Poisson distribution. These were distributed at random amongst the six neighbouring cells. One infective unit was regarded as sufficient to infect a cell, subsequent infective units having no effect. The model used discrete-time intervals corresponding to the generation time of the infective agents. Schwöbel *et al.* employed the simulation approach to estimate the probability of extinction as a function of the basic Poisson parameter λ. It was also found that there was a linear relationship between the radius of the plaque formed and the duration of the process, the actual rate of formation depending on λ. This corresponds to the linear spread of Bailey's simple epidemic in two dimensions already discussed above.

Simulation studies of a somewhat analogous carcinogenic growth process in two dimensions have also been the subject of detailed investigation by Williams and Bjerknes (1971, 1972). The essential biological picture is that the generative mass in the epithelium is situated in the basal layer, above which are the differentiated cells. When a basal cell divides, both daughter cells remain in the basal layer, a neighbouring cell chosen at random being displaced upward. Two kinds of cells are postulated: normal cells and abnormal cells, the latter leading to the development of a tumour. The tumour cells divide at a faster rate than the normal cells, say κ (> 1) times as fast, and so the clone of developing cancer cells gradually invades the whole basal layer. Williams and Bjerknes worked with a continuous-time process, assuming negative exponential distribution for both normal and abnormal cells. They were primarily concerned with cells located on a hexagonal lattice, but the broad qualitative implications were also found to be true for square and triangular lattices (the average rates of spread of the abnormal cells being respectively in the ratios of 1·00:0·80: 0·72 for the three types of lattice).

If we now change the time variable, t say, to $\tau = \kappa t$ and let $\kappa \to \infty$, we obtain a continuous-time, two-dimensional, simple epidemic process (for which Bailey's model above is a discrete-time analogue with a slight modification in the definition of "nearest neighbours"). Thus theoretical developments obtained for the carcinogenic process may, suitably interpreted, have some relevance to epidemic processes. Williams and Bjerknes found empirically that, independent of the value of κ, the periphery of the clone of abnormal cells appeared to have a greater crinkliness than would have been expected, corresponding to a dimensionality of approximately 1·1 instead of unity. The conjecture that this empirical result might hold as a general rule has been disputed by Mollison (1972).

Williams and Bjerknes (1972) present computer printouts giving typical configurations when there are, for the first time, totals of 100, 400, 900 and 1600 abnormal cells, for three special values of κ, namely 1·1, 2 and infinity. Even with modern computers the simulation of such processes could be prohibitively time-consuming, but a considerable saving was made by retaining in the computer memory only a list of peripheral points for the abnormal clone. Since configuration changes could occur only on this periphery, it was necessary to scan only the periphery and update the list when changes had occurred, instead of scanning the whole array as in Bailey's (1967a) investigation.

10
Carrier models

10.1 Introduction

As already indicated in Chapter 3, a major complication of many diseases is the existence of so-called carriers, i.e. individuals who, although apparently healthy themselves, are already infected and are capable of transmitting the infection to others. Diseases such as poliomyelitis, tuberculosis, or typhoid are typical examples. Some carriers may continue to be infectious for a very long time. Others may become clear of infection more quickly. In either case the carriers are effectively removed from circulation, but as they are not ill and exhibit no normal symptoms of disease, they are not themselves usually recognized as actual cases. On the other hand, carriers may be suspected because of the existence of an otherwise inexplicable occurrence of scattered cases. This may lead to a deliberate search for carriers, and some or all of them may be identified through the use of special tests. The practical situation is therefore liable to be somewhat complicated. In Chapter 16 we shall consider some specific models for tuberculosis and typhoid. The investigations described will be deterministic in character, though the multi-compartmental models used will have a fair degree of realism. In the present chapter we shall examine some of the simpler models in more theoretical detail. Sections 10.2 and 10.3 introduce the basic deterministic and stochastic models of Weiss (1965), further studied by Dietz (1966) and Downton (1967b). An extension of the stochastic model to deal with the possibility of time-dependent parameters (Dietz, 1967) is discussed in Section 10.4. A more realistic model (Dietz and Downton, 1968), involving the introduction of new susceptibles and carriers from outside the population, is developed in Section 10.5. Further modifications are briefly indicated in the final section. These include the creation of new carriers by cross-infection within the population (Downton, 1968; Gillian Denton, 1972); a large-population approximation to a model involving both clinically recognizable infectives and subclinically infected carriers (Pettigrew and Weiss, 1967); and the multigroup model with variations in susceptibility and infectiousness by Becker (1973).

10.2 Basic deterministic model

In this basic, somewhat simplified, model we concentrate attention on only two types of individuals, susceptibles and carriers. It is assumed that only carriers are responsible for the actual spread of infection. When a susceptible is infected he is supposed to exhibit symptoms sufficiently quickly to be effectively recognized and removed from circulation before he can transmit the disease to others. This implies reasonably efficient public health control, in that recognizable cases amongst susceptibles are removed more or less instantly after occurrence. The elimination of carriers, on the other hand, proceeds at some finite rate, which may depend on both spontaneous recovery and public health detection.

Let us suppose that at time t we have x susceptibles and y carriers. The number of new infections in time Δt is taken to be $\beta xy \, \Delta t$, where β is the infection-rate, while the number of carriers removed in Δt is assumed to be $\alpha y \, \Delta t$, where α is the removal rate for the carriers. (Weiss (1965) actually defined α and β in the alternative sense, but we have chosen to retain β as the infection-rate, in conformity with earlier chapters.) The deterministic process is accordingly characterized by the equations

$$\left.\begin{aligned}
\frac{dx}{dt} &= -\beta xy, \\[2mm]
\frac{dy}{dt} &= -\alpha y,
\end{aligned}\right\} \tag{10.1}$$

the initial conditions being

$$x = n, \quad y = b, \quad t = 0, \tag{10.2}$$

if we start with n susceptibles and b carriers at time $t = 0$.

The solution of (10.1), subject to (10.2), can be found almost immediately by solving directly, first for y and then for x, giving

$$\left.\begin{aligned}
y &= b \, e^{-\alpha t}, \\[2mm]
x &= n \exp\left\{ \frac{\beta b}{\alpha} (e^{-\alpha t} - 1) \right\}.
\end{aligned}\right\} \tag{10.3}$$

The ultimate number of unaffected susceptibles, as $t \to \infty$, is thus $x_\infty = n \, e^{-\beta b/\alpha}$, and the total size w of the observed epidemic is

$$w = n(1 - e^{-\beta b/\alpha}). \tag{10.4}$$

In the following section we shall develop the corresponding stochastic theory. So far as total average epidemic size is concerned, it appears that the deterministic and stochastic results are essentially the same when $\beta b/\alpha$ is small. But when $\beta b/\alpha$ is not small, the deterministic theory overestimates the expected size of epidemic.

10.3 Basic stochastic model

We can develop the deterministic model of the last section to provide a probability treatment in the usual way. Thus the numbers of susceptibles and carriers at time t are represented by the random variables $X(t)$ and $U(t)$. The chance of one new infection occurring in time Δt is taken to be $\beta XU \Delta t$. When this event happens X decreases by one unit, and U remains unchanged. Again, we assume that the chance of one carrier being removed in Δt is $\alpha U \Delta t$. In this case U is decreased by one unit, but X is unchanged.

It is convenient, as in Section 6.3 dealing with the general stochastic epidemic, to define the *relative removal-rate* $\rho = \alpha/\beta$, and to change to the time-scale given by $\tau = \beta t$. Let the probability of there being r susceptibles and u carriers at time τ be $p_{ru}(\tau)$, and let us introduce the joint probability-generating function $P(x, y, \tau)$ defined by

$$P(x, y, \tau) = \sum_{r, u} p_{ru}(\tau) x^r y^u. \tag{10.5}$$

Use of the standard "random variable" technique of Bailey (1964a, Sec. 7.4) then yields immediately the partial differential equation

$$\frac{\partial P}{\partial \tau} = (x^{-1} - 1) xy \frac{\partial^2 P}{\partial x\, \partial y} + \rho(y^{-1} - 1) y \frac{\partial P}{\partial y}$$

$$= (1 - x) y \frac{\partial^2 P}{\partial x\, \partial y} + \rho(1 - y) \frac{\partial P}{\partial y}, \tag{10.6}$$

subject to the initial condition

$$P(x, y, 0) = x^n u^b, \tag{10.7}$$

assuming, as in the deterministic model, that the process starts with n susceptibles and b carriers. (The problem of dealing with an arbitrary initial distribution has been considered by Severo (1967b) using his recursive approach.)

Weiss' (1965) initial treatment of this problem was largely restricted to the distribution of the ultimate size of the epidemic, though he did investigate the time-dependent aspect of the process in the special case $b = 1$. Dietz (1966) subsequently obtained an explicit solution of (10.6) using the method of Gani (1965a) already described in Section 6.3 for handling the general stochastic epidemic. A considerable amount of algebra was involved in this derivation, and a much shorter treatment was given by Downton (1967b), who started from the differential-difference equations

$$\frac{dp_{ru}}{d\tau} = (r + 1) u p_{r+1, u} - (r + \rho) u p_{ru} + \rho(u + 1) p_{r, u+1}, \tag{10.8}$$

which may be obtained directly in the usual way by considering the transitions between adjacent states, or alternatively by substituting (10.5) into (10.6).

Another way of solving (10.6) quite easily is to tackle it directly by means of the method of separating variables. (This was done for the simple stochastic epidemic at the end of Section 5.4, though in that case the identification of the constants d_j in (5.70) turned out to be somewhat intricate.) Let us look therefore for solutions of the form

$$P(x, y, \tau) = X(x)\, Y(y)\, T(\tau). \tag{10.9}$$

Substitution in (10.6), and division by XYT, gives

$$\frac{T'}{T} = (1-x)y\frac{X'Y'}{XY} + \rho(1-y)\frac{Y'}{Y} = -\lambda, \text{ say,} \tag{10.10}$$

where λ is a suitable constant.

From the first and third elements of (10.10) we have

$$T = e^{-\lambda\tau}. \tag{10.11}$$

The equation given by the second and third elements of (10.10) can be re-arranged to give

$$(1-x)\frac{X'}{X} = -\frac{\rho(1-y)}{y} - \frac{\lambda Y}{yY'} = -j, \text{ say,} \tag{10.12}$$

where j is some suitable constant. Thus all three variables, x, y and τ, can be separated. The two equations in (10.12) can be solved almost immediately, to give

$$X \propto (1-x)^j, \quad Y \propto \left(y - \frac{\rho}{\rho+j}\right)^{\frac{\lambda}{\rho+j}}. \tag{10.13}$$

Now we know that $P(x, y, \tau)$ must be a polynomial of degree n in x and b in y. Hence j must be a non-negative integer in the range $0 \leqslant j \leqslant n$, and $\lambda/(\rho+j)$ must be a non-negative integer k in the range $0 \leqslant k \leqslant b$. The permissible eigenvalues are accordingly

$$\lambda_j = k(\rho+j), \quad 0 \leqslant j \leqslant n. \tag{10.14}$$

The general solution of (10.6) can thus be written as

$$P(x, y, \tau) = \sum_{j=0}^{n}\sum_{k=0}^{b} c_{jk}\, e^{-k(\rho+j)\tau}\,(x-1)^j \left(y - \frac{\rho}{\rho+j}\right)^k, \tag{10.15}$$

where the constants c_{jk} can be determined from the initial condition in (10.7).

In fact, we can put $\tau = 0$, $x = \xi + 1$ and $y = \eta + \rho/(\rho+j)$ in (10.15), substitute into (10.7) and equate coefficients of $\xi^j \eta^k$ on both sides. This immediately gives

$$c_{jk} = \binom{n}{j}\binom{b}{k}\left(\frac{\rho}{\rho+j}\right)^{b-k}. \tag{10.16}$$

Since an obvious binomial expansion is now involved on the right of (10.15) we can simplify this expression by summing over k to yield

$$P(x, y, \tau) = \sum_{j=0}^{n} \binom{n}{j} (x-1)^j \left\{ \frac{\rho}{\rho+j} + \left(y - \frac{\rho}{\rho+j} \right) e^{-(\rho+j)\tau} \right\}^b. \qquad (10.17)$$

The individual probabilities p_{ru} can now be obtained from (10.17) by picking out the coefficient of $x^r y^u$, namely

$$p_{ru}(\tau) = \binom{n}{r}\binom{b}{u} \sum_{j=r}^{n} (-)^{j-r} \binom{n-r}{j-r} \left(\frac{\rho}{\rho+j} \right)^{b-u} e^{-u(\rho+j)\tau} (1 - e^{-(\rho+j)\tau})^{b-u}. \qquad (10.18)$$

Stochastic means and higher moments can be readily derived from the joint probability-generating function in (10.17). First, for the marginal distribution of carriers remaining at any time, we put $x = 1$ to give

$$P(1, y, \tau) = (1 - e^{-\rho\tau} + y\, e^{-\rho\tau})^b, \qquad (10.19)$$

the only term surviving from (10.17) being that for which $j = 0$. This is, of course, precisely the probability-generating function for a simple death process with parameter ρ, as follows in any case from the original definition of the process. The individual probabilities have the binomial form

$$p_{.u} = \binom{b}{u} e^{-\rho\tau u} (1 - e^{-\rho\tau})^{b-u}. \qquad (10.20)$$

In particular the stochastic mean $\bar{u}$ is given by

$$\bar{u}(\tau) = b\, e^{-\rho\tau}. \qquad (10.21)$$

This is identical with the deterministic value given in (10.3), allowing for the fact that $\tau = \beta t$.

Next, the marginal distribution of the number of susceptibles remaining at any time is found by setting $y = 1$ in (10.17), giving

$$P(x, 1, \tau) = \sum_{j=0}^{n} \binom{n}{j} (x-1)^j \left(\frac{\rho + j\, e^{-(\rho+j)\tau}}{\rho+j} \right)^b. \qquad (10.22)$$

Picking out the coefficient of x^r gives the individual probabilities

$$p_{r.} = \sum_{j=r}^{n} (-)^{j-r} \binom{n}{j}\binom{j}{r} \left(\frac{\rho + j\, e^{-(\rho+j)\tau}}{\rho+j} \right)^b$$

$$= \binom{n}{r} \sum_{j=r}^{n} (-)^{j-r} \binom{n-r}{j-r} \left(\frac{\rho + j\, e^{-(\rho+j)\tau}}{\rho+j} \right)^b, \qquad (10.23)$$

where the summation now starts at $j = r$, since for smaller values of j there are no terms involving x^r arising from $(x - 1)^j$.

The stochastic mean $\bar{r}$ is most quickly obtained from the corresponding factorial moment-generating function. If we put $x = \xi + 1$ in (10.22) and pick out the coefficient of ξ, we have immediately

$$\bar{r}(\tau) = n \left(\frac{\rho + e^{-(\rho+1)\tau}}{\rho + 1} \right)^b . \tag{10.24}$$

In particular, as $\tau \to \infty$, the limiting value of $\bar{r}$ is

$$\bar{r}(\infty) = n \left(1 + \frac{1}{\rho} \right)^{-b} , \tag{10.25}$$

and the average epidemic size $\bar{w}$ is given by

$$\bar{w} = n - \bar{r}(\infty) = n \left\{ 1 - \left(1 + \frac{1}{\rho} \right)^{-b} \right\} . \tag{10.26}$$

Comparison with (10.4) shows that, as already remarked, the stochastic mean of the total epidemic size is always less than the deterministic value, but for small b/ρ the difference is negligible.

Variances and other higher moments may be derived in a similar fashion, starting from (10.17), though they are in general more complicated to write down.

The complete probability distribution of total epidemic size can easily be dealt with by letting $\tau \to \infty$ in (10.22) or (10.23). In particular, the probability P_w of an epidemic of size w is given by

$$P_w = \lim_{\tau \to \infty} \rho_{n-w,.}$$

$$= \binom{n}{n-w} \sum_{j=n-w}^{n} (-)^{j-n+w} \binom{w}{j-n+w} \left(\frac{\rho}{\rho+j} \right)^b$$

$$= \binom{n}{w} \sum_{i=0}^{w} (-)^i \binom{w}{i} \left(\frac{\rho}{\rho+n-w+i} \right)^b ,$$

where in the last line we have used the substitution $i = j - n + w$.

Again, an explicit expression for the duration time of the epidemic is also available. It is reasonable to consider that the epidemic is terminated either by the removal of all carriers or by the infection of all susceptibles before the carriers are removed. This means that the process is considered to have terminated if it has arrived at any one of the states given by $(r, 0)$, $0 \leqslant r \leqslant n$ and $(0, u)$, $0 \leqslant u \leqslant b$, where it is important to notice that the single state $(0, 0)$ is here included twice. Since these states are absorbing, it follows that the distribution function $F(\tau)$ for the duration time is given by

$$F(\tau) = p_{.0}(\tau) + p_{0.}(\tau) - p_{00}(\tau)$$

$$= (1 - e^{-\rho\tau})^b + \sum_{j=0}^{n} (-)^j \binom{n}{j} \left(\frac{\rho + j\,e^{-(\rho+j)\tau}}{\rho+j} \right)^b$$

$$- \sum_{j=0}^{n} (-)^j \binom{n}{j} \left(\frac{\rho}{\rho+j} \right)^b (1 - e^{-(\rho+j)\tau})^b,$$

using (10.18), (10.20) and (10.23),

$$= (1 - e^{-\rho\tau})^b$$

$$+ \sum_{j=0}^{n} (-)^j \binom{n}{j} \left\{ \left(\frac{\rho + j\,e^{-(\rho+j)\tau}}{\rho+j} \right)^b - \left(\frac{\rho(1 - e^{-(\rho+j)\tau})}{\rho+j} \right)^b \right\}.$$

(10.27)

The Laplace transform of $F(\tau)$, and hence the transform of the frequency function $f(\tau)$, can be derived straightforwardly from (10.27). This can be used to obtain moments in the usual way, though compact formulae are not so far available. The stochastic mean $\bar{\tau}$ can be deduced a little more simply using the standard result

$$\bar{\tau} = \int_0^\infty \{1 - F(\tau)\} d\tau.$$

Substituting from (10.27), and integrating the binomial expansions term by term, gives

$$\bar{\tau} = \sum_{k=1}^{b} \binom{b}{k} \frac{(-)^{k-1}}{\rho k} - \sum_{j=0}^{n} \binom{n}{j} \frac{(-)^j}{(\rho+j)^{b+1}} \sum_{k=1}^{b} \binom{b}{k} \frac{\rho^{b-k} j^k - (-)^k \rho^b}{k}.$$

(10.28)

In the special case $b = 1$, when the epidemic is started by a single carrier, we have

$$\bar{\tau} = \frac{1}{\rho} - \sum_{j=0}^{n} \binom{n}{j} \frac{(-)^j}{\rho+j}$$

$$= \frac{1}{\rho} - \frac{n!}{\rho(\rho+1)\dots(\rho+n)},$$

(10.29)

the summation in the first line being an easily verified partial fraction expansion of the product term in the second line. For large n we have, using Stirling's approximation, the asymptotic form

$$\bar{\tau} = \frac{1}{\rho}\left(1 - \frac{\Gamma(n+1)\Gamma(\rho+1)}{\Gamma(n+\rho+1)}\right)$$

$$\sim \frac{1}{\rho}\left(1 - \frac{\Gamma(\rho+1)}{n^\rho}\right). \tag{10.30}$$

10.4 Time-dependent parameters

Throughout the foregoing discussion we first assumed both β and α (and thereafter ρ) to be constant. Dietz (1967), however, has shown how this restriction may be relaxed to cover the more general case of time-dependent parameters. We may, for example, want to have the removal-rate $\alpha(t)$ increasing with time to reflect the growing efficiency of public health measures during the course of an epidemic. Working in τ time, we replace (10.6) by

$$\frac{\partial P}{\partial \tau} = (1-x)y\frac{\partial^2 P}{\partial x\,\partial y} + \rho(\tau)(1-y)\frac{\partial P}{\partial y}, \tag{10.31}$$

subject to the same initial condition as before, namely (10.7).

Naturally, the solution of (10.31) is more difficult to handle than in the constant parameter case. Dietz used the following approach to obtain an expression for the mean total epidemic size.

Let us write the probability-generating function $P(x, y, \tau)$ in the following form:

$$P(x,y,\tau) \equiv \sum_{r=0}^{n}\sum_{u=0}^{b} p_{ru}(\tau)x^r y^u \tag{10.32}$$

$$= \sum_{j=0}^{n}\binom{n}{j}(x-1)^j f_j(y,\tau), \tag{10.33}$$

where the functions $f_j(y, \tau)$ are to be determined. This device is similar to that appearing in (6.34) in connection with the general stochastic epidemic. The present form has some advantages, especially in calculating the mean number of susceptibles. Substituting (10.33) in (10.31) and equating coefficients of $(x-1)^j$ gives a simple linear first-order partial differential equation for $f_j(y, \tau)$, namely

$$\frac{\partial f_j}{\partial \tau} + \{(j+\rho)y - \rho\}\frac{\partial f_j}{\partial y} = 0. \tag{10.34}$$

The solution of (10.34) is obtained by first forming the subsidiary equations

$$\frac{d\tau}{1} = \frac{dy}{(j+\rho)y - \rho} = \frac{df_j}{0}. \tag{10.35}$$

We now find two independent integrals of (10.35). One obvious solution is

$$f_j = \text{const.} \tag{10.36}$$

Another solution can be found from

$$\frac{dy}{d\tau} = (j + \rho)y - \rho. \tag{10.37}$$

Multiplying through (10.37) by the integrating factor

$$\theta_j(\tau) = \exp\left(-\int_0^\tau \{j + \rho(v)\}dv\right)$$

$$= \exp\left(-j\tau - \int_0^\tau \rho(v)dv\right) \tag{10.38}$$

leads to a second integral

$$y\theta_j(T) + \int_0^\tau \rho(z)\theta_j(z)dz = \text{const.} \tag{10.39}$$

From (10.36) and (10.39) we can write the general solution of (10.34) as

$$f_j = \Phi\left(y\theta_j + \int_0^\tau \rho\theta_j\, dz\right), \tag{10.40}$$

where Φ is an arbitrary function that can be determined from the initial conditions $P(x, y, 0) = x^n y^b$ in (10.7). Since

$$P(x, y, 0) = x^n y^b$$

$$= \{1 + (x - 1)\}^n y^b$$

$$= \sum_{j=0}^{n} \binom{n}{j}(x - 1)^j y^b, \tag{10.41}$$

comparison with (10.32) shows that

$$f_j(y, 0) = y^b. \tag{10.42}$$

If we put $\tau = 0$ in (10.40) we obtain

$$\Phi(y) = f_j(y, 0) = y^b, \tag{10.43}$$

using (10.42) and the fact that $\theta_j(0) = 1$. Hence the solution given by (10.40) must take the form

$$f_j(y, \tau) = \left(y\theta_j(\tau) + \int_0^\tau \rho(z)\theta_j(z)dz\right)^b, \tag{10.44}$$

where $\theta_j(\tau)$ is defined in (10.38). The required probability-generating function is thus given by (10.32) where the f_j have now been determined.

The stochastic mean number of susceptibles $\bar{r}$ can be obtained, as in the time-homogeneous case, from the factorial moment-generating function of the marginal distribution. We put $y = 1$ and $x = \xi + 1$ in (10.32), and simply pick out the coefficient of ξ. This gives

$$\bar{r}(\tau) = n f_1(1, \tau)$$

$$= n \left(\theta_1(\tau) + \int_0^\tau \rho(z)\theta_1(z)dz \right)^b. \tag{10.45}$$

In the limiting case $\tau \to \infty$, we have

$$\bar{r}(\infty) = n \left(\int_0^\infty \rho(z)\theta_1(z)dz \right)^b, \tag{10.46}$$

since, from (10.38), $\theta_1(\infty) = 0$. Special cases can now be evaluated from (10.46). Suppose, for example, that in the original time-scale t, the infection-rate $\beta(t) \equiv \beta$ but $\alpha(t) = \alpha + \gamma t$. Thus the infection mechanism is not time-dependent, but the removal-rate increases linearly with time. Writing the relative removal-rate as

$$\rho(\tau) = \rho + \sigma\tau, \tag{10.47}$$

we see from (10.38) that

$$\theta_1(z) = \exp\{-(1+\rho)z - \tfrac{1}{2}\sigma z^2\}. \tag{10.48}$$

Straightforward evaluation then yields

$$\bar{r}(\infty) = n \left[1 - \left(\frac{2\pi}{\sigma} \right)^{\frac{1}{2}} \left\{ 1 - \phi\left(\frac{1+\rho}{\sigma^{\frac{1}{2}}} \right) \right\} \exp\{(1+\rho)^2/2\sigma\} \right]^b, \tag{10.49}$$

where

$$\phi(v) = (2\pi)^{-\frac{1}{2}} \int_{-\infty}^v e^{-\frac{1}{2}\xi^2} d\xi. \tag{10.50}$$

Similarly, we might try the function

$$\rho(\tau) = \rho - \frac{\eta}{1+\tau}, \tag{10.51}$$

which also increases with time, but at a decreasing rate.

This time we have

$$\theta_1(z) = (1+z)^\eta e^{-(1+\rho)z}. \tag{10.52}$$

After a little algebra we arrive at the result

$$\bar{r}(\infty) = n \{1 - (1+\rho)^{-\eta-1} e^{1+\rho} \Gamma(\eta+1, \rho+1)\}^b, \tag{10.53}$$

where we use the incomplete gamma function defined by

$$\Gamma(a, v) = \int_v^\infty \xi^{a-1} e^{-\xi} d\xi. \tag{10.54}$$

As a check, we note that if $\eta = 0$ then (10.53) reduces to (10.25).

10.5   Immigration of susceptibles and carriers

The models of the previous three sections can be made more realistic (Dietz and Downton, 1968) by relaxing the restriction of a limited stock of susceptibles and carriers, and admitting the possibility of new susceptibles and carriers being introduced. Of course these could be generated from within the community by birth and infection processes, respectively. And in fact there is a variety of models that could be investigated. In the present section we shall suppose that new susceptibles appear at a constant rate μ (this covers both immigration and generation from within the community, which is supposed to be of constant size), and that new carriers are introduced at a constant rate ν.

The deterministic equations are therefore

$$\left. \begin{aligned} \frac{dx}{dt} &= -\beta x y + \mu, \\ \frac{dy}{dt} &= -\alpha y + \nu, \end{aligned} \right\} \tag{10.55}$$

subject to the initial conditions

$$x = n, \quad y = b, \quad t = 0, \tag{10.56}$$

these being identical with (10.2). We observe straightaway that an equilibrium state is possible. Setting the differential coefficients equal to zero gives

$$x_0 = \frac{\alpha\mu}{\beta\nu}, \quad y_0 = \frac{\nu}{\alpha}. \tag{10.57}$$

However, even for time-dependent parameters, equations (10.55) can clearly be integrated in a formal way by elementary means, solving first for y and then for x. When the parameters are constant, we have the simplest results. The y-equation can be solved immediately to give

$$y = \frac{\nu}{\alpha} + \left(b - \frac{\nu}{\alpha}\right) e^{-\alpha t}. \tag{10.58}$$

Substitution of (10.58) in the x-equation of (10.55) leads to the somewhat awkward form

$$x = n \exp\left\{-\frac{\beta\nu}{\alpha}t - \frac{\beta}{\alpha}\left(b - \frac{\nu}{\alpha}\right)(1 - e^{-\alpha t})\right\}$$

$$+ \frac{\mu}{\alpha} \exp\left\{-\frac{\beta\nu}{\alpha}t + \frac{\beta}{\alpha}\left(b - \frac{\nu}{\alpha}\right)e^{-\alpha t}\right\} \int_{e^{-\alpha t}}^{1} \xi^{-\frac{\beta\nu}{\alpha^2} - 1 - \frac{\beta}{\alpha}\left(b - \frac{\nu}{\alpha}\right)} d\xi. \quad (10.59)$$

A stochastic model can be constructed as in Section 10.3, except that we now incorporate the random Poisson arrival of new susceptibles and new carriers with rates μ and ν, respectively. Retaining the original t-time-scale, we can easily write down the appropriate partial differential equation for the probability-generating function as

$$\frac{\partial P}{\partial t} = \beta(1 - x)y \frac{\partial^2 P}{\partial x\, \partial y} + \alpha(1 - y)\frac{\partial P}{\partial y} + \{\mu(x - 1) + \nu(y - 1)\}P,$$
$$(10.60)$$

where $P(x, y, t)$ is given by

$$P(x, y, t) = \sum_{r,u} p_{ru}(t) x^r y^u, \quad (10.61)$$

and the initial condition can be taken to be

$$P(x, y, 0) = x^n y^b, \quad (10.62)$$

as before in (10.7).

A fair amount of analysis is possible, as with the deterministic model, even when the parameters are time-dependent (see Dietz and Downton, 1968). However, we shall confine ourselves to the time-homogeneous case for simplicity, Let us use the approach previously adopted in Section 10.4, writing

$$P(x, y, t) = \sum_{j=0}^{\infty} (x - 1)^j f_j(y, t), \quad (10.63)$$

which is closely analogous to (10.33). Substituting (10.63) in (10.60) and equating coefficients of $(x - 1)^j$ gives

$$\frac{\partial f_j}{\partial t} + \{(j\beta + \alpha)y - \alpha\}\frac{\partial f_j}{\partial y} + \nu(1 - y)f_j = \mu f_{j-1}. \quad (10.64)$$

In principle, the set of linear partial differential equations in (10.64) can be solved recursively. A few interesting results can, however, be obtained directly very quickly.

The marginal probability-generating function of the number of carriers is

$$P(1, y, t) = f_0(y, t), \quad (10.65)$$

and the relevant partial differential equation with $j = 0$ is

$$\frac{\partial f_0}{\partial t} + \alpha(y-1)\frac{\partial f_0}{\partial y} = \nu(y-1)f_0, \tag{10.66}$$

the term in f_{-1} being absent. Intermediate integrals are easily found to be

$$(y-1)e^{-\alpha t} = \text{const.}, \quad f_0 e^{-\nu y/\alpha} = \text{const.} \tag{10.67}$$

Thus

$$f_0(y, t) = e^{\nu y/\alpha}\, \Phi\{(y-1)e^{-\alpha t}\}, \tag{10.68}$$

where Φ is an arbitrary function to be determined from the initial conditions. From (10.62) and (10.65) we have

$$f_0(y, 0) = y^b. \tag{10.69}$$

Putting $t = 0$ and $y - 1 = \eta$ in (10.68), and using (10.69), shows that

$$\Phi(\eta) = (1 + \eta)^b\, e^{-\nu(1+\eta)/\alpha}. \tag{10.70}$$

We can now evaluate (10.68) explicitly to give the required marginal probability-generating function as

$$f_0(y, t) = \{1 + (y-1)e^{-\alpha t}\}^b\, \exp\left\{\frac{\nu}{\alpha}(y-1)(1-e^{-\alpha t})\right\}. \tag{10.71}$$

In particular, the average number of carriers $\bar{u}$ is

$$\bar{u} = \frac{\nu}{\alpha} + \left(b - \frac{\nu}{\alpha}\right)e^{-\alpha t}. \tag{10.72}$$

Comparison with (10.58) shows that the stochastic mean number of carriers is identical with the deterministic value. Again, as $t \to \infty$, (10.71) becomes

$$f_0(y, \infty) = \exp\left\{\frac{\nu}{\alpha}(y-1)\right\}, \tag{10.73}$$

so that the carrier distribution tends to a Poisson distribution with parameter ν/α.

Next, we consider the distribution of susceptibles. The stochastic mean is obtained fairly easily by the following argument. The factorial moment-generating function for the marginal distribution of susceptibles is $F(x, t) = P(x + 1, 1, t)$. Hence, from (10.63), we have

$$F(x, t) = \sum_{j=0}^{\infty} x^j f_j(1, t). \tag{10.74}$$

The required stochastic mean $\bar{r}$ is therefore immediately identified as

$$\bar{r} = f_1(1, t). \tag{10.75}$$

Putting $j = 1$ in (10.64) gives the equation for $f_1(y, t)$ as

$$\frac{\partial f_1}{\partial t} + \{(\beta + \alpha)y - \alpha\}\frac{\partial f_1}{\partial y} + \nu(1 - y)f_1 = \mu f_0, \qquad (10.76)$$

where f_0 is given by (10.71). This simple linear partial differential equation can be integrated straightforwardly, but a somewhat complicated expression results. We shall content ourselves here with obtaining the limiting solution as $t \to \infty$. In (10.76) we then have $\partial f_1/\partial t = 0$ to give

$$\{(\beta + \alpha)y - \alpha\}\frac{\partial f_1}{\partial y} + \nu(1 - y)f_1 = \mu\, e^{\nu(y-1)/\alpha}. \qquad (10.77)$$

We can integrate (10.77) by dividing through by the coefficient of $\partial f_1/\partial y$, multiplying by the integrating factor

$$\exp\left\{\int \frac{\nu(1 - y)dy}{(\beta + \alpha)y - \alpha}\right\},$$

and integrating. This leads to

$$f_1(y)\left(y - \frac{\alpha}{\beta + \alpha}\right)^{\frac{\nu\beta}{(\beta+\alpha)^2}} \exp\left(-\frac{\nu y}{\beta + \alpha}\right) =$$

$$\frac{\mu \exp(-\nu/\alpha)}{\beta + \alpha} \int_C^y \left(y - \frac{\alpha}{\beta + \alpha}\right)^{\frac{\nu\beta}{(\beta+\alpha)^2}-1} \exp\left(\frac{\beta\nu u}{\alpha(\beta + \alpha)}\right)du. \qquad (10.78)$$

The constant C, for the lower limit of integration on the right-hand side, is easily seen to be

$$C = \frac{\alpha}{\beta + \alpha}, \qquad (10.79)$$

since both sides of the equation must vanish when $y = \alpha/(\beta + \alpha)$.

We now put $y = 1$, and make the transformation

$$u = \frac{\alpha + \beta v}{\beta + \alpha} \qquad (10.80)$$

in the integral on the right of (10.78). After rearranging we have

$$f_1(1) = \frac{\mu\, e^{-\eta}}{\beta + \alpha} \int_0^1 e^{\eta v}\, v^{\frac{\alpha\eta}{\beta}-1}\, dv, \qquad (10.81)$$

where

$$\eta = \frac{\nu\beta^2}{\alpha(\beta + \alpha)^2}. \qquad (10.82)$$

In terms of the confluent hypergeometric distribution given by

$$M(a,c;x) = \frac{\Gamma(c)}{\Gamma(a)\,\Gamma(c-a)} \int_0^1 e^{xv} v^{a-1}(1-v)^{c-a-1}\, dv, \qquad (10.83)$$

we can rewrite $f_1(1)$ to yield

$$\bar{r}(\infty) = f_1(1) = \frac{\mu(\beta+\alpha)\,e^{-\eta}}{\beta v}\, M\!\left(\frac{\alpha\eta}{\beta}, \frac{\alpha\eta}{\beta}+1;\eta\right). \qquad (10.84)$$

An alternative expression is possible in terms of the incomplete gamma function, if this is preferred.

It has not so far proved possible to reduce (10.84) to simpler terms. However, one important result is readily deduced. Since $e^{v-1} \geqslant v$, it follows that

$$\bar{r}_\infty = \frac{\mu(\beta+\alpha)\,e^{-\eta}}{\beta v}\, \frac{\alpha\eta}{\beta} \int_0^1 e^{v\eta}\, v^{\frac{\alpha\eta}{\beta}-1}\, dv$$

$$\geqslant \frac{\mu(\beta+\alpha)}{\beta v}\, \frac{\alpha\eta}{\beta} \int_0^1 v^{\frac{\eta(\beta+\alpha)}{\beta}-1}\, dv$$

$$= \frac{\alpha\mu}{\beta v}. \qquad (10.85)$$

Thus the stochastic mean number $\bar{r}(\infty)$ of susceptibles ultimately remaining in the population is at least as large as the corresponding deterministic value x_0 shown in (10.57). As shown by the computations of Dietz and Downton (1968), the value of the ratio $\bar{r}(\infty)/x_0$ can in fact be considerably greater than unity for certain values of the parameters, notably when the "adjusted immigration rate" η and the relative removal-rate α/β are both small. In such circumstances therefore a deterministic model could be very misleading.

As already mentioned, more general methods of analysis are possible, permitting the investigation of non-homogeneous processes in finite terms, and allowing the easier calculation of higher moments of the number of susceptibles. In particular, it can be shown that the function

$$F_j(y,t) = \sum_{r=0}^\infty \sum_{u=0}^\infty p_{ru}(t)\, r^{(j)}\, y^u \qquad (10.86)$$

satisfies the equation

$$\frac{\partial F_j}{\partial t} + \{(j\beta+\alpha)y - \alpha\}\frac{\partial F_j}{\partial y} + v(1-y)F_j = j\mu F_{j-1}, \qquad (10.87)$$

with boundary condition

$$F_j(0,y) = r^{(j)}y^b, \qquad (10.88)$$

where

$$r^{(j)} = r(r-1) \dots (r-j+1), \qquad (10.89)$$

that is, the jth factorial power of r. Equation (10.87) is similar to, but not identical with, equation (10.64).

A formal recursive solution to (10.87) can be found by making an appropriate change in the variable y. For details, see Dietz and Downton (*loc. cit.*). The advantage of this approach, which can be useful for solving similar problems, is that $F_0(y, t)$ is the generating function of the marginal probability distribution of carriers, and $F_j(1, t)$ is the jth factorial moment of the number of susceptibles. Further examples of the use of the technique is handling generalizations of the present models are given in Becker (1970b).

10.6   Modifications and extensions

In the last section we considered in some detail the possibility of modifying the basic carrier models of Sections 10.2 and 10.3 by introducing the immigration of both susceptibles and carriers. Another feature which can be incorporated is the creation of new carriers within the population by cross-infection. Downton (1968) has studied this problem in some detail, with special reference to the ultimate size of the epidemic, ignoring the possibility of migration. Although we shall not examine the details here, it is worth pointing out that there appear to be appreciable differences between the deterministic and stochastic versions. The former clearly exhibits threshold behaviour of the type already noted in Section 6.2 for the general deterministic epidemic. On the other hand, the stochastic carrier model does not seem to show such a phenomenon in any obvious way, although the general stochastic epidemic does have its own threshold theorem, as shown in Section 6.5.

Further developments in the analysis of Downton's stochastic model have been made by Gillian Denton (1972), who has shown how a time-dependent solution can be obtained using the technique of Gani (1967) already described in Section 6.3. Again, Severo (1969b) has extended his recursive methods to cover an extension of the general stochastic epidemic allowing for the removal of susceptibles as well as infectives. This extension, when appropriately interpreted, can in fact be shown to apply to Downton's model.

Another model, including the immigration of susceptibles and the creation of new carriers by a birth process, has been studied by Dietz (1969). A somewhat more general model has also been developed and analysed in detail by Becker (1970b).

We should also mention the work of Pettigrew and Weiss (1967), which deals with the situation involving two kinds of infectives, namely clinically recognizable infectives and subclinically infected carriers, but which ignores immigration and supposes that the population is large enough and the numbers of infected individuals small enough for us to assume that the stock of susceptibles remains constant. This large-population approach is similar to that of Bailey (1964b) and Morgan (1964) mentioned in Section 6.9 in the context of non-carrier models. In contrast to the latter studies, Pettigrew and Weiss show that it is quite possible to obtain unimodal epidemic curves without recourse to the additional complications of non-zero latent periods or non-exponentially distributed infectious periods.

Another extension by Becker (1973) of Weiss's original model incorporates several different groups of individuals so as to allow for variations in susceptibility and infectivity. It is shown that the mean epidemic size is a minimum when the individuals are homogeneous.

Again, Griffiths (1973a) discusses the application of rather general multivariate birth-and-death processes to large population approximations of epidemic processes, using in particular branching process representations. Carrier models can then be treated as special cases of the generalized theory.

It should also be noted that an extension of Bartlett's approach (see Section 9.4) to the initial geographical spread of an epidemic has been made to carrier-borne diseases by Radcliffe (1973).

The extent to which additional refinements of carrier models are really worthwhile is a question of great interest and importance, perhaps to be settled only by fitting different models to data on specific diseases.

11

Host-vector and venereal disease models

11.1 Introduction

This chapter introduces two new topics which, in certain important instances, are practically isomorphic so far as the broad population structure of the models is concerned. The first topic is the problem of diseases that involve host-vector relationships, such as plague, typhus, malaria, schistosomiasis, etc. There are of course many variations to be found in practice. Thus in some cases, e.g. plague, we may be faced with an animal reservoir of disease. This maintains the existence of the disease, which once having been transferred to a human population can continue to spread through the latter according to the kind of models already discussed. In other cases, e.g. malaria, it is obligatory for the parasite to spend part of its life cycle inhabiting the vector, so that the infection switches back and forth between host and vector, and the rate of infection in any one of the populations depends in some way on both the number of susceptibles in that population and the number of infectives in the other population.

The second topic deals with the problems of venereal diseases, e.g. syphilis and gonorrhoea, which, at least in situations of heterosexual spread, also involve the obligatory switching of infection back and forth between two distinct, identifiable populations. To this extent, therefore, the two groups of models have the same structure if we restrict attention to the broader aspects of the population dynamics.

In the present chapter we shall review some of the general theory of such models, which admittedly ignore many of the finer details that may well have to be taken into account if we are studying a specific disease in greater depth. A particular instance of this is malaria, for which there exist models exhibiting a considerable degree of biological realism. These applications will be discussed later in Chapter 17 on parasitic disease models. Again, in gonorrhoea there are many special features that would have to be incorporated in any practically orientated model, such as the absence of immunity in recovered infectives, the

fact that the majority of infected females are without overt symptoms, and
the circumstance that the diagnosis of infection in females often depends
primarily on the occurrence of disease in male contacts.

Of course, the treatment of two interacting populations can be regarded as
special cases of the deterministic or stochastic models referred to in Sections
5.10 and 6.9, respectively. However, most of these discussions are either too
formal or too algorithmic to provide much insight into the structure of the
phenomena concerned. There is therefore some advantage in examining in their
own right a few simple models of the type indicated, where there is cross-
infection between groups but none within groups.

In Section 11.2 we introduce the basic deterministic modelling for epidemics, and go on to consider some aspects of the stochastic analogue in Section 11.3. If we confine our attention to small epidemics in large populations,
or the opening stages of major epidemics in large populations, then somewhat
more tractable models can be developed. The work of Griffiths (1972, 1973a)
is accordingly reviewed in Section 11.4. Finally, some introductory comments
are made in Section 11.5 to the study of endemic models.

11.2 Deterministic epidemics

First, we consider the formulation of the basic deterministic epidemic model.
Comparatively little work seems to have been done in this area, although
Kermack and McKendrick (1927) devoted some discussion to one of the simplest models possible over 45 years ago, and obtained a generalization of their
single-population Threshold Theorem already discussed in Section 6.2. Ignoring
here the complication of variable infection- and recovery-rates, we may set out
the basic ideas as follows.

We suppose that there are two populations, one of humans and one of the
intermediate host or vector. The numbers of susceptibles, infectives and removals in the former population at time t are given by (x, y, z), where
$x + y + z = n$; and the corresponding quantities for the latter population are
(x', y', z'), with $x' + y' + z' = n'$. Since we wish the human susceptibles to acquire infection from infectious vectors, and conversely, we assume that the
numbers of new infections in time Δt are $\beta xy' \, \Delta t$ for humans and $\beta' x'y \, \Delta t$ for
vectors. The corresponding quantities for removals are simply $\gamma y \, \Delta t$ and
$\gamma' y' \, \Delta t$. Instead of equations (6.1) which arise when a single population is involved, we now have the two sets given by

$$
\left.
\begin{aligned}
\frac{dx}{dt} &= -\beta xy', & \frac{dx'}{dt} &= -\beta' x'y, \\[2mm]
\frac{dy}{dt} &= \beta xy' - \gamma y, & \frac{dy'}{dt} &= \beta' x'y - \gamma' y', \\[2mm]
\frac{dz}{dt} &= \gamma y, & \frac{dz'}{dt} &= \gamma' y',
\end{aligned}
\right\}
\qquad (11.1)
$$

where the initial states when $t = 0$ are $(x_0, y_0, 0)$ and $(x'_0, y'_0, 0)$. Dividing the first equation on the left by the third on the right, yields, after integration,

$$-\log(x/x_0) = \beta z'/\gamma'. \tag{11.2}$$

Similarly,

$$-\log(x'/x'_0) = \beta' z/\gamma. \tag{11.3}$$

Following the notation of Section 6.2, and writing the specifications of the two populations at $t = \infty$ as $(n - ni, 0, ni)$ and $(n' - n'i', 0, n'i')$, we have from equations (11.2) and (11.3)

$$\left.\begin{array}{l} \beta n'i'/\gamma' = -\log(1 - i), \\ \beta' ni/\gamma = -\log(1 - i'), \end{array}\right\} \tag{11.4}$$

where we take y_0 and y'_0 as negligibly small, so that x_0 and x'_0 are approximately equal to n and n'. If we expand the logarithmic expressions in (11.4), retain the first two terms only, and then multiply corresponding sides of the two equations so obtained, we have

$$\frac{\beta\beta' nn' ii'}{\gamma\gamma'} \doteqdot (i + \tfrac{1}{2}i^2)(i' + \tfrac{1}{2}i'^2).$$

After cancellation of the factor ii', rearrangement gives

$$\frac{nn'}{\rho\rho'} - 1 = \tfrac{1}{2}(i + i'), \tag{11.5}$$

where we have ignored the second-order term in ii', and have written ρ and ρ' for the two relative removal-rates. It is evident from (11.5) that, since i and i' must both be positive or zero, we must have $nn' > \rho\rho'$ for a true epidemic to occur. There are not in fact separate thresholds for man and vector, but there is the joint threshold product of relative removal-rates, $\rho\rho'$.

Let us write π for the product of numbers of susceptibles in the two populations, so that $\pi = xx'$. We then have $\pi_0 \doteqdot nn'$, and therefore

$$\pi_\infty = x_\infty x'_\infty$$

$$\doteqdot \pi_0(1 - i - i'), \tag{11.6}$$

neglecting the product ii'. Substituting for $i + i'$ from (11.5) and writing

$$\pi_0 = \rho\rho' + \epsilon, \tag{11.7}$$

then gives

$$\pi_0 - \pi_\infty \doteqdot 2\epsilon. \tag{11.8}$$

The result in (11.8) is the modified form of the Threshold Theorem, as obtained by Kermack and McKendrick, and shows that if there is an epidemic the product of the numbers of susceptibles is reduced to a value as far below the threshold as it originally was above it.

The exact values of the individual intensities, i and i', are of course given by the solutions of (11.4). Approximate values for small epidemics are easily found by solving the equations obtained by retaining only the first two terms of the logarithmic expansions. We find

$$i \doteq \frac{2\epsilon}{n\left(n' + \dfrac{\gamma'}{\beta}\right)}, \quad i \doteq \frac{2\epsilon}{n'\left(n + \dfrac{\gamma}{\beta'}\right)}, \tag{11.9}$$

where we have made use of the fact that $\rho\rho' \doteq nn' - \epsilon$.

Of course, the above treatment is somewhat heuristic in nature, and in any case deals only with first approximations. It would, therefore, be worthwhile investigating the situation more exactly along the lines of Section 6.2.

For the time being, we first note the general feature of the existence of a threshold, which determines whether or not a true epidemic outbreak occurs. This is clearly related to the need for public health authorities to be able to manipulate human and vector densities, and the relevant contact and removal parameters, so as to maintain the populations in sub-threshold conditions. These remarks apply not only to the handling of parasitic diseases, but also to the control of venereal diseases where contact-rates and removal-rates can be influenced to some extent through administrative policies relating to health education.

However, a word of warning is necessary about the interpretation of thresholds, especially in regard to the implications for possible interventions. If the parameters β, β', γ and γ' in the above model are independent of n and n', then we can consider in a straightforward way the effect of changing some of them by public health action so as to ensure that $nn' < \rho\rho'$ or, better still, $nn' \ll \rho\rho'$. Thus, reducing the size of the vector population n' is always a step in the direction of preventing disease.

But suppose that some of the parameters depend on n or n'. In malaria, for example, according to commonly accepted ideas (see Chapter 17 for further details), we may suppose that the mosquito vector exhibits a certain man-biting rate b'. Then in unit time x' susceptible mosquitoes bite $b'x'$ people, of whom $(b'x')(y/n)$ are affected by malaria. Let f be the proportion of the latter who are actually infectious. Then the rate at which newly infected mosquitoes occur is $b'fx'y/n$. In other words, $\beta' = b'f/n$. Similarly, in unit time y' infected mosquitoes, of whom a proportion f' are infectious, bite $b'y'$ people, of whom $(b'y')(x/n)$ are susceptible. The rate at which newly infected people occur is thus $b'f'xy'/n$, i.e. $\beta = b'f'/n$.

This is of course a departure from homogeneous mixing as previously conceived. Nevertheless, equations (11.1) still hold with the above definitions of β and β'. But the condition $nn' > \rho\rho'$, necessary for a true epidemic to occur, becomes, on substituting for β and β', $nn' > \gamma\gamma'n^2/b'^2ff'$ or $n'/n > \gamma\gamma'/b'^2ff'$. Thus it is now the *ratio* of the vector population to the host population that is the critical quantity, and not the product. This threshold result, applicable to malaria, goes back to the original work of Ross (1911), long before the studies of Kermack and McKendrick (1927). For a more detailed discussion of malaria modelling, see Chapter 17.

Similar restrictions on homogeneous mixing are also required in any but the most superficial approaches to the modelling of venereal diseases. Suppose for example that we have a freely mixing community of n males and n' females. Let the rate of sexual contacts between males and females be c per unit time. Then in unit time x' susceptible females contact cx' males, of whom $(cx')(y/n)$ are infected. Let the probability of infection passing from an infected male to a susceptible female during a single contact be g. The rate at which new female infections occur is thus $cgx'y/n$, i.e. $\beta' = cg/n$. Similarly, the rate of occurrence of new male infections is $cg'xy'/n'$, where g' is the probability of infection passing from an infected female to a susceptible male during a single contact, i.e. $\beta = cg'/n'$.

This time the condition $nn' > \rho\rho'$, necessary for a true epidemic to occur, becomes $nn' > \gamma\gamma'nn'/c^2gg'$ or $c^2gg' > \gamma\gamma'$. The population sizes are now irrelevant, but a clear indication is given of what balance must be maintained between social behaviour and the more specifically medical factors if epidemic outbreaks are to be avoided. Of course this discussion is couched in rather general terms. For any given disease a more detailed investigation would be desirable, taking into account any special features that may be present, e.g. the absence of immunity in recovered cases of gonorrhoea.

11.3 Stochastic epidemics

There is no difficulty in formulating a stochastic version of the deterministic model of the previous section. We can introduce the random variables $X_1(t)$ and $Y_1(t)$ to represent the numbers of susceptibles and infectives, respectively, for the first population, with corresponding variables $X_2(t)$ and $Y_2(t)$ for the second population. The probability of a new infection occurring in the first population in time Δt is $\beta_1 X_1 Y_2 \Delta t$. When this transition occurs, X_1 decreases by one unit and Y_1 increases by one unit. Again, the probability of a removal in Δt is $\gamma_1 Y_1 \Delta t$, with Y_1 decreasing by one unit and X_1 remaining unchanged. Similar considerations apply to the second population *mutatis mutandis*. We also define the relative removal-rates $\rho_1 = \gamma_1/\beta_1$, $\rho_2 = \gamma_2/\beta_2$.

Let $p(r_1, s_1; r_2, s_2; t)$ be the probability of there being r_1 susceptibles and s_1 infectives in the first population, and r_2 susceptibles and s_2 infectives in the second population, at time t. We define the probability-generating function as

$$P(x_1, y_1; x_2, y_2; t) = \sum_{r_1, s_1} \sum_{r_2, s_2} p(r_1, s_1; r_2, s_2; t) x_1^{r_1} y_1^{s_1} x_2^{r_2} y_2^{s_2}. \tag{11.10}$$

Using the standard methods adopted in earlier chapters (e.g. Bailey, 1964a, Sec. 7.4), we can write down immediately the partial differential equation satisfied by the probability-generating function, namely

$$\frac{\partial P}{\partial t} = \beta_1 y_2 (y_1 - x_1) \frac{\partial^2 P}{\partial x_1 \partial y_2} + \gamma_1 (1 - y_1) \frac{\partial P}{\partial y_1}$$

$$+ \beta_2 y_1 (y_2 - x_2) \frac{\partial^2 P}{\partial x_2 \partial y_1} + \gamma_2 (1 - y_2) \frac{\partial P}{\partial y_2}, \qquad (11.11)$$

with initial condition

$$P(x_1, y_1; x_2, y_2; 0) = x_1^{n_1} y_1^{a_1} x_2^{n_2} y_2^{a_2}, \qquad (11.12)$$

assuming that the epidemic starts with n_1 susceptibles and a_1 infectives in the first population, and n_2 susceptibles and a_2 infectives in the second population.

So far, no explicit analysis is available of this stochastic formulation, which no doubt presents considerable difficulties. A threshold theorem can however be obtained, corresponding to the single population case treated in Section 6.5. Unfortunately, we cannot as yet achieve the degree of sophistication present in Whittle's theorem, but must confine ourselves to an approximate discussion of the type mentioned at the beginning of Section 6.5, originally due to Bartlett (1955, p. 129) and extended by him to the present host-vector model (Bartlett, 1964, 1966).

According to this approach, we assume that the initial populations of susceptibles, n_1 and n_2, are sufficiently large for the populations of infectives to be approximately subject to a bivariate birth-and-death process. The probability of a new infection occurring in the first population in Δt is now $\beta_1 n_1 Y_2 \Delta t$, and the probability of a removal is $\gamma_1 Y_1 \Delta t$. The corresponding quantities for the second population are $\beta_2 n_2 Y_1 \Delta t$ and $\gamma_2 Y_2 \Delta t$. Even this simplified linear process is not readily soluble, but the extinction phenomena can be treated by viewing the model as a continuous-time branching process. Standard theorems can then be applied (e.g. Sevastyanov, 1951; Mode, 1971).

From the branching process point of view, the "offspring" arising from a single infective individual of the first population in Δt may be classified as follows. Let the numbers of infectives newly formed in the first and second populations be S_1 and S_2, respectively. If the individual is removed, with probability $\gamma_1 \Delta t$, we have $S_1 = 0 = S_2$. If an infection of a susceptible from the second population occurs, with probability $\beta_2 n_2 \Delta t$, we have two individual infectives, one from each population, so that $S_1 = 1 = S_2$. The balance of probability, $1 - (\beta_2 n_2 + \gamma_1) \Delta t$, is allotted to the case when no transition occurs, with the original infective simply remaining, and then $S_1 = 1$, $S_2 = 0$. We then form the expectation

$$\mathop{E}_{\Delta t} y_1^{S_1} y_2^{S_2} = f_1(y_1, y_2)$$

to give the joint probability-generating function for the numbers of "offspring" in the two populations arising in Δt from one infective of the first population. A similar argument applies to "offspring" of infectives in the second population. It is easily seen that the functions so defined are explicitly given by

$$f_1(y_1, y_2) = y_1 + \{\gamma_1 - (\beta_2 n_2 + \gamma_1)y_1 + \beta_2 n_2 y_1 y_2\}\Delta t,$$
$$f_2(y_1, y_2) = y_2 + \{\gamma_2 - (\beta_1 n_1 + \gamma_2)y_2 + \beta_1 n_1 y_1 y_2\}\Delta t.$$
(11.13)

We now define the extinction probability $p_1(t)$ to be the probability that the epidemic process is already over at time t, i.e. $s_1(t) = 0 = s_2(t)$, given that the process started at $t = 0$ with $a_1 = 1$ and $a_2 = 0$. Conversely, we define $p_2(t)$ to be the probability of extinction at time t, given the starting point at $a_1 = 0$ and $a_2 = 1$.

Actually, it is quite possible to write down the backward differential equations for p_1 and p_2, using elementary probability considerations. These simultaneous equations can be solved quite easily in the limiting case of $dp_1/dt = 0 = dp_2/dt$, giving two roots for each variable. Unfortunately, this method does not tell us which roots to choose. The branching process theory, on the other hand, specifies that the probabilities of ultimate extinction, $p_1(\infty)$ and $p_2(\infty)$, are given by the *smallest* non-negative solutions of the equations

$$g_1(y_1, y_2) = 0, \quad g_2(y_1, y_2) = 0,$$
(11.14)

where

$$f_1 = y_1 + g_1 \Delta t, \quad f_2 = y_2 + g_2 \Delta t.$$
(11.15)

Substituting from (11.15) into (11.11) shows that equations (11.14) are

$$\beta_2 n_2 y_1 y_2 - (\beta_2 n_2 + \gamma_1)y_1 + \gamma_1 = 0,$$
$$\beta_1 n_1 y_1 y_2 - (\beta_1 n_1 + \gamma_2)y_2 + \gamma_2 = 0.$$
(11.16)

Explicit solutions are readily found to be

$$p_1(\infty) = 1 \text{ or } \frac{\gamma_1(\beta_1 n_1 + \gamma_2)}{\beta_1 n_1(\beta_2 n_2 + \gamma_1)};$$
$$p_2(\infty) = 1 \text{ or } \frac{\gamma_2(\beta_2 n_2 + \gamma_1)}{\beta_2 n_2(\beta_1 n_1 + \gamma_2)}.$$
(11.17)

It follows from (11.17) that for $p_1(\infty) < 1$ we must have $n_1 n_2 > \rho_1 \rho_2$, and the same condition for $p_2(\infty) < 1$. Otherwise we have $p_1(\infty) = 1 = p_2(\infty)$. Thus the chance of ultimate extinction of the process stemming from any given initial infective is unity if $n_1 n_2 \leqslant \rho_1 \rho_2$. And so extinction is certain for any process starting with a_1 infectives in the first population and a_2 infectives in the second population if $n_1 n_2 \leqslant \rho_1 \rho_2$. The threshold value, involving the joint product $\rho_1 \rho_2$ of the relative removal-rates, is thus identical with the deterministic result obtained in Section 11.2.

When $n_1 n_2 > \rho_1 \rho_2$, on the other hand, the chance of the process not becoming extinct, starting from the initial values (a_1, a_2) is

$$1 - \left\{ \frac{\gamma_1(\beta_1 n_1 + \gamma_2)}{\beta_1 n_1(\beta_2 n_2 + \gamma_1)} \right\}^{a_1} \left\{ \frac{\gamma_2(\beta_2 n_2 + \gamma_1)}{\beta_2 n_2(\beta_1 n_1 + \gamma_2)} \right\}^{a_2}$$

$$= 1 - \left(\frac{\rho_1}{n_1}\right)^{a_1} \left(\frac{\rho_2}{n_2}\right)^{a_2} \left(\frac{\beta_1 n_1 + \gamma_2}{\beta_2 n_2 + \gamma_1}\right)^{a_1 - a_2}. \tag{11.18}$$

This expression is therefore the approximate chance of a major epidemic building up. Note that (11.18) cannot be written solely as a function of ρ_1 and ρ_2 or of $\rho_1 \rho_2$, though if we define "cross" relative removal-rates

$$R_1 = \frac{\gamma_1}{\beta_2}, \quad R_2 = \frac{\gamma_2}{\beta_1}, \tag{11.19}$$

then (11.18) can be put in the form

$$1 - \left(\frac{R_1}{n_1}\right)^{a_1} \left(\frac{R_2}{n_2}\right)^{a_2} \left(\frac{n_1 + R_2}{n_2 + R_1}\right)^{a_1 - a_2}, \tag{11.20}$$

which is in terms of R_1 and R_2 only, but not of $R_1 R_2$.

The foregoing discussion probably represents the simplest and most straight-forward approach to the stochastic modelling of host-vector and venereal diseases. However, it may be of importance for practical applications to look more closely at the departures from homogeneous mixing mentioned at the end of Section 11.2, in connection with the more detailed modelling of malaria, for example, or of venereal disease. In the deterministic case, the basic equations are unchanged in essence, though some redefinition of parameters may be necessary. If total population sizes remain constant, the same kind of adjustments should be valid for the stochastic versions as well. But if the totals vary, some rethinking of the mixing and contact mechanisms may be necessary.

Some further work has been done recently by Radcliffe (1973) on the initial spread of a host-vector type of disease over a geographical area, using an extension of Bartlett's approach (see Section 9.4).

11.4 Small epidemics in large populations

The bivariate birth-and-death approximation used in the previous section to obtain a simple stochastic threshold theorem may also be applied to study processes which entail only small epidemics in large populations, or perhaps the early stages of major epidemics in large populations. We might, for example, want to examine the consequences of introducing a parasitic disease involving a vector, or some form of venereal disease, into a region or population previously unaffected.

As already mentioned, this means that we can regard the first population of infectives as subject to a birth-and-death process with probabilities of a birth or death in Δt being $\beta_1 n_1 Y_2 \Delta t$ and $\gamma_1 Y_1 \Delta t$, respectively, the corresponding values for the second population being $\beta_2 n_2 Y_1 \Delta t$ and $\gamma_2 Y_2 \Delta t$. In this case

(Griffiths, 1972) the differential equation (11.11) reduces to

$$\frac{\partial P}{\partial t} = \{\beta_2 n_2 y_1 (y_2 - 1) + \gamma_1 (1 - y_1)\} \frac{\partial P}{\partial y_1} + \{\beta_1 n_1 y_2 (y_1 - 1) + \gamma_2 (1 - y_2)\} \frac{\partial P}{\partial y_2},$$

(11.21)

with initial condition $P(y_1, y_2; 0) = y_1^{a_1} y_2^{a_2}.$ (11.22)

Although (11.21) is not readily soluble, mean values are easily found. If we put $y_1 = e^{\theta_1}$ and $y_2 = e^{\theta_2}$ in (11.21), we obtain the following partial differential equation for the moment-generating function M:

$$\frac{\partial M}{\partial t} = \{\beta_2 n_2 (e^{\theta_2} - 1) + \gamma_1 (e^{-\theta_1} - 1)\} \left|\frac{\partial M}{\partial \theta_1}\right| + \{\beta_1 n_1 (e^{\theta_1} - 1) + \gamma_2 (e^{-\theta_2} - 1)\} \left|\frac{\partial M}{\partial \theta_2}\right|.$$

(11.23)

Alternatively, equation (11.23) may be written down directly by the usual standard procedure.

Now let $\mu_1(t)$ and $\mu_2(t)$ be the stochastic means of $Y_1(t)$ and $Y_2(t)$, respectively. Equating coefficients of θ_1 and θ_2 on both sides of (11.23) then gives

$$\left. \begin{aligned} \frac{d\mu_1}{dt} &= \beta_1 n_1 \mu_2 - \gamma_1 \mu_1, \\ \frac{d\mu_2}{dt} &= \beta_2 n_2 \mu_1 - \gamma_2 \mu_2. \end{aligned} \right\}$$

(11.24)

These equations are of course precisely the same as the corresponding deterministic equations for the approximating process being considered, as expected for a linear system.

Now let us assume that extinction is certain, i.e. that $n_1 n_2 \beta_1 \beta_2 \leqslant \gamma_1 \gamma_2$ (see Section 11.3). Eliminating μ_2 from (11.24) gives

$$\frac{d^2\mu_1}{dt^2} + (\gamma_1 + \gamma_2) \frac{d\mu_1}{dt} + (\gamma_1 \gamma_2 - n_1 n_2 \beta_1 \beta_2) \mu_1 = 0,$$

(11.25)

the quantity μ_2 obviously satisfying the same equation. The required solution of (11.25) can be written in the form

$$\mu_1(t) = A_1 e^{\lambda_1 t} + A_2 e^{\lambda_2 t},$$

(11.26)

where λ_1 and λ_2 ($\lambda_1 \geqslant \lambda_2$, say) are the roots of

$$\lambda^2 + (\gamma_1 + \gamma_2)\lambda + (\gamma_1 \gamma_2 - n_1 n_2 \beta_1 \beta_2) = 0.$$

(11.27)

Now at $t = 0$ we have

$$\mu_1(0) = a_1, \quad \mu_2(0) = a_2.$$

(11.28)

And substituting (11.28) in (11.24) gives

$$\frac{d\mu_1(0)}{dt} = \beta_1 n_1 a_2 - \gamma_1 a_1. \tag{11.29}$$

The initial conditions (11.28) and (11.29) enable us to calculate the constants A_1 and A_2 in (11.26). We easily find

$$A_1 = \frac{-(\lambda_2 + \gamma_1)a_1 + \beta_1 n_1 a_2}{\lambda_1 - \lambda_2}, \quad A_2 = \frac{(\lambda_1 + \gamma_1)a_1 - \beta_1 n_1 a_2}{\lambda_1 - \lambda_2}. \tag{11.30}$$

The stochastic mean $\mu_1(t)$ is thus expressed by (11.26), where the constants A_1 and A_2 are defined in (11.30), and λ_1 and λ_2 are the roots of (11.27). The corresponding expression for $\mu_2(t)$ is obviously derived simply by interchanging the suffixes 1 and 2.

The average total epidemic sizes can also be obtained fairly easily. In stochastic terms, we introduce random variables $Z_1(t)$ and $Z_2(t)$ to represent the total number of removals in each of the two populations at time t. It is then quite straightforward to write down an extension of (11.23) for the joint moment-generating function of Y_1, Y_2, Z_1 and Z_2. Equating the coefficients of the linear terms in the dummy variables then yields two equations in addition to (11.24). If we write $\nu_1(t)$ and $\nu_2(t)$ for the stochastic mean numbers of removals, we find

$$\frac{d\nu_1}{dt} = \gamma_1 \mu_1, \quad \frac{d\nu_2}{dt} = \gamma_2 \mu_2. \tag{11.31}$$

Once again, these are identical with the deterministic values and could be written down immediately since the process is still linear.

We quickly find

$$\begin{aligned} \nu_1(\infty) &= \gamma_1 \int_0^\infty \mu_1(t)dt \\ &= -\frac{\gamma_1(A_1\lambda_2 + A_2\lambda_1)}{\lambda_1\lambda_2}, \quad \text{using (11.26),} \\ &= \frac{\gamma_1\gamma_2 a_1 + n_1\beta_1\gamma_1 a_2}{\gamma_1\gamma_2 - n_1 n_2 \beta_1 \beta_2}, \end{aligned} \tag{11.32}$$

using (11.30) and (11.27).

Let us define

$$\phi_1 = \frac{\gamma_1}{n_2\beta_2}, \quad \phi_2 = \frac{\gamma_2}{n_1\beta_1}. \tag{11.33}$$

Substitution in (11.32) gives

$$\nu_1(\infty) = \frac{\phi_1\phi_2 a_1 + \phi_1 a_2}{\phi_1\phi_2 - 1}. \tag{11.34}$$

Similarly,

$$\nu_2(\infty) = \frac{\phi_2 a_1 + \phi_1\phi_2 a_2}{\phi_1\phi_2 - 1}. \tag{11.35}$$

Thus the mean epidemic sizes, w_1 and w_2, not counting the initial numbers of infectives a_1 and a_2, are given by

$$w_1 = v_1(\infty) - a_1 = \frac{a_1 + \phi_1 a_2}{\phi_1 \phi_2 - 1},$$

$$\left.\begin{array}{l} \\ \\ \end{array}\right\} \quad (11.36)$$

$$w_2 = v_2(\infty) - a_2 = \frac{\phi_2 a_1 + a_2}{\phi_1 \phi_2 - 1}.$$

These values correspond with those given by Griffiths (1972, equation (22)) for the special case $a_1 = 1, a_2 = 0$.

Actually, Griffiths gives a more extensive discussion based on an associated discrete-time branching process. In this case it is possible to obtain an expression for the whole joint probability-generating function of the cumulative, i.e. removed, population sizes.

When, alternatively, $n_1 n_2 \beta_1 \beta_2 > \gamma_1 \gamma_2$, extinction is not certain. There is then no overall limiting distribution of epidemic sizes, though, as pointed out by Griffiths, we may be interested in those realizations that do become extinct. Applying the results of Section 5 of Waugh (1958), Griffiths shows that the instantaneous transition probabilities of the given process *conditional upon extinction* are obtained by replacing the rates $n_1 \beta_1$, $n_2 \beta_2$, γ_1 and γ_2, by $\gamma_1 \omega$, γ_2/ω, $n_1 \beta_1/\omega$ and $n_2 \beta_2 \omega$, respectively, where

$$\omega = \frac{n_1 \beta_1 + \gamma_2}{n_2 \beta_2 + \gamma_1}. \quad (11.37)$$

With these substitutions, therefore, we can apply the foregoing results to epidemic processes that do not become extinct, at least so far as the behaviour of only minor outbreaks is concerned.

Further discussion of some of these problems is given by Griffiths (1973a) in his development of multivariate birth-and-death processes as large population approximations to epidemic processes, using especially branching process representations.

As in the two previous sections, we might find it necessary in certain more specific applications to redefine the parameters of the above model so as to allow for some kinds of nonhomogeneous mixing.

11.5   Endemic models

In both host-vector diseases and venereal diseases one is concerned, not only with the behaviour of individual epidemic outbreaks, but also with a possible endemic situation. It is a fairly straightforward matter to generalize to the case of two populations the model already introduced in Section 7.2, or to extend by the introduction of new susceptibles the model of Section 11.2. Thus, in an obvious notation, equations (7.1) and (11.1) are replaced by

$$\frac{dx}{dt} = -\beta xy' + \mu, \quad \frac{dx'}{dt} = -\beta' x'y + \mu',$$

$$\frac{dy}{dt} = \beta xy' - \gamma y, \quad \frac{dy'}{dt} = \beta' x'y - \gamma' y'. \tag{11.38}$$

Little work seems to have been done on this kind of theoretical model, whether in the above deterministic form or in a suitable stochastic analogy. Of course, equilibrium values are given in the usual way by equating the differential coefficients to zero, yielding the endemic levels

$$x_0 = \mu\gamma'/\beta\mu', \quad x_0' = \mu'\gamma/\beta'\mu,$$

$$y_0 = \mu/\gamma, \qquad y_0' = \mu'/\gamma'. \tag{11.39}$$

Small oscillations about equilibrium could be investigated as in Section 7.2.

Although it is reasonable to explore deterministic models of this sort as a preliminary undertaking, it should be remembered that they were not entirely satisfactory in the simpler case involving no vector. The success achieved by a stochastic approach to the problem of recurrent outbreaks of measles (Sections 7.4 and 7.5) suggests that a similar investigation would be worth carrying out in the present two-population situation.

However, we should again bear in mind the restrictions, first mentioned at the end of Section 11.2, that are necessary to ensure an adequate degree of realism in models of at least some parasitic or venereal diseases. Considerable care should therefore be taken in setting up appropriate stochastic models before extensive mathematical investigations are embarked on. As indicated at the end of Section 11.3, special attention may have to be given to the mixing and contact mechanisms if the total population sizes vary.

A generalization of equation (11.38) has been made by Goffman and Newill (1964), involving the direct removal of susceptibles in addition to the other transitions already included. Although there is some relevance here to host-vector problems, the authors' main concern is with applications to the transmission and spread of ideas.

12

The purposes of general theory

Now that we have completed our survey of the general mathematical theory of epidemics, as opposed to the more specific applications to be attempted in Part 3, the time has come to make a critical evaluation of the importance and purpose of such investigations. As indicated at the end of Chapter 1, the spirit of the present book is inimical to a concentration on matters of purely academic mathematical interest, but is strongly in favour of theoretical work which is liable to provide insights of practical consequence. Of course, a mathematician *qua* mathematician is entitled to devote whatever time he has available to any problems he finds personally interesting. But we should be deluding ourselves if we imagined we were working on the theory of actual diseases in the real world when we were merely absorbed in the abstract intricacies of problems derived from, but not intimately related to, practical needs.

In the light of such criteria we can ask, for example, what is the justification for the enormous amount of effort devoted to analysing the properties of the simple stochastic epidemic, as described in Chapter 5? That these studies have an intrinsic mathematical fascination is undeniable. But what about the practical insights and implications? It can be argued, probably correctly, that very realistic models are difficult to handle, and that it is reasonable to start at the beginning with the easiest problems and gradually introduce additional modifications as the ability to manipulate various techniques increases.

From this point of view, the investigation of probability-generating functions, moment-generating functions, epidemic curves, duration times, asymptotic approximations, estimation problems, etc., can all be seen as essential precursors to the more serious study of general epidemics in Chapter 6. Although some of the methods unfortunately do not in fact lend themselves to easy extension to more complex models, the attempts are orientated in the right direction.

The general epidemic models, both deterministic and stochastic, certainly have a greater aura of realism about them. Although admittedly oversimplified, they incorporate a number of factors of major importance. And the threshold theorems, epidemic curves and distributions of total epidemic size, appear to provide quite good qualitative explanations of observed phenomena, so far as they go. Again, the attempts to develop approximating stochastic systems and asymptotic approximations not only help to exhibit further useful properties of the models themselves, but also contribute to refining the techniques that may be adaptable to more sophisticated but realistic models. The problems of parameter estimation in the latter are becoming increasingly difficult. More emphasis is therefore being placed on the role of computational methods, and their implications both for direct numerical calculation and for the utilization of simulation studies.

A partial synthesis of all these approaches can be seen in Chapter 7, where a wide range of mathematical and computational techniques have been enlisted in the elucidation of many difficult problems arising in the interpretation of public health measles data. This applies, for example, to the occurrence of an undamped series of outbreaks, and to the phenomenon of fade-out of infection in communities below a certain critical size.

Large populations are almost always extremely complex and heterogeneous, and any epidemic that occurs is unlikely to be repeated under identical conditions. Nevertheless, a good deal of practical insight has been obtained into the mechanisms that underlie the observed phenomena, although we may in general be unable to achieve anything sufficiently precise to justify formal statistical tests of goodness-of-fit. The future development of public health control programs should proceed more effectively because of the existence of this large body of general theory.

There are of course many obviously realistic aspects and factors which are hard to incorporate in general theory. For example, most continuous-time models make rather drastic oversimplications of biological detail in the cause of mathematical tractability. Thus it is common to assume a zero latent period, so that newly infected individuals become immediately infectious to others. While broad population theory may be rather insensitive to such details, this is not true of processes in small groups such as individual households. Discrete-time chain-binomial models are a great improvement in handling this type of data. *Ad hoc* statistical applications are dealt with later in Chapter 14, but in recent years some general theory, as described in Chapter 8, has begun to be developed. This may in due course provide more powerful tools for practical applications as well. Certain kinds of discrete-time theory are also important in the interpretation of results obtained when continuous-time computer simulations are replaced by discrete-time approximations for ease of calculation.

Again, the factor of the spatial distribution of large populations can have a major impact on the pattern of spread of disease through a community, being responsible for significant departures from the simple assumption of random homogeneous mixing. Chapter 9 discusses theoretical treatments that indicate the existence of appropriately modified threshold theorems, as well as simulation studies that enable one to build up a picture of the way in which an epidemic wave spreads from an initial focus.

As is well known, many diseases involve the existence of disease carriers who do not exhibit obvious clinical systems. This fact can have appreciable repercussions on the construction and interpretation of appropriate models, for diseases such as typhoid fever, for example. Chapter 10 reviews some of the theory now available, and shows how various additional aspects such as the immigration of new susceptibles and carriers, or the genesis of new carriers within the community, etc., can be taken into account. While the simpler theoretical treatments tend to show the qualitative consequences of the existence of carriers, it can also be seen how the addition of extra factors, ostensibly increasing realism, tends to obscure the structure of observable phenomena.

Finally, in Chapter 11, there was a preliminary investigation into models, that are developed in much greater detail in Chapter 17, involving both host and vector, like malaria, or two obligatory populations as in venereal disease. Again, there are threshold results that can be obtained, and various other theoretical properties that hold for the general models studied, and which might also hold for any specific models that were developed for individual diseases.

In most of the work mentioned above, one starts off by assuming infection-rates, removal-rates, etc. to be constant, though in many cases this restriction can subsequently be relaxed to allow for time-dependent rates. This naturally makes for greater generality, but usually results at the same time in vastly increased difficulties of analysis. Many other modifications can also be considered, such as more general assumptions as to the rates of contact between individuals, or the introduction of several possibly heterogeneous groups.

The precise implications of all these extensions are indicated in more detail in the discussions of the individual technical results. In the present chapter we are concerned more with the overall conclusions of the general theory than with the mathematical minutiae. It certainly appears that the general theory has a number of practical consequences. And this justifies a fair amount of effort being put into developing a well-organized corpus of knowledge to be used as background for facilitating down-to-earth interventions such as disease control programs.

However, the recitation of these generalities is still not entirely satisfactory. The question remains: can it be said in broad terms just what the advantages of the general theory are? Can we in fact list the features that clearly relate to an improved handling of practical applications? Naturally, expert opinions, if solicited, would be bound to differ as to what were the major contributions. Moreover, there could be endless disputes about the importance of any single theoretical result. The following summary therefore attempts to list the main theoretical developments that are, in the writer's opinion, of direct relevance to the issues of disease prevention and control in the real world.

   To begin with, as we shall see more explicitly in Part 3, appropriate quantitative modelling is of immediate value to epidemiological and public health
work. For example, scientific hypotheses can be tested, biologically significant
parameters can be estimated, and alternative intervention strategies can be
evaluated.

   In order to undertake such modelling expeditiously, we need a body of
knowledge to guide us. We must know what models are already available, what
their properties are, how mathematically tractable they are, whether convenient
approximations exist, what computational methods are required, what expectations there are of exact mathematical results, whether simulation studies are
likely to be useful, how to choose between deterministic and stochastic formulations, whether to include spatial factors, whether the models are reasonably
robust to possible oversimplifications in the assumptions, whether commonly
held epidemiological ideas are consistent with and follow from the common-
sense assumptions usually made, whether modifications proposed in models
for greater realism would in fact lead to appreciably different results, etc.

   We also expect the general theory to indicate where the main gaps in our
knowledge lie, what would be the most fruitful areas for new practice-orientated
research, what kind of analytical and computational techniques need to be
developed in order to save time and effort, what might be the consequences
for theoretical work of new developments in computer technology, etc.
Conversely, we expect some indications of what is *not* worth doing, what
would be mathematical refinement purely for its own sake, what kind of
theorems valid only under very severe restrictions would have little practical
consequences, what sort of statistical data would be inherently uninformative
and therefore useless as a basis for further analysis, etc.

   No doubt the reader will add further items to the above list according to
his inclinations; and may have his own views as to which individual models
are realistic and useful, and which are hopelessly oversimplified; or which
theorems provide genuine insight, and which are of only academic interest.
Nevertheless the broad purposes of the general theory remain clear, and should
be borne in mind when we come to the more practically orientated discussions
of Part 3.

Part 3

Specific Applications

13

The detection of infectiousness

13.1 Introduction

In the preceding chapters we have been largely concerned with investigating mathematical models for infectious diseases, in order, for example, to gain insight into large-scale phenomena or to estimate parameters from observed data. Most mathematical research has in fact assumed that the disease in question was already recognized as infectious, and has started by looking for an appropriate model having sufficient mathematical simplicity without being too remote from epidemiological reality. In some cases the adequacy of the model could be tested by fitting to actual data. This general situation is no doubt ascribable to the widespread occurrence of infectious disease and the vast unexplored field available for mathematical investigation. Accordingly, comparatively little has been done on testing whether case-to-case infection is an important element in any given disease. The epidemiologist naturally has his own methods of research, and these have indeed proved extremely effective. However, the question to be considered now is to what extent these standard procedures can be refined and made more precise by the use of statistical significance tests. We should expect such methods, if adequately developed, to allow epidemiologists to detect the existence of infectiousness more readily in situations where opinion was uncertain, because of the complexity or paucity of the data, for example, Of course, it goes without saying that evidence for the infectious nature of many diseases is so overwhelming that statistical tests are unnecessary.

But suppose that there is an outbreak, or at least an increase, of diarrhoeal disease in an Indian village, say. Certain organisms are identifiable, but they are often present anyway. There seems to be a clustering of cases in some households, but many buildings are in close proximity, individual rooms often being shared by families, and larger freely mixing units may be formed from children's playgroups. It may therefore be extremely difficult to say whether the distribution of cases throughout the village over several months involves a major case-to-case transmission element of the kind considered in this book,

225

or whether the observed pattern is largely the results of an intricate interaction
of environmental and sociological factors. A satisfactory solution of such complex problems has yet to be reached, though some simpler situations can be
handled statistically.

In Section 13.2 we shall look briefly at the kind of methods normally
employed by epidemiologists, and shall then go on to survey in a broad way
the sort of statistical tests that are appropriate to different types of data. In
Section 13.3 we discuss the analysis of household distributions of cases, and in
Section 13.4 the possibilities of examining time-interval distributions are reviewed. Finally, Section 13.5 refers to some of the work that has been done
on space—time interactions.

It is not our intention here to go into these matters very deeply, although
there is a huge statistical literature on the detection of nonrandomness. Departures from random distributions in space or time, or both, may occur for a
wide variety of reasons, and are not automatically evidence for the existence
of infectiousness. Moreover, there are to date few if any conclusive examples
of the existence of an infectious element being established mainly by statistical
investigation. This could however well happen in the future when more refined
and sensitive methods have been developed.

13.2   Standard epidemiological approaches

Since this book is devoted primarily to mathematical theory, we shall not
enter upon a full discussion of the various arguments which an epidemiologist
might employ to establish the infectiousness of any given disease, but shall
merely indicate briefly those aspects which are already susceptible of exact
mathematical analysis or seem at any rate capable of it in the foreseeable
future.

Any new disease which exhibited a strongly marked epidemiological pattern
such as that of measles would be quickly recognized as infectious. Typical
characteristics are a tendency for cases to occur in household groups; a relatively
well-defined time-interval between cases not occurring within a day or two of
each other; and the possibility of tracing most cases to contact with a previous
case. With less immediately obvious patterns, suitably drawn-up tables and
graphs might well reveal the infectious nature of the disease. Thus with a series
of cases in a village it might be noticed that the graph of notifications showed
several regularly spaced peaks suggestive of an infectious disease with serial
interval equal to the time-interval between peaks. Careful field-work might
establish a pattern of contacts between cases fitting in with this supposition. It
might be possible to supplement such studies with clinical tests based on, say,
throat-swabs or blood-samples. A search for healthy carriers might fill gaps in
the general picture, and so on. All this is commonplace to the epidemiologist,
and such methods are widely used and have had many notable successes.

Suppose now that the situation is less satisfactory: the data, though perhaps suggestive of infectiousness, do not absolutely rule out a purely random incidence. We might hope to perform some statistical significance test that would assist the drawing of inferences. However, a major difficulty arises if the data are largely anecdotal in nature, as frequently happens. Although this is not serious from a general scientific point of view if hypotheses suggested by the data can be tested subsequently, it often prevents satisfactory statistical analysis because the data have been accumulated in a more or less opportunist and haphazard way, so that no basic sampling scheme can be discerned. To collect the right data in the right way is quite essential to the adequate development of many types of analysis. This is abundantly clear from investigations in terms of latent periods and infectious periods, for instance, to be described in Chapter 14. It is of course not always practicable to collect data in ways that permit simple methods of numerical assessment. If, however, the actual process of collection, though not ideal, can be specified fairly exactly, then it may be possible to extract reliable conclusions by a more searching mathematical study. We shall confine our discussion below to significance tests appropriate to observations that have been accumulated according to certain simple rules.

Some mention should perhaps be made of the use of maps showing the geographical distribution of cases of disease, as in the studies of Cruickshank (1940, 1947) on tuberculosis and cancer. Mathematical analysis of so-called "statistical maps" was undertaken by Moran (1948), but is apparently applicable only where the basic geographical units are fairly large. We do not yet know how to test for independence the spatial pattern of individual cases in a heterogeneous community like a small town.

Further progress was made, however, by the pioneer work of Knox, who started to examine not merely the time-intervals between successive events, but also the time-intervals between all possible pairs of events. This approach was first applied to congenital tracheo-oesophageal fistula and oesophageal atresia (Knox, 1959). However, the technique could equally well be used for distribution in space as well, where of course the notion of successive events is meaningless. The extension was made not only to the cleft lip and palate data (Knox, 1963a, b, c), but also to childhood leukaemia (Knox, 1964a). Significant space—time clustering was found for both of these conditions. That this result was not merely an artefact of the statistical method is suggested by the fact that non-significant results were obtained for several other diseases (Knox, 1965).

Knox's technique, further described in Knox (1964b, 1965), was to set certain arbitrary definitions of adjacency in space and time, and then to exhibit the data in the form of a 2×2 contingency table. As a first approximation it was assumed that if both dichotomies were highly asymmetrical then the number of pairs occurring in the smallest cell of the table would have a Poisson distribution, with the usual 2×2 table expectation, thus leading to an obvious significance test. This conjecture turned out to be substantially correct, though other tests based on larger contingency tables were not so satisfactory.

A more extensive discussion of space–time interaction methods is reserved for Section 13.5. There is no doubt that appropriately developed statistical tests of this kind can be very sensitive to departures from strict randomness that may be of great epidemiological interest and importance. However, even when such interactions are established, there are still many problems in determining their nature, in particular in disentangling infectious factors from other concomitant influences.

13.3   Household distribution of cases

Let us suppose that records of cases of a particular disease have been collected from some community over a certain period of time. Let us also assume that for households of any given size we can classify the data so as to give an observed frequency distribution for the number of households having any specified number of cases. For the moment we suppose that information on the dates of onset is either lacking or uncertain. What conclusions can be drawn from the observed distributions as to the possible infectiousness of the disease? The answer to this question depends partly on certain further details about the data available, and partly on any alternative explanations we have in mind. The problem is mathematically similar to that arising in genetics (see Bailey, 1951, for classification of methods and references) where we try to estimate the segregation ratio for a recessive abnormality which is sufficiently rare for most marriages to be between heterozygous individuals. In some circumstances, therefore, forms of analysis used in genetics could be applied directly to epidemic data, making of course the necessary changes in interpretation. We shall list below some of the chief situations that seem to require consideration in epidemiology.

13.31   Random incidence of cases: zero class present

First let us see what should occur if cases of a disease occur effectively at random. We should in fact expect the total number of cases arising in households of a given size over a particular period of time to have a distribution which is binomial if the disease confers immunity, when repeated attacks are not possible, and Poisson if it does not confer immunity, when repeated attacks are possible. Suppose that for n households of total size k there are a_j with j cases, so that

$$n = \sum_{j=0} a_j.$$

We assume here that the class $j = 0$, containing a_0 households, is actually observed. When the disease confers immunity, let the chance that any given person is attacked be $p = 1 - q$. Thus the probability, P_j, of any household having exactly j cases is given by the binomial expression

$$P_j = \binom{k}{j} p^j q^{k-j}, \quad j = 0, 1, ..., k. \tag{13.1}$$

As all classes are observable, the maximum-likelihood estimate of p is

$$\left. \begin{array}{l} \hat{p} = \dfrac{1}{nk} \displaystyle\sum_{j=1}^{k} ja_j = \dfrac{\bar{\jmath}}{k}, \\[4mm] \bar{\jmath} = \dfrac{1}{n} \displaystyle\sum_{j=1}^{k} ja_j. \end{array} \right\} \tag{13.2}$$

where

Substituting for p from (13.2) into (13.1) quickly gives fitted expectations, nP_j, from which a goodness-of-fit χ^2 can be calculated in the usual way.

If the disease does not confer immunity, (13.1) would be replaced by the Poisson series

$$P_j = e^{-m} m^j / j!, \quad j = 0, 1, 2, ..., \tag{13.3}$$

where m is the expected number of cases per family. The estimate of m is now

$$\left. \begin{array}{l} \hat{m} = \bar{\jmath}. \\[4mm] \bar{\jmath} = \dfrac{1}{n} \displaystyle\sum_{j=1}^{\infty} ja_j. \end{array} \right\} \tag{13.4}$$

where

Unless the disease is very prevalent, there may in practice be little to choose between the two alternative distributions.

13.32 Random incidence of cases: zero class absent

Let us now suppose that we have information only on those households containing at least one case, i.e. the class $j = 0$ is missing. This is quite common in practice, though it should sometimes be possible to estimate a_0 with sufficient accuracy from census data or other survey material. The distributions corresponding to (13.1) and (13.2) are, respectively, the truncated binomial

$$P_j = \binom{k}{j} \frac{p^j q^{k-j}}{1-q^k}, \quad j = 1, 2, ..., k, \tag{13.5}$$

and the truncated Poisson

$$P_j = \frac{m^j}{(e^m - 1)j!}, \quad j = 1, 2, ... \tag{13.6}$$

The unknown parameters p or m are readily estimated by maximum likelihood. If we now write

$$n = \sum_{j=1} a_j,$$

and still define $\bar{j}$ formally as in (13.2), the likelihood for the binomial case can be put in the form

$$e^L \propto \prod_{j=1}^{k} \left\{\frac{p^j q^{k-j}}{1-q^k}\right\}^{a_j}$$

$$= \frac{p^{n\bar{j}} q^{nk-n\bar{j}}}{(1-q^k)^n}. \tag{13.7}$$

Taking logs and differentiating gives, after a little algebra, the following expression for the score:

$$S_p \equiv \frac{dL}{dp} = \frac{n}{q}\left(\frac{\bar{j}}{p} - \frac{k}{1-q^k}\right). \tag{13.8}$$

The equation $S_p = 0$ is easily solved by successive approximation as in ordinary maximum-likelihood scoring. With p large and q small a convenient starting value is $p_0 = \bar{j}/k$. On the other hand, if p is small, a better starting value can be obtained by taking the first three terms in the expansion of $q^k = (1-p)^k$, as pointed out to the writer by A. M. Walker. This leads to the value $p_0 = 2(\bar{j}-1)/(k-1)$.

Similarly, in the Poisson case, we find

$$e^L \propto \prod_{j=1}^{\infty} \left\{\frac{m^j}{e^m-1}\right\}^{a_j}$$

$$= \frac{m^{n\bar{j}}}{(e^m-1)^n}, \tag{13.9}$$

leading to
$$S_m \equiv \frac{dL}{dm} = n\left(\frac{\bar{j}}{m} - \frac{1}{1-e^{-m}}\right). \tag{13.10}$$

This time, convenient starting values, m_0, are $\bar{j}$ for large m and $2(1-\bar{j}^{-1})$ for small m. The calculation of expectations and testing goodness-of-fit then proceed as before.

13.33 Infectious disease: no cross-infection

Another important but simple possibility is that the disease is caused by an infective agent to which all members of a household are equally exposed. For example, the milk supply of a group of households might have become infected by a typhoid-carrier. The first crop of cases would be expected to follow a binomial distribution, though in this example there might also be further secondary cases later due to cross-infection within households. If all infected milk could be traced we should have data, with zero class present, to which a complete binomial could legitimately be fitted. In general, however, when the true nature of the situation is unknown we should have to employ the truncated binomial method given above. It is perhaps worth pointing out that the present type of explanation with no cross-infection would be specially indicated if, for all households of given size in the population, we obtained a bad fit when the zero class were present, but an adequate fit if the zero class were omitted.

13.34   Miscellaneous complications

Now it might happen that the chance of a household being brought into the record depended on the number of cases it contained — such a contingency is briefly referred to again in Section 14.46 under the heading of *ascertainment*. There has been extensive discussion of such problems in the genetical literature (see Bailey, 1951), and this should be consulted for methods of investigating more complicated situations. We may, for example, have two parameters, namely, the chance of any individual having the character in question and the chance of his being selected; and in one study the total number of families sampled also enters as an unknown parameter to be estimated. When the chance of selection, i.e. of entering the record, is appreciable, each affected individual in a family may either be recorded in his own right or only because other members of the family were under investigation first. Similar considerations apply in the present context. Really adequate data should therefore enable one to say not only how many cases a household contains, but also how many independent selections are involved. In the special case, where the chance of selection is small and each household is selected through only one member, the analysis simplifies. We have a binomial distribution, without truncation, of all cases not counting the selected one, and the methods of Section 13.31 then apply.

The above remarks are of course valid only for diseases conferring immunity. When there is no immunity we must resort to the Poisson model. Thus if the chance of selection is small, we should expect a complete Poisson distribution of all cases not counting the first one. But if multiple selections of households were involved, we should have to re-work some of the genetical applications referred to above with a Poisson instead of a binomial as the basic distribution.

It would be advisable to sound a note of warning here with regard to the likely contingency of heterogeneous data. Consider a disease which is not subject to case-to-case transmission but whose incidence is related to environmental conditions. We might obtain binomial or Poisson distributions in restricted geographical areas or within distinct social classes, although finding significant departures using pooled data. Before tentatively adopting the hypothesis of infectiousness we should make an attempt to subdivide the data into reasonably homogeneous groups. The tests recommended above should then be carried out on each group separately. In some circumstances it might be appropriate to make allowance for a variable incidence using, for example, the method applied to chain-binomials in Section 14.4. This would be suitable if there was good reason to expect a variable incidence, but no homogeneous groups could be isolated.

An alternative approach by Mathen and Chakraborty (1950) to the use of data on the household concentration of disease should perhaps be mentioned here. These authors recommended examining the distribution of the total number of households affected for a given number of cases in a community of given size. It is not clear that this procedure would be superior to those described above, especially as it seems to presuppose rather more knowledge about the population than we often have at our disposal, and further makes no direct use of the variable number of cases within the several households.

13.35   Illustrative example

As a brief illustration of the application of a significance test to actual data, let us consider some of the Providence measles material to be analysed further in Chapter 14. We are here concerned only with the distribution of the total number of cases per household. The appropriate observations for households of three are shown in Table 13.1, as given again later in Table 14.10.

Table 13.1   *Total number of cases for households of three*

Total number of cases j	Observed number of households	Providence measles data	Fitted values		
			Truncated binomial $(k=3)$	Complete binomial $(k=2)$	Chain binomial
1	a_1	34	7·9	6·5	24·7
2	a_2	25	76·7	79·9	36·0
3	a_3	275	249·4	247·6	273·3
Total	n	334	334·0	334·0	334·0

We do not in this case have full data showing how many households of three were completely unaffected: we cannot therefore apply the method of Section 13.31. Since the zero class is absent, we turn to Section 13.32 and use equation (13.8) appropriate to the truncated binomial with $k = 3$. Ignoring the factor n/q, we must solve

$$\frac{2·7215}{p} - \frac{3}{1-q^3} = 0,$$

from which we readily obtain the approximation $\hat{p} = 0·907$. Expectations, calculated from (13.5), are shown in the fourth column of Table 13.1. It is clear that the fit is quite inadequate, and in fact $\chi^2 = 124$ on one degree of freedom. We can also try the suggestion made in Section 13.34, appropriate in certain circumstances, of seeing whether we could fit a complete binomial to the data ignoring one case in each household. The analysis of Section 13.31

now applies with $k = 2$, but we must remember to replace the quantities a_1, a_2 and a_3 in the second column of Table 13.1 by a_0, a_1 and a_2, respectively. Equation (13.2) then yields $\hat{p} = 575/668 = 0.861$. Expectations calculated from the frequencies in (13.1) are given in the fifth column of Table 13.1. The fit is now even worse with $\chi^2 = 157$ on one degree of freedom. The last column of the Table shows the chain-binomial expectations obtained in Section 14.32; these, too, are unsatisfactory. It is interesting to remark that the only adequate representation we have been able to find so far is a chain-binomial allowing for variations between households in the chance of infection. Moreover, as shown in Section 14.42, such a model will fit the data so far available even when the individual links of the chains are analysed.

13.4 Distribution of time-intervals

We have seen in Section 13.3 how to make use of the household distribution of cases to test whether various hypotheses not involving case-to-case infection could adequately explain the data. Moreover, it appears from the small amount of observational material actually analysed that there is quite a good chance of discriminating between such hypotheses and the alternatives supplied by chain-binomial theory. These methods, however, make no use of the actual time-intervals between successive cases, though as indicated in Section 13.2, epidemiologists do in fact find graphs showing dates of notifications extremely helpful. Further, with diseases having fairly constant serial intervals and in conditions where contacts are easily traceable, even a small amount of data will exhibit a regular pattern of incidence strongly indicative of infectious spread. We should therefore be able to draw tentative conclusions from cases which appear at first sight merely sporadic and which show no obvious tendency to concentration in household groups. In order to reach decisions when the situation is less clear-cut, we require the assistance of appropriate statistical tests. The basic problem is to test whether a series of events occurring in time is in some sense random or not. There is a large literature on this subject, and Pyke (1965, 1972) should be consulted for extensive discussion and references. We shall in the following section give a single easily applied test that seems quite adequate in the present context.

13.41 An interval test for randomness

Suppose that for some given disease we have the recorded dates of onset of each case (or perhaps of some other more suitable measuring point: see Hope Simpson, 1948), and we ask whether this observed series could be regarded as a set of random events, i.e. whether we have a Poisson process. This problem was first considered in the context of epidemic disease by Greenwood (1946), who suggested a test, based on the sum of squares of intervals between success-ive events, which was later investigated more fully by Moran (1946, 1951b). However, an alternative procedure put forward by Bartlett in the discussion on

Greenwood's paper seemed more promising, and this was subsequently confirmed by Moran (1951b). The basic idea is as follows. If successive events occur at random in time, then the intervals between them, say $t_1, t_2, ..., t_k$, must have identical independent negative exponential distributions, namely

$$dF = \beta e^{-\beta t_i} dt_i, \quad i = 1, 2, ..., k, \tag{13.11}$$

where β is some unknown scale parameter. Now the distribution in (13.11) implies that $2\beta t_i$ is distributed like χ^2 with two degrees of freedom. We could therefore treat the t_i as sample estimates of variance, each based on two degrees of freedom, and then use Bartlett's test for the homogeneity of variances. Moran (1951b) showed that this is in fact the likelihood ratio test relative to the alternative hypothesis that $2\beta t_i$ is distributed like χ^2 with 2ν degrees of freedom, where $\nu \neq 1$. This is quite a reasonable alternative hypothesis, as with ν large the intervals will tend to have the same relative size corresponding to a constant serial interval, while small ν corresponds to greater clustering than expected from a random distribution.

The appropriate form of Bartlett's test (cf. Rao, 1952, pp. 226–9), suitably modified to allow for the small number of degrees of freedom, i.e. two, corresponding to each interval, is to use the approximation indicated by

$$\frac{12k}{(7 + 1/k)} \left[\log_e \left\{ \frac{1}{k} \sum_{i=1}^{k} t_i \right\} - \frac{1}{k} \sum_{i=1}^{k} \log_e t_i \right] \sim \chi^2_{k-1}. \tag{13.12}$$

Thus the left-hand side of (13.12) is distributed approximately as χ^2 with $k - 1$ degrees of freedom, and so significance may be judged in the usual way.

The test just given is valid for communities of any size, large or small, if a given individual can suffer repeated attacks of the disease in question. On the other hand, the test will be satisfactory only for large communities if repeated attacks are not possible. The reason for this is that the stock of susceptibles at risk is then continually depleted by successive cases. Thus if we start with n individuals at risk there are only $n - i$ at risk after the first i cases. It is therefore $(n - i)t_i$, rather than t_i itself, that is now proportional to a χ^2 with two degrees of freedom. All that we need do is simply to modify the test in (13.12) by substituting $(n - i)t_i$ for t_i.

13.42   General remarks on time-distribution of cases

It will be realized that in applying the foregoing test the null hypothesis assumes that the process considered is homogeneous in time. Appreciable seasonal fluctuations alone would be likely to give significant results in series that were in other respects quite random. Again, marked departures from randomness could easily arise in a long series when there were isolated crops of cases due entirely to environmental causes. Care is therefore needed in the interpretation of significant findings. Although these may well be important pointers, confirmation of an infectious case-to-case type of spread must be sought either in a well-established epidemiological pattern of events in a whole community or in the fitting of acceptable models to family data.

The time-interval type of test seems most likely to be useful when we have data on apparently sporadic cases extending over not too long a period of time. With greater incidence and multiple cases in households, tests based on household distributions seem preferable, although of course the two types of analysis are not strictly equivalent.

If we try to apply the test in (13.12) to relatively abundant data we may run into difficulty if the returns are grouped by, say, days or weeks. For then we may have two or more cases occurring in the same group giving intervals of zero, for which χ^2 will be infinite. We should then have to use some alternative test. Instead of examining intervals for departures from a negative exponential distribution, we could test the times of onset for departures from a rectangular distribution over the whole period of observation. To this end we could use χ^2 to compare the observed and expected histograms for goodness-of-fit, or, alternatively, Smirnov's ω^2 or Kolmogorov's D_n to test agreement between the observed and expected distribution functions (see, for example, Barnard, 1953; Maguire *et al.*, 1953).

13.5   Space—time interactions

We have already introduced the notion of investigating space—time interactions in Section 13.2, where we were discussing the problems as they arose directly out of an epidemiological context. To give a specific illustration, let us consider the childhood leukaemia data of Knox (1964a) derived from Northumberland and Durham over the years 1951—60, as shown in Table 13.2.

Table 13.2   *Distribution of 96 cases of leukaemia by types of space—time pairs*

	Up to 1 km	Over 1 km	Totals
Up to 60 days	5	147	152
60 days or more	20	4388	4408
Totals	25	4535	4560

The dichotomies in space and time have been based on dividing points at one km and 60 days, respectively. There were 96 cases in all, giving a total of $\frac{1}{2}.95.96 = 4560$ separate though not independent pairs. Knox calculates the expectation of the upper left-hand cell as $(25 \times 152)/4560 = 0.83$, and notes that the probability of observing a Poisson variable with this mean having a value of five or more is less than 1/750. Pike (discussion to Knox, 1965) confirmed the essential significance of this result by quoting a Monte Carlo randomization study which showed that the relevant probability was at any rate less than 1/500. Barton and David (1966), using a graph-theoretic specification, subsequently demonstrated that the conjecture of a Poisson distribution for low-level epidemicity was in fact justified to a good approximation. A more extensive investigation of this whole approach was made by Barton *et al.* (1967).

To put the matter a little more formally, let us suppose that there are N points (x_i, y_i, t_i), where (x_i, y_i) are the space coordinates, and t_i is the time-value. It is convenient to define

$$\left. \begin{aligned} d_{ij}^2 &= (x_i - x_j)^2 + (y_i - y_j)^2, \\ t_{ij} &= |t_i - t_j|, \end{aligned} \right\} \tag{13.13}$$

where $i \neq j$. Two arbitrary standards, δ and τ, are chosen, so that (x_i, y_i, t_i) and (x_j, y_j, t_j) are defined as adjacent in space if $d_{ij} < \delta$ and adjacent in time if $t_{ij} < \tau$. We then classify all $\frac{1}{2}N(N-1)$ pairs of points according to whether they are adjacent or not in time or space, or both. Let N_{1S} be the total number of adjacencies in space, and N_{1T} the number of adjacencies in time, while n_{ST} denotes the number of adjacencies in both space and time. Then, on the hypothesis of randomness, it can be shown that

$$\left. \begin{aligned} E(n_{ST}) &= \frac{2N_{1S}N_{1T}}{N(N-1)}, \\ E(n_{ST}^2) &= \frac{2N_{1S}N_{1T}}{N^{(2)}} + \frac{4N_{2S}N_{2T}}{N^{(3)}} + \frac{4(N_{1S}^{(2)} - 2N_{2S})(N_{1T}^{(2)} - 2N_{2T})}{N^{(4)}}, \end{aligned} \right\} \tag{13.14}$$

where N_2 refers to the number of pairs of adjacencies with a common point, and $N^{(r)} = N(N-1) \dots (N-r+1)$. Moreover, as stated above, in conditions of low epidemicity n_{ST} is an approximately Poisson variable.

Barton *et al.* (1967) showed that Knox's test is in fact quite powerful for a Neyman-type contagious model, for which each secondary point is supposed to be essentially coincident with the primary point from which it is derived. We might therefore expect that the test would be useful in indicating at least the existence of an infectious factor in the occurrence of the disease, although the actual epidemiology might be more complicated than the model implied.

Various generalizations are possible. Thus instead of merely counting adjacent points, we might take appropriate functions of the d_{ij} and t_{ij}, and form a test-statistic such as

$$R = \sum_{n_{ST}} f(d_{ij})g(t_{ij}). \tag{13.15}$$

Again, in order to be independent of the criteria δ and τ, we might prefer

$$R = \sum_{i>j} f(d_{ij})g(t_{ij}), \tag{13.16}$$

where convenient choices of the indicated functions might be $f(d_{ij}) = d_{ij}$, $g(t_{ij}) = t_{ij}$; or $f(d_{ij}) = d_{ij}^2$, $g(t_{ij}) = t_{ij}^2$, etc. Barton et $al.$ indicate how the distributions under randomization can be obtained, and how a choice can be made of the most sensitive tests.

These kinds of tests seem likely to display significant space–time inter-= actions when a disease has a marked infectious aspect, and when the serial interval between successive cases is fairly short. If the serial interval is long, on the other hand, a reformulation of the approach is required. Pike and Smith (1968) have extended Barton and David's (1966) graph-theoretic treatment of Knox's approach so as to deal with this more general situation.

More recently, Abe (1973) has made a new review of Knox's tests, in particular the use by Knox (1963a) of polychotomous divisions of time and space yielding the familiar type of contingency table, which can then be subjected to the usual χ^2 test. While this to some extent mitigates the bias introduced by arbitrary dichotomies, the classical test-statistic

$$X^2 = \sum_{i,j} \frac{(O_{ij} - E_{ij})^2}{E_{ij}}, \qquad (13.17)$$

where O_{ij} and E_{ij} are the observed and expected values in the cell indicated by (i, j), does not have the expectation $(h - 1)(k - 1)$, which occurs when the observations are independently assigned to a table with h rows and k columns (or vice versa).

An amended statistic proposed by Abe can be derived as follows. Let the number of pairs occurring in the ith and jth column be n_{ij}, the expectation in a familiar notation being $e_{ij} = n_{i.}\, n_{.j}/n$. Let us put

$$x_{ij} = n_{ij} - e_{ij}, \qquad (13.18)$$

for the individual deviations of the observed number of pairs in any cell from the expected value. By examining in detail the variances and covariances of the n_{ij}, Abe shows how to calculate the covariance matrix $\mathbf{V}$ of the set of all x_{ij} represented as a column vector $\mathbf{x}$. An appropriate test-statistic is now

$$Q = \mathbf{x}'\mathbf{V}^{-1}\mathbf{x}, \qquad (13.19)$$

which may be referred to the χ^2 distribution with $(h - 1)(k - 1)$ degrees of freedom. This approximation is likely to be a great improvement, especially if the n_{ij} are not too small. In any case Q has the correct expectation, which X^2 in (13.17) does not have in this particular application.

Several other writers have also examined these problems of detecting epidemiologically significant clusters. Thus Pinkel and Nefzger (1959) discussed the space–time distribution of leukaemia, though they did not distinguish the different aspects very clearly, and, as pointed out by Ederer, Myers and Mantel (1964), the statistical analysis was unsatisfactory. The latter authors presented a method of studying temporal clusters within spatial units, using occupancy theory to provide appropriate significance tests. Again, use has been made of Bross's (1958) ridit analysis, and also of the "persisting high rates" approach of Mustacchi (1965). A comparative analysis has been made of these three last methods by Mustacchi, David and Fix (1967). Mantel (1967) has used a generalized regression approach. Finally, we mention a recent paper by Larsen, Holmes and Heath (1973), giving a new combinatorial test for measuring uni-modal clustering that can also be used to examine evidence from neighbouring census tracts for space–time interactions.

For further details of these various techniques the interested reader should consult the sources cited. The major problem about all these analyses is that it seems very difficult to make any substantive advances as a result of carrying out the various kinds of cluster analyses. Sometimes significant space–time associations are revealed, and sometimes they are not. Moreover, it is very easy for spurious effects to arise. Thus an unusually enthusiastic physician operating in a limited locality could easily increase the reporting rate and generate an apparent space–time interaction. A similar result could occur over a wider area, e.g. the several states of the United States, when a disease is notifiable in some areas but not others. The extent to which such phenomena occur also depends on the intervals chosen in the space–time grid. Again, any population which grows at different rates in different parts of the area studied can exhibit space–time interactions which have no special significance. Further, even when a genuine clustering occurs this still might be due to genetic or environmental effects rather than an infectious mechanism.

Because of these uncertainties of interpretation the topic of the present section has been treated in outline rather than in detail. The best method of establishing an infectious type of spread is still probably to show that one model, inherently plausible from a biological and epidemiological point of view, will explain the data while alternatives are unsatisfactory.

14

Chain-binomial models

14.1　Introduction

In Part 2 we mostly considered epidemic processes occurring in continuous
time. Relatively little general theory exists for discrete-time models, but an
introduction to this subject was made in Chapter 8. The treatment was concentrated largely on the theory of the so-called "chain-binomial" type of model,
problems of statistical applications to specific epidemiological data, mostly on
measles, being reserved for the current chapter. We shall therefore start the
present detailed discussions *de novo*, repeating for convenience the basic
definitions of the chain-binomial type of model, and giving an expanded
account of the epidemiological context.

We have already seen how continuous-time stochastic models can be used
both for the general analysis of large-scale phenomena, and also for the analysis
of household data (see Section 6.8). In the latter event, conditions were liable
to be more exacting because of the possibility of using standard methods of
estimation and goodness-of-fit tests. Some diseases, such as perhaps scarlet
fever or diphtheria, might legitimately be investigated in this way because the
continuous-infection assumption is probably not too far removed from reality.
But other infectious diseases, such as measles, mumps or chickenpox, where
the incubation and latent periods may be less variable and infectivity is thought
to be confined to a relatively short period of time, clearly require a rather
different treatment. The natural thing is to consider as a first approximation a
model in which the latent and incubation periods are constant, the period of
infectiousness is reduced to a single point, and a single attack confers immunity. If, therefore, an epidemic is started in a group of susceptibles by a single
case, or by several simultaneously infectious cases, the whole process will continue in a series of stages or generations, separated by intervals equal to the
latent period, until either there are no more susceptibles to be infected or else
at some point it happens by chance that there are no fresh infections to keep
the process going.

Representations of this type seem to have been first used in the USA by

239

Lowell J. Reed and Wade Hampton Frost (see Wilson and Burke, 1942; Abbey, 1952; Maia, 1952; Elveback and Varma, 1965) round about 1928, though they did not apparently publish anything themselves. Their theoretical analyses seem to have been virtually deterministic, but the essentially probabilistic nature of the epidemic was illustrated for teaching purposes by means of a mechanical model that mixed up together appropriately coloured balls in a trough. The first published reference to a fully stochastic model of this type appears in Lidwell and Sommerville (1951), and the following year Helen Abbey (1952) made a special investigation of the Reed—Frost theory. A slightly different variant was put forward in England as early as 1931 by Greenwood, who was primarily interested in analysing data from several families of a given size, in contradistinction to Reed and Frost, who were mainly concerned with the course of a single epidemic in a fairly large group of susceptibles.

At each stage in the epidemic there are certain numbers of infectives and susceptibles, and it is reasonable to suppose that the latter will yield a fresh crop of cases at the next stage distributed in a binomial series. We thus have a *chain* of binomial distributions, the actual probability of a new infection at any stage depending on the numbers of infectives and susceptibles at the previous stage. The exact mathematical form of the probabilities involved will be given in the next section, and these depend to some extent on the mechanism of infection envisaged. However, the probability of any particular pattern of events can, at any rate for the simplest model, always be put in terms of a single basic parameter p, which measures the chance of contact between any two individuals of the group sufficient to produce a new infection, if one is an infective and one a susceptible.

An important point that arises in connexion with the practical application of chain-binomial theory is the question of correctly identifying the links of the chain. Substantial departures from the assumptions of constant incubation and latent periods and very short infectious period will of course render invalid the chain-binomial models considered here, though the modified set-up discussed in Chapter 15 may be useful. It might happen, however, that the strict chain-binomial mechanism was operative so far as the process of infection was concerned (constant latent period and short infectious period), but that we failed to pick out the links in the chain properly because actual symptoms developed in an erratic way some time after the infectious point (highly variable incubation period). A similar state of affairs has already been discussed in connexion with the continuous-infection model investigated in Section 6.8. One way out of the difficulty is to base our analysis on the *total* number of cases only occurring during the course of the epidemic, as this can usually be determined with much greater reliability, though of course we lose precision when we come to estimate the parameters involved.

We shall introduce the basic Greenwood and Reed—Frost models in Section 14.2 and shall discuss the estimation of the relevant parameter, together with testing goodness-of-fit, in Section 14.3. The two following sections, 14.4 and 14.5, deal with the modifications necessary for taking account of possible heterogeneity between households and between individuals. Various errors that may arise in counting susceptibles are treated in Section 14.6, while the problem of extra-household infections is introduced in Section 14.7. The final Section 14.8 is devoted to a short discussion.

It should perhaps be mentioned here that, when an electronic computer is available, certain computational processes can be greatly facilitated. This point has already been discussed more extensively in Chapter 4. When explicit solutions to maximum-likelihood equations are available, sophisticated computing is usually unnecessary. But when, as in Section 14.4, a full scoring procedure is appropriate on a desk machine, it may be easier to maximize the log likelihood directly. Since the likelihoods occurring in the present chapter all have a fairly simple multiplicative form, no special discussion has been devoted to computer programming aspects which can easily be handled *ad hoc*.

14.2 Basic models

Let us take the Reed–Frost formulation of the theory first. We suppose that the epidemic is started in a homogeneously mixing group of susceptibles by one infective or by several simultaneously infectious persons, as the case may be. The latent period can be taken as the unit of time. Then let r_t be the number of uninfected susceptibles just prior to time t, and let s_t be the number of infected individuals just prior to time t who will become infectious at that instant. If $p = 1 - q$ is the chance of adequate contact between any two specified members of the group at time t, then q^{s_t} is the chance that any given susceptible will have adequate contact with none of the s_t infectives. Accordingly, $1 - q^{s_t}$ is the probability of adequate contact with at least one, which is what we require for infection to take place. The conditional probability of exactly s_{t+1} freshly infected persons, who will in turn become infectious at time $t + 1$, is therefore

$$\Pr\{s_{t+1} | r_t, s_t\} = \frac{r_t!}{s_{t+1}! r_{t+1}!} (1 - q^{s_t})^{s_{t+1}} q^{s_t r_{t+1}}, \qquad (14.1)$$

as previously stated in (8.3). The conditional probability distribution for the number of new cases at each stage of the epidemic is given by binomial expressions like (14.1), the process ceasing as soon as any stage produces no new cases.

Greenwood's variant is slightly simpler mathematically in that he assumed that the chance of infection was not influenced by the number of infectives available to transmit the disease. Thus in this case the probability of a given susceptible being infected at time t can be simply written as p instead of

$1 - q^{s_t}$. The corresponding form of (14.1) is then

$$\Pr\{s_{t+1}|r_t, s_t\} = \frac{r_t!}{s_{t+1}! r_{t+1}!} p^{s_{t+1}} q^{r_{t+1}}. \qquad (14.2)$$

For families of two or three with only a single primary case these two models are indistinguishable, but in other situations there is a difference. If we prefer to use the simpler Greenwood version then we can either regard this as a convenient approximation to the more exact Reed–Frost specification, or as precisely appropriate to a disease in which the transmission of infection, when the latter is present at all, depends largely on factors internal to the susceptibles themselves. This would occur if, for example, infectious material were widely spread through a household by an infectious person, but actual infection only occurred when an individual susceptible's resistance was sufficiently reduced.

We usually assume that the disease in question is sufficiently rare in the community at large for there to be only a negligible chance of more than one member of a household being *independently* infected from outside (but see Section 14.7). Multiple introductions, on the other hand, which occur when several members are infected simultaneously by an outside contact, present no special difficulty as they all become infectious together and the assumption of distinct stages made above will be fulfilled.

14.21 Frequency distribution of types of chain

The whole course of any one epidemic in a particular community can be characterized quite unambiguously simply by noting how many simultaneous introductions there are at the start and how many fresh cases occur at each stage. Thus, if in a group of susceptibles we have one initial case followed after the elapse of the incubation period by two further cases, these in turn being succeeded by just one new case at each of the next two stages, we can write this as $1 \rightarrow 2 \rightarrow 1 \rightarrow 1$ or, more shortly, $\{121^2\}$ in a quasi-partitional notation. The first figure to appear in the set of symbols gives the number of introductions, and the remaining figures refer to the numbers of new cases arising at each stage. To complete the specification we must also know the total number of individuals in the group.

The probability of any particular type of chain can be obtained quite easily by multiplying together the probabilities appropriate to each stage given by (14.1) or (14.2). Thus, if we have the chain $\{121^2\}$ in a household of five, the relevant values of r_t and s_t are

t	r_t	s_t
0	4	1
1	2	2
2	1	1
3	0	1
4	0	0

The table terminates with the line in which s_t first becomes zero, and it is important to notice that r_t will still be positive at this point if not all susceptibles have been infected. In the Greenwood model the required probability is

Table 14.1   *Individual chains for households of two*

Type of chain	Frequency
$\{1\}$	q
$\{1^2\}$	p

Table 14.2   *Individual chains for households of three*

Type of introduction	Type of chain	Frequency	
		Reed—Frost	Greenwood
Single	$\{1\}$	q^2	
	$\{1^2\}$	$2pq^2$	
	$\{1^3\}$	$2p^2q$	
	$\{12\}$	p^2	
Double	$\{2\}$	q^2	q
	$\{21\}$	$1-q^2$	p

Table 14.3   *Individual chains for households of four*

Type of introduction	Type of chain	Frequency	
		Reed—Frost	Greenwood
Single	$\{1\}$	q^3	q^3
	$\{1^2\}$	$3pq^4$	$3pq^4$
	$\{1^3\}$	$6p^2q^4$	$6p^2q^4$
	$\{12\}$	$3p^2q^3$	$3p^2q^2$
	$\{1^4\}$	$6p^3q^3$	$6p^3q^3$
	$\{1^2 2\}$	$3p^3q^2$	$3p^3q^2$
	$\{121\}$	$3p^3q(1+q)$	$3p^3q$
	$\{13\}$	p^3	p^3
Double	$\{2\}$	q^4	q^2
	$\{21\}$	$2pq^3(1+q)$	$2pq^2$
	$\{21^2\}$	$2p^2q^2(1+q)$	$2p^2q$
	$\{2^2\}$	$p^2(1+q)^2$	p^2
Triple	$\{3\}$	q^3	q
	$\{31\}$	$1-q^3$	p

quickly found to be $12p^4q^3$, while the Reed–Frost version gives $12p^4q^4(1 + q)$. Tables 14.1 to 14.4 give the frequency distributions of all types of chains, with both single and multiple introductions, for groups having a total size of up to five individuals. Apart from groups of two, and groups of three with only a single initial case, the Greenwood and Reed–Frost models always lead to different sets of probabilities.

Table 14.4 *Individual chains for households of five*

Type of introduction	Type of chain	Frequency	
		Reed–Frost	Greenwood
Single	{1}	q^4	q^4
	{1²}	$4pq^6$	$4pq^6$
	{1³}	$12p^2q^7$	$12p^2q^7$
	{12}	$6p^2q^6$	$6p^2q^4$
	{1⁴}	$24p^3q^7$	$24p^3q^7$
	{1²2}	$12p^3q^6$	$12p^3q^5$
	{121}	$12p^3q^5(1+q)$	$12p^3q^4$
	{13}	$4p^3q^4$	$4p^3q^2$
	{1⁵}	$24p^4q^6$	$24p^4q^6$
	{1³2}	$12p^4q^5$	$12p^4q^5$
	{1²21}	$12p^4q^4(1+q)$	$12p^4q^4$
	{121²}	$12p^4q^4(1+q)$	$12p^4q^3$
	{12²}	$6p^4q^2(1+q)^2$	$6p^4q^2$
	{1²3}	$4p^4q^3$	$4p^4q^3$
	{131}	$4p^4q(1+q+q^2)$	$4p^4q$
	{14}	p^4	p^4
Double	{2}	q^6	q^3
	{21}	$3pq^6(1+q)$	$3pq^4$
	{21²}	$6p^2q^6(1+q)$	$6p^2q^4$
	{2²}	$3p^2q^4(1+q)^2$	$3p^2q^2$
	{21³}	$6p^3q^5(1+q)$	$6p^3q^3$
	{212}	$3p^3q^4(1+q)$	$3p^3q^2$
	{2²1}	$3p^3q^2(1+q)^3$	$3p^3q$
	{23}	$p^3(1+q)^3$	p^3
Triple	{3}	q^6	q^2
	{31}	$2pq^4(1+q+q^2)$	$2pq^2$
	{31²}	$2p^2q^3(1+q+q^2)$	$2p^2q$
	{32}	$p^2(1+q+q^2)^2$	p^2
Quadruple	{4}	q^4	q
	{41}	$1-q^4$	p

When enumerating such probabilities systematically there is an advantage in using a slightly more general procedure. Thus the probability of the Greenwood chain $(s_0, s_1, s_2, ..., s_k)$, where s_k is the last non-zero s-value, is

$$\Pr\{s_0, ..., s_k\} = \prod_{t=0}^{k} \frac{r_t!}{s_{t+1}! r_{t+1}!} p^{s_{t+1}} q^{r_{t+1}}$$

$$= \frac{r_0!}{s_1! s_2! ... s_k! r_{k+1}!} p^{\sum\limits_{i=1}^{k} s_i} q^{\sum\limits_{j=1}^{k+1} r_j}, \qquad (14.3)$$

and the corresponding Reed—Frost analogue is

$$\Pr\{s_0, ..., s_k\} = \frac{r_0!}{s_1! s_2! ... s_k! r_{k+1}!} q^{\sum\limits_{j=0}^{k} s_j r_{j+1}} \prod_{i=0}^{k-1} (1 - q^{s_i})^{s_{i+1}}. \qquad (14.4)$$

Table 14.5 *Total size of epidemic for households of three*

Type of introduction	Number of cases	Frequency	
		Reed—Frost	Greenwood
Single	1	q^2	
	2	$2pq^2$	
	3	$p^2(1 + 2q)$	
Double	2	q^2	q
	3	$1 - q^2$	p

Table 14.6 *Total size of epidemic for households of four*

Type of introduction	Number of cases	Frequency	
		Reed—Frost	Greenwood
Single	1	q^3	q^3
	2	$3pq^4$	$3pq^4$
	3	$3p^2 q^3(1 + 2q)$	$3p^2 q^2(1 + 2q^2)$
	4	$p^3(1 + 3q + 6q^2 + 6q^3)$	$p^3(1 + 3q + 3q^2 + 6q^2)$
Double	2	q^4	q^2
	3	$2pq^3(1 + q)$	$2pq^2$
	4	$p^2(1 + q)(1 + q + 2q^2)$	$p^2(1 + 2q)$
Triple	3	q^3	q
	4	$1 - q^3$	p

With comparatively small groups of individuals such as we find in ordinary households, analyses based on complete enumeration of all possible chains are quite appropriate, and the questions of estimation and goodness-of-fit that arise

Table 14.7 *Total size of epidemic for households of five*

Type of introduction	Total no. of cases	Frequency	
		Reed–Frost	Greenwood
Single	1	q^4	q^4
	2	$4pq^6$	$4pq^6$
	3	$6p^2q^6(1+2q)$	$6p^2q^4(1+2q^3)$
	4	$4p^3q^4(1+3q+6q^2+6q^3)$	$4p^3q^2(1+3q^2+3q^3+6q^5)$
	5	$p^4(1+4q+10q^2+20q^3+30q^4+36q^5+24q^6)$	$p^4(1+4q+6q^2+16q^3+12q^4+12q^5+24q^6)$
Double	2	q^5	q^3
	3	$3pq^6(1+q)$	$3pq^4$
	4	$3p^2q^4(1+q)(1+q+2q^2)$	$3p^2q^2(1+2q^2)$
	5	$p^3(1+q)(1+2q+4q^2+6q^3+6q^4+6q^5)$	$p^3(1+3q+3q^2+6q^3)$
Triple	3	q^6	q^2
	4	$2pq^4(1+q+q^2)$	$2pq^2$
	5	$p^2(1+q+q^2)(1+q+q^2+2q^3)$	$p^2(1+2q)$
Quadruple	4	q^4	q
	5	$1-q^4$	p

will be discussed later in Section 14.3. If we wanted to deal with large populations, a rather more general theory would probably be necessary to handle the matter in a manageable way, although Abbey (1952) succeeded in applying the Reed—Frost model, without enumeration of chains, to fairly big groups of schoolchildren (see also Section 14.33 below).

14.22 Distribution of total number of cases

As already mentioned in the introductory remarks at the beginning of this chapter, the chain-binomial model might be basically correct, although we were not able to identify the links of the chain with any certainty, having accurate data only on the total number of cases that occurred. For group sizes up to five, we can obtain the required frequencies merely by amalgamating the appropriate elements in Tables 14.2 to 14.4. Thus a total of four cases in a group of five with a single primary case might have arisen from any of the chains $\{1^4\}$, $\{1^22\}$, $\{121\}$ or $\{13\}$. The probabilities obtained in this way are shown in Tables 14.5 to 14.7.

The attempt to use analyses of the total number of cases in a household has another disadvantage apart from the loss of statistical precision when estimating parameters. This is that if we cannot identify the links of the chain with much confidence, we are also likely to be uncertain about the type of introduction involved. In practice, however, there may in some instances be good independent reasons for thinking that multiple introductions are fairly uncommon, and if this is so we can base the analysis on the assumption of single introductions. Again, if the chaining is only mildly confused by, for example, moderate variations in the latent and incubation periods, then it is likely that the earlier links and the type of introduction will be fairly clear, while only the later elements of the chain will be really indistinguishable.

If the size of the group under consideration is at all large it is probably better to calculate the frequencies of the total number of cases more directly, instead of deriving them from the probabilities of the individual chains as suggested above. Although at present no explicit general formulae exist, we can obtain recurrence relations fairly easily as follows. Consider first the Greenwood model. Let us write $_aP_{nj}$ for the probability that a group of *total* size n will have a *total* of j cases when there are a introductions, where $a \leq j \leq n$. Since the distribution at each stage is binomial, the chance of k cases at $t = 1$ is

$$\binom{n-a}{k} p^k q^{n-a-k}.$$

There are then k cases and $n - a - k$ uninfected susceptibles. Thus the probability of a further $j - a$ new cases (including the k) to make j in all is

$_k P_{n-a,\,j-a}$. We therefore have

$$
_a P_{nj} = \sum_{k=1}^{j-a} \binom{n-a}{k} p^k q^{n-a-k}\, _k P_{n-a,\,j-a},
$$

where, in particular,

$$
_a P_{na} = q^{n-a}.
$$

$$\left.\begin{array}{c}\\ \\ \\ \\ \end{array}\right\}\quad(14.5)$$

This is more or less equivalent to a formula given by Greenwood (1931) but is generalized here to cover multiple introductions. The analogous result for the Reed–Frost model, obtained in an entirely similar manner, is

$$
_a P'_{nj} = \sum_{k=1}^{j-a} \binom{n-a}{k} (1-q^a)^k\, q^{a(n-a-k)}\, _k P'_{n-a,\,j-a}
$$

with

$$
_a P'_{na} = q^{a(n-a)},
$$

$$\left.\begin{array}{c}\\ \\ \\ \\ \end{array}\right\}\quad(14.6)$$

where primes are used to distinguish this model from the Greenwood one. Actually, a more convenient recurrence procedure can be obtained for the Reed–Frost model since we can show that $_a P'_{nj}$ is proportional to $_a P'_{jj}$. Suppose we compare two groups, one with n individuals and one with j individuals, each having a introductory cases of the disease. Then epidemics of total size j will have the same set of constituent chains in each group. By considering (14.4) it is easy to see that the probability of occurrence of any chain in the first group is

$$
\binom{n-a}{j-a} q^{j(n-j)}
$$

times the corresponding probability for the second group, and that this factor is independent of chain-type. Hence

$$
_a P'_{nj} = \binom{n-a}{j-a} q^{j(n-j)}\, _a P'_{jj},
\tag{14.7}
$$

which is a generalization of an essentially similar formula given by Lidwell and Sommerville (1951). A similar argument applied to Greenwood's model does not simplify so readily, since in this case the multiplying factor varies with the number of links in each chain.

14.3   Estimating the chance of adequate contact

It is a fairly straightforward matter to use the foregoing results, in particular the frequency distributions appearing in Tables 14.1 to 14.7, for estimating the basic parameter p from data on several households by means of the method of maximum likelihood. In the case of chained data for the Greenwood model it is always possible to find explicit formulae for the estimate of p and its large-sample variance, but otherwise, with chained Reed—Frost data or with total epidemic sizes for either model, it is usually best to resort to the more general maximum-likelihood scoring procedure. The illustrative examples given below should make clear what is involved. It is also possible, of course, to estimate p from data on a *single* large group using (14.3) or (14.4). This is discussed in Section 14.33.

14.31   Use of individual chains

Consider first the observed and expected numbers for Greenwood or Reed—Frost chains in households of three with a single introduction shown in Table 14.8. The probabilities are taken from Table 14.2 above. Application of the usual maximum-likelihood procedure gives the efficient estimate

$$\hat{p} = \frac{b + 2c + 2d}{2a + 3b + 3c + 2d},$$

with variance

$$\mathrm{var}\,(\hat{p}) = \frac{pq}{2n(1 + pq)}.$$

(14.8)

The fairly extensive investigation of Wilson, Bennett, Allen and Worcester (1939) into measles epidemics occurring in Providence, Rhode Island, during 1929—34, provides suitable material for analysis. These authors discussed many different ways of examining their data. The figures shown in Table 14.8 are based on households of three, with a single primary case and just two other susceptibles at risk between the ages of 7 months and 10 years. This particular

Table 14.8   *Greenwood or Reed—Frost chains for households of three*

Type of chain	Expected number of households	Observed number of households	Providence measles data	Fitted values
{1}	nq^2	a	34	14·9
{1²}	$2npq^2$	b	25	23·5
{1³}	$2np^2q$	c	36	87·7
{12}	np^2	d	239	207·9
Total	n	n	334	334·0

classification seems most likely to give reasonably homogeneous data. Application of (14.8) gives $\hat{p} = 0.789 \pm 0.015$. Fitted values are shown in the last column of the table. It is clear from inspection that the fit is unsatisfactory, and this is borne out by the high value of χ^2 obtained, namely 59·8 on 2 degrees of freedom, for which $P < 0.001$.

In Table 14.9 similar material is set out for households of four. This time we must distinguish between the Greenwood and Reed—Frost models. For the

Greenwood version we have the estimate

$$\hat{p} = \frac{b + 2(c + d) + 3(e + f + g + h)}{3a + 5b + 6c + 4d + 6e + 5f + 4g + 3h} \equiv \frac{A}{B},$$

with

$$\text{var}(\hat{p}) = \frac{\hat{p}q}{B},$$

(14.9)

where B is the denominator of the fractional expression for $\hat{p}$. Substituting the numerical values of Table 14.9 in equation (14.9) gives $\hat{p} = 0.791 \pm 0.022$. Again, one can see that there is only poor agreement between observation and hypothesis.

Table 14.9   *Greenwood and Reed–Frost chains for households of four*

Type of chain	Expected number of households		Observed number of households	Providence measles data	Fitted values	
	Greenwood	Reed–Frost			Greenwood	Reed–Frost
$\{1\}$	nq^3	nq^3	a	4	0.9	1.2
$\{1^2\}$	$3npq^4$	$3npq^4$	b	3	0.4	0.7
$\{1^3\}$	$6np^2q^4$	$6np^2q^4$	c	1	0.7	1.0
$\{12\}$	$3np^2q^2$	$3np^2q^3$	d	8	8.2	2.2
$\{1^4\}$	$6np^3q^3$	$6np^3q^3$	e	4	2.7	3.4
$\{1^2 2\}$	$3np^3q^2$	$3np^3q^2$	f	3	6.5	7.3
$\{121\}$	$3np^3q$	$3np^3q(1 + q)$	g	10	31.0	38.7
$\{13\}$	np^3	np^3	h	67	49.6	45.5
Total	n	n	n	100	100.0	100.0

Estimation for the Reed–Frost model is a little more involved, and is most easily accomplished using maximum-likelihood scoring. As there is only one parameter to be estimated, all we require is the score

$$S'_p = \frac{b + 2c + 2d + 3e + 3f + 3g + 3h}{p}$$

$$- \frac{3a + 4b + 4c + 3d + 3e + 2f + g}{q} - \frac{g}{1 + q},$$

(14.10)

using a prime to distinguish the score in this model from the previous one. We have to solve the equation $S'_p = 0$, and although this is actually a quadratic in p it is probably simpler in practice to take a few trial values and interpolate inversely, especially as this gives the amount of information automatically. For example, we find

$$S_{p=0.76} = 17.81 \quad \text{and} \quad S_{p=0.77} = -1.41.$$

Hence the required estimate is $\hat{p} = 0.769$ and the amount of information is $100(17.81 + 1.41) = 1922$ units, giving a standard error of 0.023. As before, the goodness-of-fit is obviously inadequate.

The possibility of a more satisfactory analysis being obtained from the total number of cases has already been mentioned, and we shall examine these data again from this point of view in the next section. However, although there are some difficulties in chaining measles data, we should hardly expect them to be so great as to lead to the discrepancies revealed above. For this reason alternative explanations are required, and these will be dealt with in due course.

14.32   Use of total number of cases

We now turn to the analysis of data based on the total number of cases only. Instead of Table 14.8 we have the material appearing in Table 14.10.

Table 14.10 *Total number of cases for households of three (Greenwood or Reed–Frost)*

Total number of cases	Expected number of households	Observed number of households	Providence measles data	Fitted values
1	nq^2	a	34	24·7
2	$2npq^2$	b	25	36·0
3	$np^2(1 + 2q)$	c	275	273·3
Total	n	n	334	334·0

The appropriate score is

$$S_p = \frac{b + 2c}{p} - \frac{2a + 2b}{q} - \frac{2c}{1 + 2q}. \qquad (14.11)$$

We obtain in the usual way the estimate $\hat{p} = 0.728 \pm 0.018$. The goodness-of-fit χ^2 with one degree of freedom is 6.85 which is significant at the 1 percent level, and still unsatisfactory.

The corresponding set-up for households of four is shown in Table 14.11. The appropriate scores are easily seen to be

$$S_p = \frac{b + 2c + 3d}{p} - \frac{3a + 4b + 2c}{q} - \frac{4cq}{1 + 2q^2} - \frac{3d(1 + 2q + 6q^2)}{1 + 3q + 3q^2 + 6q^3}, \qquad (14.12)$$

for the Greenwood model, and

$$S_p' = \frac{b + 2c + 3d}{p} - \frac{3a + 4b + 3c}{q} - \frac{2c}{1 + 2q} - \frac{3d(1 + 4q + 6q^2)}{1 + 3q + 6q^2 + 6q^3}, \qquad (14.13)$$

for the Reed—Frost model. Proceeding as before, we find the estimates $\hat{p} = 0.709 \pm 0.031$ and $\hat{p}' = 0.653 \pm 0.029$, respectively. The goodness-of-fits are here quite unexceptionable. Pooling the first two classes in the Greenwood model, we obtain a χ^2 of 4·74 with 2 degrees of freedom, while for the Reed—Frost version the fit happens by chance to be very nearly exact.

14.33 Application to a single chain

We have, in Sections 14.31 and 14.32, been considering the estimation of p from data on either chains or total epidemic sizes, where the number of households involved is relatively large. If we had only a few households of the sizes under discussion little statistical information would be available. On the other hand, we might be concerned with a single large group such as a school or classroom. In this event we can write down the likelihood of the observed pattern of events — always supposing of course that we can chain the data reasonably accurately — in terms of (14.3) or (14.4). The parameter p can then be estimated by maximum likelihood in the obvious way, as was done by Abbey (1952) for quite large groups of schoolchildren. Thus the score for the Greenwood model is

$$S_p = \frac{1}{p}\sum_{i=1}^{k} s_i - \frac{1}{q}\sum_{j=1}^{k+1} r_j, \tag{14.14}$$

while for the Reed—Frost model we have

$$S'_p = \sum_{i=0}^{k-1} \frac{s_i s_{i+1}}{q(q^{-s_i}-1)} - \frac{1}{q}\sum_{j=0}^{k} s_j r_{j+1}. \tag{14.15}$$

As this is virtually equivalent to basing the estimate of p on information drawn from the binomial distributions occurring at the various stages, we should expect the application of maximum likelihood to be approximately valid for a large group. Goodness-of-fit can be tested by amalgamating the contributions to χ^2 obtained by comparing the observed and expected numbers of susceptibles and infectives at each stage. Thus, on the Reed—Frost model, the expected numbers at the jth stage corresponding to the observed r_j and s_j are $r_{j-1}(1-q^{s_{j-1}})$ and $r_{j-1}q^{s_{j-1}}$, respectively; and the analogous Greenwood expectations are pr_{j-1} and qr_{j-1}. Stages involving small expectations are omitted. Those that are included each contribute one degree of freedom to χ^2. A special study of this procedure was carried out by Joyce Almond (1954), who concluded that it is quite satisfactory, provided that the number of susceptibles at each stage is sufficiently large, and provided that we remove one degree of freedom to allow for the parameter estimated. So far as Abbey's analysis of the school data is concerned, it may be mentioned here that it was unfortunately impossible to obtain satisfactory values of χ^2, even when allowance was made for errors in counting the numbers of susceptibles. However, there are obviously severe difficulties with very large

Table 14.11 *Total number of cases for households of four*

Total number of cases	Expected number of households		Observed number of households	Providence measles data	Fitted values	
	Greenwood	Reed–Frost			Greenwood	Reed–Frost
1	nq^3	nq^3	a	4	2·5	4·2
2	$3npq^4$	$3npq^4$	b	3	1·5	2·8
3	$3np^2 q^2 (1 + 2q^2)$	$3np^2 q^3 (1 + 2q)$	c	9	14·9	9·0
4	$np^3 (1 + 3q + 3q^2 + 6q^3)$	$np^3 (1 + 3q + 6q^2 + 6q^3)$	d	84	81·1	84·0
Total	n	n	n	100	100·0	100·0

groups in picking out chains that are likely to be at all realistic, and a more searching investigation designed to take account of the many causes of variation is clearly called for.

14.4   Variations between households

While simple chain-binomial models can sometimes be made to fit measles data so far as total size of household epidemic is concerned (e.g. Providence data above for households of four, and more generally in Greenwood, 1931), the theory is liable to break down when individual links of chains are taken into account. There is often difficulty in analysing measles records into the correct constituent chains owing to obvious variations in latent and incubation periods or uncertainty in distinguishing multiple primaries, but this hardly seems sufficient to explain the present discrepancy. Greenwood (1949) considered the possibility of variation in p, which is *a priori* quite likely on general epidemiological grounds. Factors such as age, sex, heredity, standards of hygiene and nutrition, etc. could all have an important influence. If p varies amongst the individuals of a given household, it can be shown that the distribution of cases at the first stage will still be binomial. But it is easily seen that this is not so in the measles data already discussed. The suggestion was therefore made by Greenwood that the explanation might well lie in variation between households. This is highly plausible, as the data in question were collected over several years and almost certainly must have involved a variety of social groups for which differences in important factors might easily be pronounced. A detailed analysis based on this idea was later made by Bailey (1953b, 1956c) and is described below. As we shall see, satisfactory agreement between hypothesis and observation can be obtained in this way, but more data are required to give real support to the theory. In particular, we might expect variation in the chance of infection to be much smaller for comparatively homogeneous groups of households, and this needs examination.

14.41   The basic model

The simplest way of taking account of possible variations in the chance of infection, p, seems to be to introduce a suitable distribution for p, and then to go through the usual process of estimating the parameters in this distribution and testing the goodness-of-fit. A convenient assumption is to suppose that p varies according to the beta-distribution,

$$dF = \frac{1}{B(x,y)} p^{x-1} q^{y-1} dp, \quad 0 \leqslant p \leqslant 1, \tag{14.16}$$

where $B(x,y)$ is the usual beta-function, and we must have $x > 0, y > 0$.

Since we are assuming that p is the same for all the members of a given household and only varies between households, the required expectations are obtained by averaging the frequencies for each kind of chain over the distribution

Table 14.12 *Modified chains for households of three (Greenwood or Reed–Frost)*

Type of chain	Expected number of households	Expected number on modified model		Observed number	Providence measles data	Fitted values
		In terms of x and y	In terms of p and z			
{1}	nq^2	$\dfrac{ny(y+1)}{(x+y)(x+y+1)}$	$\dfrac{nq(q+z)}{(1+z)}$	a	34	34·9
{1²}	$2npq^2$	$\dfrac{2nxy(y+1)}{(x+y)(x+y+1)(x+y+2)}$	$\dfrac{2npq(q+z)}{(1+z)(1+2z)}$	b	25	22·7
{1³}	$2np^2q$	$\dfrac{2nx(x+1)y}{(x+y)(x+y+1)(x+y+2)}$	$\dfrac{2npq(p+z)}{(1+z)(1+2z)}$	c	36	37·6
{12}	np^2	$\dfrac{nx(x+1)}{(x+y)(x+y+1)}$	$\dfrac{np(p+z)}{(1+z)}$	d	239	238·8
Total	n	n	n	n	334	334·0

in (14.16). This then exhibits the expectations as functions of the parameters x and y. As all the frequencies in Greenwood and Reed–Frost chains are, at most, linear sums of quantities like $p^u q^v$, it is convenient to work out the expectation of this item separately. Thus

$$
\begin{aligned}
E(p^u q^v) &= \frac{1}{B(x,y)} \int_0^1 p^{x+u-1} q^{y+v-1} dp \\
&= \frac{B(x+u, y+v)}{B(x,y)} \\
&= \frac{x(x+1)\ldots(x+u-1)y\,(y+1)\ldots(y+v-1)}{(x+y)\,(x+y+1)\ldots(x+y+u+v-1)} .
\end{aligned}
\tag{14.17}
$$

If u or v is zero, then the factors in the numerator on the right of (14.17) involving x or y, respectively, are absent. Applying these results to the expressions in Table 14.8 for households of three gives the derived values shown in Table 14.12.

14.42   Estimation of parameters from chains

We could now proceed directly with the maximum-likelihood estimation of x and y, but there is a certain disadvantage in doing so. The reason is that if the variation in p is small, x and y are both very large, indeed infinite in the limit when p is constant. This is a nuisance when one wants to perform a significance test for the existence of variation in p. Armitage (in discussion on Bailey, 1955) suggested using the reciprocals $x' = x^{-1}$ and $y' = y^{-1}$, but even here maximum-likelihood scoring fails in the limit as x' and y' tend to zero because the scores contain terms proportional to $(x')^{-1}$ and $(y')^{-1}$. It follows from (14.16) that the average value of p is given by

$$
\bar{p} = \frac{x}{x+y} = \frac{y'}{x'+y'} ,
\tag{14.18}
$$

and one solution of the difficulty would be to use $\bar{p}$ as one parameter, and x' or y' as the other. It turns out, however, to be considerably simpler algebraically to use the parameters

$$
p = \frac{x}{x+y} , \quad z = \frac{1}{x+y} ,
\tag{14.19}
$$

where, for convenience, we have dropped the bar from $\bar{p}$.

Households of three

Table 14.12 also gives the alternative form of the expectations for households of three in terms of p and z. These yield the scores

$$
\left.\begin{array}{l}
S_p = \dfrac{b+c+d}{p} - \dfrac{a+b+c}{q} + \dfrac{c+d}{p+z} - \dfrac{a+b}{q+z}, \\[2mm]
S_z = -\dfrac{n}{1+z} - \dfrac{2(b+c)}{1+2z} + \dfrac{c+d}{p+z} + \dfrac{a+b}{q+z},
\end{array}\right\} \quad (14.20)
$$

while the observed information functions are

$$
\left.\begin{array}{l}
I_{pp} = \dfrac{b+c+d}{p^2} + \dfrac{a+b+c}{q^2} + \dfrac{c+d}{(p+z)^2} + \dfrac{a+b}{(q+z)^2}, \\[2mm]
I_{pz} = \dfrac{c+d}{(p+z)^2} - \dfrac{a+b}{(q+z)^2}, \\[2mm]
I_{zz} = -\dfrac{n}{(1+z)^2} - \dfrac{4(b+c)}{(1+2z)^2} + \dfrac{c+d}{(p+z)^2} + \dfrac{a+b}{(q+z)^2}.
\end{array}\right\} \quad (14.21)
$$

The quantities given in (14.20) and (14.21) can be evaluated quite rapidly in practice for arbitrary values of p and z, as the quotients appearing in each line can be accumulated directly on a calculating machine, the squares of denominators in information functions being read directly from *Barlow's Tables*.

A convenient way of obtaining initial values of p and z, with which to commence maximum-likelihood scoring, is to amalgamate the second and third classes in Table 14.12 and equate observations to expectations, giving the estimates

$$
\left.\begin{array}{l}
\breve{p} = \dfrac{b+c+2d}{2n}, \\[2mm]
\breve{z} = \dfrac{4ad-(b+c)^2}{2n(b+c)}.
\end{array}\right\} \quad (14.22)
$$

These are in fact maximum-likelihood estimates based on the first stage of the epidemic only.

Using the estimates given by (14.22) for the Providence measles data we find the initial values

$$\breve{p} = 0.807, \quad \breve{z} = 0.706,$$

for which the scores are $S_p = -4.3511$ and $S_z = +1.0265$. The information and covariance matrices are

$$
\mathbf{I} = \begin{bmatrix} 3204.2 & 47.129 \\ 47.129 & 36.432 \end{bmatrix}, \quad \mathbf{V} = 10^{-4} \times \begin{bmatrix} 3.1814 & -4.1155 \\ -4.1155 & 279.80 \end{bmatrix}.
$$

The adjustments to be made to $\breve{p}$ and $\breve{z}$ are therefore -0.002 and $+0.031$, giving 0.805 and 0.737, respectively. A further stage of iteration makes only

Table 14.13   *Modified Greenwood chains for households of four*

Type of chain	Expected nos. on Greenwood model	Expected nos. on modified model	Observed nos.	Providence measles data	Fitted values
{1}	nq^3	$\dfrac{nq(q+z)(q+2z)}{(1+z)(1+2z)}$	a	4	4·9
{1²}	$3npq^4$	$\dfrac{3npq(q+z)(q+2z)(q+3z)}{(1+z)(1+2z)(1+3z)(1+4z)}$	b	3	2·6
{1³}	$6np^2q^4$	$\dfrac{6npq(p+z)(q+z)(q+2z)(q+3z)}{(1+z)(1+2z)(1+3z)(1+4z)(1+5z)}$	c	1	2·0
{12}	$3np^2q^2$	$\dfrac{3npq(p+z)(q+z)}{(1+z)(1+2z)(1+3z)}$	d	8	5·2
{1⁴}	$6np^3q^3$	$\dfrac{6npq(p+z)(p+2z)(q+z)(q+2z)}{(1+z)(1+2z)(1+3z)(1+4z)(1+5z)}$	e	4	2·1
{1²2}	$3np^3q^2$	$\dfrac{3npq(p+z)(p+2z)(q+z)}{(1+z)(1+2z)(1+3z)(1+4z)}$	f	3	3·1
{121}	$3np^3q$	$\dfrac{3npq(p+z)(p+2z)}{(1+z)(1+2z)(1+3z)}$	g	10	13·8
{13}	np^3	$\dfrac{np(p+z)(p+2z)}{(1+z)(1+2z)}$	h	67	66·3
Total	n	n	n	100	100·0

a small change to give finally, after recalculation of the information and co-variance matrices,

$$\check{p} = 0.805 \pm 0.018, \quad \check{z} = 0.738 \pm 0.176.$$

Casual inspection shows that the fit is now quite good, as is verified by the calculated value of 0.32 for χ^2 with one degree of freedom. The corresponding values of x and y are 1.091 and 0.264, respectively. Since y is less than unity, this means that the beta-distribution in (14.16) is J-shaped with an infinite ordinate at $p = 1$.

Households of four

A similar analysis may be undertaken for households of four individuals. The appropriate expectations and observations are set out in Table 14.13 for the modified form of the Greenwood model. The corresponding Reed—Frost version is a little more complicated and perhaps not worth dealing with in detail at present. For reasons of space the expected frequencies are given only in terms of p and z.

The required maximum-likelihood scores are now

$$
\left.
\begin{aligned}
S_p &= \frac{n-a}{p} - \frac{n-h}{q} + \frac{n-a-b}{p+z} + \frac{e+f+g+h}{p+2z} - \frac{n-g-h}{q+z} \\
&\quad - \frac{a+b+c+e}{q+2z} - \frac{b+c}{q+3z}, \\
S_z &= -\frac{n}{1+z} - \frac{2n}{1+2z} - \frac{3(n-a-h)}{1+3z} - \frac{4(b+c+e+f)}{1+4z} \\
&\quad - \frac{5(c+e)}{1+5z} + \frac{n-a-b}{p+z} + \frac{2(e+f+g+h)}{p+2z} \\
&\quad + \frac{n-g-h}{q+z} + \frac{2(a+b+c+e)}{q+2z} + \frac{3(b+c)}{q+3z},
\end{aligned}
\right\} (14.23)
$$

with observed information functions as overleaf.

$$I_{pp} = \frac{n-a}{p^2} + \frac{n-h}{q^2} + \frac{n-a-b}{(p+z)^2} + \frac{e+f+g+h}{(p+2z)^2} + \frac{n-g-h}{(q+z)^2}$$

$$+ \frac{a+b+c+e}{(q+2z)^2} + \frac{b+c}{(q+3z)^2},$$

$$I_{pz} = \frac{n-a-b}{(p+z)^2} + \frac{2(e+f+g+h)}{(p+2z)^2} - \frac{n-g-h}{(q+z)^2} - \frac{2(a+b+c+e)}{(q+2z)^2} - \frac{3(b+c)}{(q+3z)^2},$$

$$I_{zz} = -\frac{n}{(1+z)^2} - \frac{4n}{(1+2z)^2} - \frac{9(n-a-h)}{(1+3z)^2} - \frac{16(b+c+e+f)}{(1+4z)^2} - \frac{25(c+e)}{(1+5z)^2}$$

$$+ \frac{n-a-b}{(p+z)^2} + \frac{4(e+f+g+h)}{(p+2z)^2} + \frac{n-g-h}{(q+z)^2} + \frac{4(a+b+c+e)}{(q+2z)^2} + \frac{9(b+c)}{(q+3z)^2}.$$

$$(14.24)$$

This time there seems to be no very satisfactory way of obtaining initial estimates, but we can always try out a few arbitrary values, selecting for the full scoring process those pairs of values which on the whole give the smallest scores. In the present case we can start with the estimates already obtained for families of three. As the scoring procedure has already been illustrated above, we need only give the final result here, which is

$$\hat{p} = 0.822 \pm 0.028, \quad \hat{z} = 0.521 \pm 0.178.$$

Again, the fitted values closely follow the observations. Grouping the first six classes into three pairs gives a total of 4 degrees of freedom. Thus there are 2 degrees of freedom for the goodness-of-fit χ^2 which is 2.16, indicating a perfectly adequate fit.

It is worth noticing that the estimates of p and z do not differ significantly between households of three and four, so we can combine the results using weighted means, where the weights are the reciprocals of the variances. This gives the rather more accurate pooled estimates

$$\hat{p} = 0.810 \pm 0.015, \quad \hat{z} = 0.630 \pm 0.125,$$

with $$\hat{x} = 1.29, \quad \hat{y} = 0.30.$$

14.43   Significance tests for variation in chance of infection

Since we may expect that sometimes the chance of infection will not vary appreciably from family to family, we shall often be interested to test whether failure of the simple model, involving p only, to fit the data could be explained by a value of $\hat{z}$ significantly different from zero. We can, of course, do this by estimating p and z jointly, as shown above, and then applying a specific test to $\hat{z}$. In general we shall want a one-sided test, since z is an essentially nonnegative quantity. It is, however, rather quicker to avoid the full scoring procedure by basing a significance test, also in general one-sided, on the distribution of the score S_z, calculated for the values $z = 0$ and $p = \hat{p}_0$, where $\hat{p}_0$ is the maximum-likelihood estimate of p when $z = 0$. Thus, for households of three, this value is given by

$$\hat{p}_0 = \frac{b + 2c + 2d}{2a + 3b + 3c + 2d}, \tag{14.25}$$

which is equation (14.8) above repeated here for convenience. The score for z is

$$S_z(\hat{p}_0, 0) = \frac{c + d}{\hat{p}_0} + \frac{a + b}{1 - \hat{p}_0} - (a + 3b + 3c + d), \tag{14.26}$$

with variance

$$\text{var } \{S_z(\hat{p}_0, 0)\} = \frac{n(3 - 7pq)}{1 + pq}. \tag{14.27}$$

The expression on the right of (14.27) is calculated from the fact that in large samples

$$\text{var } \{S_z(\hat{p}_0, 0)\} = [I_{zz} - I_{pz}^2/I_{pp}]_{z=0}. \tag{14.28}$$

For the data in Table 14.12 we have $\hat{p}_0 = 0.789$ and $S_z = 172 \pm 23$, giving a highly significant result as expected. If this result had not been significant we could hardly have expected the failure of fit with p only to be explained by variation in infectiousness of the type envisaged and so could have avoided the full procedure of estimating both p and z.

With families of four the test is not quite so simple, but we can still test the significance of z without using the full scoring technique. This time we have

$$\hat{p}_0 = \frac{b + 2(c + d) + 3(e + f + g + h)}{3a + 5b + 6c + 4d + 6e + 5f + 4g + 3h}, \tag{14.29}$$

i.e. the same as (14.9), and

$$S_z(\hat{p}_0, 0) = \frac{(c + d) + 3(e + f + g + h)}{\hat{p}_0} + \frac{3(a + e) + 6(b + c) + (d + f)}{1 - \hat{p}_0}$$

$$- (3a + 10b + 15c + 6d + 15e + 10f + 6g + 3h). \tag{14.30}$$

We must calculate the variance of this score directly, using (14.28), where

$$I_{pp} = \frac{b + 2(c + d) + 3(e + f + g + h)}{\hat{p}_0^2} + \frac{3(a + e) + 4(b + c) + 2(d + f) + g}{(1 - \hat{p}_0)^2},$$

$$I_{pz} = \frac{(c + d) + 3(e + f + g + h)}{\hat{p}_0^2} - \frac{3(a + e) + 6(b + c) + (d + f)}{(1 - \hat{p}_0)^2},$$

$$I_{zz} = \frac{(c + d) + 5(e + f + g + h)}{\hat{p}_0^2} + \frac{5(a + e) + 14(b + c) + (d + f)}{(1 - \hat{p}_0)^2}$$

$$- \{5(a + h) + 30(b + f) + 55(c + e) + 14(d + g)\},$$

(14.31)

since there does not appear to be any simplified formula corresponding to
(14.27). Applying these results to the data of Table 14.13 gives $\hat{p}_0 = 0.791$
and $S_z = 157 \pm 41$, again a strongly significant finding.

14.44   Estimation of parameters from total size of epidemic

If, following the line of thought already mentioned in several places, we
preferred to base the estimation of p and z on the distribution of total size
of epidemic, then we should require basic tables of expectations and observations formed from Tables 14.12 and 14.13, for example, by amalgamating
the appropriate lines. Maximum-likelihood estimation would be straightforward though rather more laborious, and hardly worth undertaking here.

14.45   Apparent change in infectiousness

It is of considerable epidemiological importance to know whether the
infectiousness of a disease changes during the course of an epidemic. Where
the community as a whole is concerned, we might estimate p from suitable
households, using batches of data relating to different periods of time during
the course of the epidemic. On the other hand, some writers (e.g. Hope
Simpson, 1952) have suggested estimating the chance of infection at each
stage of the chain-binomial process within households. Although this may
sometimes be valid there is a danger of being misled if p varies from household to household. For example, consider Table 14.12. The expected numbers of households with 0, 1 and 2 cases at the first stage are $nq(q + z)/(1 + z)$,
$2npq/(1 + z)$ and $np(p + z)/(1 + z)$, respectively, for which the expected
number of new cases is easily seen to be $2np$. With two susceptibles at
risk, this means that the ordinary "susceptible-exposure attack-rate" estimated by $(b + c + 2d)/2n$ will on average be exactly p. But the corresponding estimate from the second stage, $c/(b + c)$, is on average $(p + z)/(1 + 2z)$,
which is always nearer to 0.5 than p itself. Similarly with larger households.
Whenever there is a chance of p varying between households, it seems advisable to test this possibility as described above before jumping to conclusions
about changes in infectiousness.

14.46   Note on ascertainment

In discussing the effect of variations in p between households we have im-
plicitly assumed that this variation occurred only in respect of the chance of
cross-infection within each household, such as might be brought about by differences in overcrowding. The chance of the first case occurring has been taken
to be the same for all households. If, on the other hand, the probability of
the first case varies, then all households do not have the same chance of entering the record. Such a state of affairs is closely analogous to that occurring in
genetics, when the chance of a family being noticed may depend on the number
of abnormal individuals it contains. This is usually referred to as *ascertainment*
(see Fisher, 1934; Bailey, 1951). In the present context we might suppose that
the chance of entering the record was proportional to p, which would only
entail replacing x or z by $x + 1$ or $(x + y + 1)^{-1}$, respectively; the estimate of
p would remain unchanged. More important is the effect of ascertainment on
the situation in which variation *between individuals* is basic. This is discussed
below in Section 14.5.

14.5   Variations between individuals

We now consider the effect of variations between individuals. This is the
kind of thing we might expect to persist even if we had succeeded in classi-
fying our data into groups which were reasonably homogeneous so far as
differences in cross-infection were concerned. For even with households sufficiently alike in social class, hygiene, nutrition, etc., there are bound to be
important differences between the members of any household with regard
to such factors as age, sex, patterns of behaviour, etc., and these may easily
affect the chance of infection being transferred between any two individuals.
Changes in immunity with age are also well known to epidemiologists. Moreover, some interesting empirical evidence on the way the chance of infection
might vary according to the type of recipient—donor pair considered, e.g.
baby—mother, was given by Heasman in the discussion on the Royal Statistical Society paper by Bailey (1955).

14.51   The basic model

We shall suppose here that p varies independently from person to person
with some, at present, unspecified frequency distribution. The question of
ascertainment is vital. For, neglecting the possibility of multiple introductions,
it is clear that households containing relatively immune individuals will contract an initial case, and so be recorded, less frequently than those with several
highly susceptible persons. Provided that the epidemic is not too prevalent in
the general community it is reasonable to assume that the probability of a
particular household having a given member as the initial case is proportional
to that member's chance of infection. Suppose we restrict attention to households of three, for which the members, in some arbitrary order, have

independent chances of infection p_1, p_2 and p_3, equal to $1 - q_1$, $1 - q_2$ and $1 - q_3$, respectively. The chance that the household enters the record through the first member being infected from outside is taken to be kp_1, where k is a small constant; and kp_2 and kp_3 for the other two members, respectively. When the first member is the initial case, the conditional distribution of the four types of chain is given by Table 14.14.

Table 14.14 *Conditional distribution of chains when first member is initial case*

Type of chain	Probability
{1}	$q_2 q_3$
{1²}	$p_2 q_3^2 + p_3 q_2^2$
{1³}	$p_2 q_3 p_3 + p_3 q_2 p_2$
{12}	$p_2 p_3$

In order to obtain the frequencies expected in a sample, we first multiply each probability in Table 14.14 by kp_1, and then add the corresponding expressions for the second and third members, after which we take expectations over the distribution of p. If we write

$$\mathrm{E}(p_i) = P = 1 - Q, \quad \mathrm{var}(p_i) = v, \tag{14.32}$$

so that

$$\mathrm{E}(p_i^2) = P^2 + v, \quad \mathrm{E}(p_i q_i) = PQ - v, \quad \mathrm{E}(q_i^2) = Q^2 + v, \\ \mathrm{E}(p_i p_j) = P^2, \text{etc.}, \tag{14.33}$$

then the required expectations, after removing a factor $3kP$ to make the frequencies sum to unity, finally take the form shown in Table 14.15.

Table 14.15 *Chains for households of three with a variable chance of infection between individuals*

Type of chain	Expected number	Observed number	Providence measles data	Fitted values
{1}	nQ^2	a	34	12·4
{1²}	$2nP(Q^2 + v)$	b	25	42·7
{1³}	$2nP(PQ - v)$	c	36	61·4
{12}	nP^2	d	239	217·5
Total	n	n	334	334·0

14.52 Estimation of parameters

The usual maximum-likelihood procedure gives

$$\hat{P} = \frac{b + c + 2d}{2n},$$

and

$$\hat{v} = \frac{(2a + b + c)\{b(b + 2d) - c(2a + c)\}}{4n^2(b + c)}. \tag{14.34}$$

Substituting in the Providence figures gives $\hat{P} = 0.807$ and $\hat{v} = 0.0418$. Inspection of the fitted values shows that this type of hypothesis does not give a satisfactory explanation of the data, and the alternative assumption of variation in the chance of infection between households is preferable. The variance of the estimate $\hat{P}$ is $PQ/2n$, but a simple formula for var (v) is not available. It could, of course, be evaluated from Fisher's formula

$$\text{var}(T) = \Sigma \bar{a}\left(\frac{\partial T}{\partial a}\right)^2 - n\left(\frac{\partial T}{\partial n}\right)^2, \tag{14.35}$$

where the observed numbers a, etc. are replaced by their expectations after differentiation. Alternatively, one could go through the full maximum-likelihood procedure of deriving the information matrix and then inverting it.

14.6 Errors in counting susceptibles

So far in the discussion of chain-binomial theory we have always assumed that the actual numbers of infectives and susceptibles are known exactly. Even when there is difficulty in recognizing different chains, we have supposed that the initial and final states of the household epidemic could be accurately recorded. In practice, there are several ways in which these assumptions may fail to be fulfilled. With a disease like measles it is usual to regard all individuals with a previous history of attack as being immune, and all those with no such history as being susceptible. However, with many diseases it is common for sub-clinical attacks to confer immunity, while overt immunizing attacks may be forgotten. Alternatively, immunity acquired in the past may be diminished or lost with the passage of time. Thus there is a distinct possibility of error in the numbers of both immunes and susceptibles. We shall show below how such errors can be allowed for.

14.61 Sub-clinical immunizations

The source of error most easily taken into account is that arising from sub-clinical immunizations, or even forgotten immunizing attacks. Abbey (1952) discussed this aspect in her investigation of Reed–Frost theory in measles epidemics, but did not give details of the analysis used. Apparently an additiona parameter was introduced to estimate the chance that a family of four, for example, really contained only two susceptibles instead of three. Unfortunately, satisfactory fits of theory to observation were not obtained. We can, however, generalize further, as is done below, and take into account the possibility of such a family containing only one susceptible or even none.

Ascertainment is again important here, as households which have a small number of true susceptibles (as opposed to apparent ones) will develop their initial case less often than those with a large number, and so come into the record less frequently. It is appropriate therefore to assume that the chance of a household entering the records is proportional to the number of susceptibles it contains, including the initial case. Let us suppose that households of a given size in the population have a binomial distribution of susceptibles with parameter α. Then households that have been actually ascertained are easily shown to yield a binomial distribution of susceptibles, with parameter α, *not counting the initial case.*

Consider households of three. The proportions of these with 0, 1 and 2 true susceptibles apart from the initial case are $(1 - \alpha)^2$, $2\alpha(1 - \alpha)$ and α^2, respectively. The first of the three types with no true susceptibles can lead only to the chain $\{1\}$. The second, with one susceptible, will yield $\{1\}$ and $\{1^2\}$ with probabilities q and p; while the third type gives rise to all four classes $\{1\}$, $\{1^2\}$, $\{1^3\}$ and $\{12\}$, with the usual probabilities q^2, $2pq^2$, $2p^2q$ and p^2. Combining these frequencies gives the expectations shown in Table 14.16.

Table 14.16   *Chains for households of three with missed immunes*

Type of chain	Expected number	Observed number
$\{1\}$	$n(1 - \alpha p)^2$	a
$\{1^2\}$	$2n\alpha p(1 - \alpha + \alpha q^2)$	b
$\{1^3\}$	$2n\alpha^2 p^2 q$	c
$\{12\}$	$n\alpha^2 p^2$	d
Total	n	n

Maximum-likelihood estimation can proceed in the usual way. If we were dealing with households of four or more, the ordinary method of calculating scores and information functions would be the only satisfactory course. With households of three, however, we can obtain explicit solutions, and can short-cut the work by noticing that the model is formally the same as that exhibited in Table 14.15. This is equivalent to thinking in terms of a variable p, taking the values 0 and p with probabilities $1 - \alpha$ and α. We can then use (14.32) to write the parameters P and v as

$$P = \alpha p, \quad v = \alpha p^2 - (\alpha p)^2, \tag{14.36}$$

from which it follows that

$$p = \frac{P^2 + v}{P}, \quad \alpha = \frac{P^2}{P^2 + v}. \tag{14.37}$$

The required estimates can then be obtained by substituting the values of $\hat{P}$ and $\hat{v}$, given by (14.34), in (14.37). General formulae for the variances are bound to be complicated. If therefore the efficient estimates $\hat{p}$ and $\hat{\alpha}$ obtained by the above method lead to a satisfactory goodness-of-fit χ^2, it is probably best to re-work the calculations on the basis of the scoring technique so as to find the variances. So far as the Providence measles data are concerned, we have already shown that the hypothesis of variations in p between individuals is inadequate. Since the present model can be regarded as a special case of this, the same poor fit would be obtained.

14.62 Lost immunity

The question of lost immunity is a little more complicated to deal with. In the absence of suitable data to investigate we shall only give a brief indication of the kind of analysis required. This should, however, suggest the form in which data involving the possible loss of immunity ought to be collected.

Let us take the simplest possible case that will lead to the calculation of estimates, namely a household of three in which there is one initial infective, one known susceptible, and one apparent immune whose chance of having lost immunity is β. We can follow the same kind of argument as in Section 14.31. We have a group of two, including a single primary case with probability $1 - \beta$, and a group of three with a single primary with probability β, according as the apparent immune is or is not really immune. It is a simple matter to combine the appropriate frequencies to give the quantities shown in Table 14.17, from which estimates of p and β can be derived if necessary.

Table 14.17   *Chains for households of three, containing one initial case, one susceptible and one apparent immune*

Type of chain	Expected number	Observed number
{1}	$nq(1 - \beta + \beta q)$	a
{1²}	$np(1 - \beta + 2\beta q^2)$	b
{1³}	$2n\beta p^2 q$	c
{12}	$n\beta p^2$	d
Total	n	n

It is hardly worth pursuing this topic further at present, but the example presents sufficiently clearly the type of data required. In practice, a fair amount of enumeration of the various types of household would be needed, and one could even envisage allowing for both lost immunity and subclinical immunization.

14.7 Extra-household infections

All the chain-binomial models discussed so far in this chapter assume that the epidemic process within any household is started off by one or more simultaneously infected primary cases, after which the introduction of fresh infections from outside is supposed to be unlikely. If the disease is highly infectious, as already observed in at least some measles data, this supposition is not unreasonable. But with a lower degree of intra-household infectiousness, the possibility of some contamination from outside the household should be considered.

Yamamoto (1959) discussed extensions, in relation to influenza, both of the Reed—Frost and Greenwood types of models, in which there is a probability p of adequate contact between any two specified members of the household, and a probability π of an introduction occurring from outside the household. There are certain difficulties in specifying such a model in a completely satisfactory way, and a more detailed treatment was given by Sugiyama (1960, 1961). He supposes that we have a sequence of basic time-periods, equal in length to the latent period. Then p is the probability that a given susceptible will be infected by a given infective during a particular time-period, while π is the probability that the susceptible will contract the disease by outdoor infection during the time-period.

Let T be the length of the basic time-period. Then we start observation of the households in a given area at time t, and record what happens at successive moments $t + T$, $t + 2T$, etc. In the case where there are only three susceptibles, Sugiyama proposes to concentrate attention on only three time-intervals. There are then 20 different types of observable outcome, depending on how many cases are recorded at each stage, including zeros. Consider for example the realization $\{1 \to 1 \to 0\}$, or $\{1^2 0\}$ in an obvious extension of our previous notation. The first case must be infected from outside, and the probability of observing one case amongst three susceptibles is $3\pi(1-\pi)^2$. In the second time-interval the probability of a susceptible escaping infection from both outside and inside is $(1-\pi)(1-p)$. Hence the binomial probability of observing just one case in the two susceptibles is $2\{1 - (1-\pi)(1-p)\}(1-\pi)(1-p)$. Lastly, the probability of no further cases in the last stage with only one susceptible remaining is just $(1-\pi)(1-p)$. The resultant probability of $\{1^2 0\}$ is thus

$$6\pi(1-\pi)^4 (1-p)^2 \{1 - (1-\pi)(1-p)\}.$$

Sugiyama enumerates all 20 outcomes with their corresponding probabilities

for the case of three-susceptible households observed for three periods, and
shows how to proceed with maximum-likelihood estimation of the parameters
p and π. The scoring approach already adopted many times in the present
chapter is quite straightforward on account of the multiplicative form of the
individual probabilities. An illustration is given by Sugiyama of an application
to A-Asia 57 influenza epidemic data from Osaka.

While the idea of investigating the importance of extra-household, or outdoor,
infections is obviously an excellent one, there is a serious unresolved problem
in setting up a sufficiently realistic model. We may quite legitimately assume
that, in diseases with a relatively stable latent period, followed by a fairly short
infectious period, the chaining of at least the early stages of a purely intra-
household epidemic will be identifiable in terms of distinct generations of appropriate binomial distributions. But there is no good reason to suppose that
any outdoor infections after the first one will be introduced synchronously with
the existing sequence of generations. In special cases of nearly constant latent
periods and very short infectious periods, it might be possible to discern a
superposed sequence of generations derived from outside that was out of phase
with an existing sequence. But in general it would seem that much more searching type of analysis would be required to handle the problem of extra-household infections.

14.8 Discussion

In view of the various modifications proposed in this chapter for rehabili-
tating the original chain-binomial models, it is worth while giving a short account
of the general implications as they appear at the time of writing.

When Greenwood (1931) originally put forward his chain-binomial model for
measles (taken from the 1926 outbreak in St Pancras), he found quite satisfactory
agreement of the theory with several bodies of data on households with totals
of 3, 4, 5 and 6 members, using an analysis based on the total number of cases.
Actually he estimated p by equating the observed and expected mean numbers
of cases. Maximum efficiency is of course achieved by the method of Section
14.32. In subsequent studies of measles epidemics in Providence, Rhode Island,
Wilson et al. (1939) observed that although such analyses, based on total epidemic size, often but not always gave reasonably adequate descriptions of the
data, the theory broke down completely when an attempt was made to account
for individual links of chains. As shown, however, in Section 14.4 above, the
situation can be saved by postulating variation in p between households. Non-
significant values of χ^2 are obtained for the two reasonably large samples on
households with totals of three and four individuals. To be satisfactorily vali-
dated the analysis needs to be repeated on more extensive material. It will be
recalled that the distribution of p implied by the investigations of Section
14.42 was a very broad one, J-shaped in fact with an infinite ordinate at $p = 1$.
While this is quite in keeping with the character of the data, which were collected

over a period of five years, and presumably entailed much important environmental variation as well, it would be a useful check in future work to try to
divide up extensive records into more homogeneous groups. If, for example,
overcrowding were an important factor in influencing the value of p, then analyses for sections of the data, in which the number of rooms per individual,
say, were relatively constant, ought to show more circumscribed distributions
of $\dot{p}$. This state of affairs would be revealed by comparatively small values of
z in each of several groups, for which estimates of p might differ widely.

Although it is freely admitted that more evidence is required, an encouraging sign is that while the model with p varying between households appears
acceptable, other alternatives, such as a straight or truncated binomial distribution of total epidemic size (see Section 13.35) or the model involving variations in chance of infection between individuals, are unequivocally rejected.
The data available are therefore sufficiently extensive to discriminate between
the alternative hypotheses so far considered.

Subsequent studies by Horiuchi *et al.* (1959) on measles confirmed the value
of the chain-binomial approach in a different epidemiological environment. Using
the model of Section 14.4, values of 0·66, 0·72 and 0·79 were obtained for $\bar{p}$
in three different Japanese cities. The x and y estimates suggested a J-shaped
distribution in one case, but a bell-shaped curve in the other two. However,
the amounts of data available, only 45 households in all, were rather too small
for very firm results to be obtained.

Application of chain-binomials, with or without modifications, to diseases
other than measles should also be the subject of further research. Lidwell and
Sommerville (1951), Heasman (discussion on Bailey, 1955), and Heasman and
Reid (1961) reported successes with the common cold. Hope Simpson and
Sutherland (1954), on the other hand, obtained somewhat ambiguous results
for influenza. Chain-binomial analyses were also used by Hope Simpson (1952)
to investigate the infectiousness of chicken-pox and mumps, as well as measles.
Although the technical niceties of a full mathematical treatment were avoided,
results of considerable interest and epidemiological importance appeared to
emerge.

In recent years there seems to have been relatively little interest in statistical
applications of chain-binomial models, with the exception of the interference
models discussed in Chapter 18. There is no doubt that this approach, though
making somewhat severely restrictive assumptions, can help to elucidate results
of epidemiological interest. However, since variable latent periods and extended
infectious periods seem to be the rule rather than the exception, it is natural
to try to construct models that are more realistic in these respects than simple
chain-binomials. In this way more information of biological and epidemiological
significance can be extracted from a given body of data. Such models, having
a more detailed structure, will be discussed in the next chapter.

15

Latent, infectious, and incubation periods

15.1 Introduction

Up to the present we have employed only two kinds of basic stochastic models for epidemic processes. The first is the continuous-infection type discussed extensively in Part 2, in which a susceptible becomes infectious immediately after the receipt of infection and continues in this state until removal from circulation by death or isolation. If the time elapsing between receiving infectious material and the development of infectiousness were short, and if the infectious period up to removal were approximately negative exponential in distribution, then such a model would be quite appropriate. Whether this closely mimics any actual disease is still uncertain, though scarlet fever and diphtheria, for example, would be strong candidates. The second model, dealt with in Chapters 8 and 14, assumes roughly constant incubation periods and very short periods of infectiousness, leading, apart from certain modifications, to basic chains of binomial distributions. For measles, at any rate, one version of this representation has met with some success, the small amount of data available passing the appropriate goodness-of-fit tests. Applications have also been made to mumps, chickenpox and the common cold.

Now in spite of the initial success of chain-binomial theory in describing household epidemics of measles, there is always a certain amount of difficulty in identifying the links of the chain. This is because the variation in time-interval between successive cases is often quite large, so that in a specific instance we are not sure whether we have a chain of, say, type $\{1^3\}$ or $\{12\}$. The same source of confusion may also leave us in doubt as to the kind of introduction involved, so that $\{1^3\}$ is mistaken for $\{21\}$. In practice it has usually been necessary to reject a certain amount of data, before a tidy classification into unambiguous chains was possible, and this of course reflects unfavourably on the resulting analysis. It is therefore worth while seeking for a model which will take into account the observed variation in time-interval between successive cases, and so enable all the data to be used. Not only should this improve the reliability of the analysis from a statistical point of view, but it might also be expected to throw more light on the nature of the biological process taking place.

We shall find it useful in the subsequent analysis to consider in more detail the notions of latency, incubation and infection already discussed generally in Chapter 3. The extent to which we shall require precise mathematical formulations of possible variations in these basic factors is considered below in Section 15.4. Here we shall merely recapitulate the main concepts.

After a susceptible individual exposed to a source of infection has actually become infected, a certain amount of biological development may be necessary before he can in turn pass the disease on to others. This interval of apparent quiescence is the latent period, which in general may be supposed to have its own frequency distribution. The latent period ends when the individual in question becomes a possible source of infection for other susceptibles. He continues in this state for the infectious period, which again may vary in length, as also may the intensity of infectiousness. During the infectious period other susceptibles at risk may become infected in accordance with some suitable probability law. When symptoms appear in the infective he is usually recognized as an actual case and withdrawn from circulation. Although he may still continue to excrete or exhale infectious material to some extent, in many diseases he is no longer a substantial risk to others. The infectious period is therefore effectively terminated as soon as symptoms are noticed. The time elapsing between receiving infection and registering symptoms is the incubation period, which is in this model the sum of the latent and infectious periods. As indicated in Chapter 3, there are several ways in which the real situation may involve further complications, such as symptoms occurring some time after the end of the infectious period, but the above description appears to represent the basic minimum required for the present discussion.

It should of course be emphasized that there is a good deal of information in the literature on incubation periods as such. See, for example, the papers and bibliographies of Sartwell (1950, 1966). However, knowledge is required, by direct observation or inference, of the time of exposure of each individual case. Sartwell found that lognormal distributions gave good descriptions of the variation in incubation periods for a considerable number of well-known diseases. Although such direct epidemiological observation can also yield information about latent and infectious periods, it is usually very difficult to obtain sufficient data for accurate estimates to be made. Moreover, inferences are often based on rather heterogeneous collections of material. The approach of the present chapter, on the other hand, is to try to construct models that will extract the maximum amount of information from appropriately collected bodies of relatively homogeneous data, thus allowing for the fact that basic biological parameters for a given disease may show appreciable variation between different communities, at different times, and under different environmental conditions.

We shall be concerned only with models that are sufficiently detailed to explain the observed epidemiological phenomena in terms of the mechanisms of population dynamics. We shall moreover confine attention to the simplest, reasonably adequate, continuous-time formulations. A somewhat different approach, already referred to in Section 8.1, is that of Bartoszyński (1967) utilizing a discrete-time Galton—Watson process. While this does incorporate variable latent and infectious periods, it neglects changes in the number of susceptibles as the epidemic develops.

Reference should also be made to more fundamental investigations in which attempts have been undertaken to relate empirical distributions of incubation periods and latent periods to the underlying pathogenic processes (Meynell and Meynell, 1958; Gart, 1965; Williams, 1965b,c; Armitage, Meynell and Williams, 1965; Puri, 1966, 1967; Meynell and Williams, 1967; Williams and Meynell, 1967; and Meynell and Maw, 1968).

We shall start by discussing in Section 15.2 the implications of some first-class data on measles in households of two susceptibles. The basic model proposed is described in Section 15.3, and the theory required for parameter estimation appears in Section 15.4 together with an application to the measles data. Section 15.5 treats various complications such as the effects of variation in the chance of infection, or making allowances for misclassified chains. Extensions to households of three are considered in Section 15.6. The improvements possible with appropriate computerization are indicated in Section 15.7, where illustrations are given for both measles and infectious hepatitis. Problems of further extension to larger groups of individuals are discussed in Section 15.8.

15.2 Preliminary analysis of data

Let us examine first the sort of data that arise in the simplest possible situation, where we have households with only two individuals, one of whom is the index case. It is at present not easy to find such material in the literature in a suitable form, although a considerable amount must be potentially available. The author is therefore greatly indebted to Dr R. E. Hope Simpson, of the Cirencester Public Health Laboratory Service, for allowing his own excellent collections of data to be used in this chapter.

Now in 264 households containing two children under the age of 15, one of whom is the index case and the other a susceptible at risk, there were 45 households with no further case and 219 with two cases in all. The distribution of time-interval between the latter two cases is shown in Table 15.1. It will be seen from the figures in the "Total" column for observed numbers of households that the distribution appears to consist of two distinct, though overlapping parts. The two parts, labelled A and B, are approximately indicated by the figures in the two adjacent columns on the left of the "Total" column. An obvious interpretation is that A arises from both susceptibles in the family

Table 15.1   *Observed and expected values for Hope Simpson's data on measles in households of two (Cirencester area 1946–52)*

Time-interval between two cases in days	Observed number of households			Expected number
	A	*B*	Total	
0	5	.	5	4·67
1	13	.	13	8·58
2	5	.	5	6·73
3	4	.	4	4·53
4	2	1	3 ⎫ 5	2·78 ⎫ 5·03
5	.	2	2 ⎭	2·25 ⎭
6	.	4	4	3·97
7	.	11	11	8·85
8	.	5	5	16·63
9	.	25	25	24·72
10	.	37	37	29·44
11	.	38	38	29·28
12	.	26	26	25·44
13	.	12	12	19·99
14	.	15	15	14·28
15	.	6	6	9·02
16	.	3	3 ⎫	4·82 ⎫
17	.	1	1 ⎪	2·09 ⎪
18	.	3	3 ⎬ 8	0·71 ⎬ 7·84
19	.	.	. ⎪	0·18 ⎪
20	.	.	. ⎪	0·04 ⎪
21	.	1	1 ⎭	0·00 ⎭
Sub-totals	29	190	219	219·00
One case only (*C*)			45	44·11
Primary and secondary (*B*)			190	190·89
Overall total (*A* + *B* + *C* = *N*)			264	264

having been infected simultaneously by contact with the same outside source of infection; and that *B* is due to cross-infection within the family.

The first modification of the strict chain-binomial model which we might try is, ignoring for the moment the possibility of variations in the chance of infection, to have a variable latent period with variance *v*, but still retaining a very short infectious period immediately followed by recognizable symptoms. On this hypothesis, *v* would be the variance of the *B*-distribution, which would reflect precisely the behaviour of the latent period. The *A*-distribution, on the other hand, arises from the absolute difference between two independently distributed latent periods, each starting at the same instant of time. It follows therefore that the second moment, V, of this distribution about the origin should be equal to $2v$. From Table 15.1 we have, ignoring the minor arbitrary decision involved in allocating observations where the two distributions overlap, estimates of 3·48 for V, based on 29 degrees of freedom, and 6·57 for v, with 189 degrees of freedom. On the assumption of a normally distributed latent period, V is significantly less than v, and the hypothesis that $V = 2v$ is quite untenable.

The next obvious choice of hypothesis is to have a variable latent period as above, followed by an extended but constant period of infectiousness. A somewhat intricate analysis is required for the investigation of this seemingly simple set-up, and this is described in detail below.

15.3 Basic model for households of two

The hypothesis mentioned at the end of the last section, namely, that the latent period is variable, with say a normal distribution, and that it is followed by an extended but constant period of infectiousness, was first suggested by Bailey in 1954, and investigated in greater detail in subsequent papers (Bailey, 1954a, 1955, 1956a, b, c). An encouraging measure of agreement has been obtained between theory and observation, and this seems to justify giving a fairly detailed description of the analysis involved. To facilitate application either to fresh measles data or to records on some other disease, a full account is provided of maximum-likelihood estimation. Section 15.4 contains all the scores and information functions required for a more or less mechanical calculation of the various parameters involved.

Let us assume that the latent period, ξ, is normally distributed with mean μ and variance σ^2, while the ensuing infectious period is of constant length α. Infection of the susceptible at risk during this time is taken to be a Poisson process such that the chance of his contracting the disease in time dt is λdt. Let the number of households observed in the A- and B-distributions be A and B, respectively, and let C be the number of households with only one case. We shall put $A + B + C = N$.

Now suppose that ω is the variable for the A-distribution. Since this is the absolute difference between two independent latent periods, the frequency distribution of ω is

$$f(\omega) = \frac{1}{\sigma\sqrt{\pi}} e^{-\omega^2/(4\sigma^2)}, \quad 0 \leqslant \omega < \infty. \tag{15.1}$$

Next, consider the $B + C$ families with either both a primary and a secondary case (B) or a single primary case only (C). The chance of the second susceptible escaping infection by the first case during the infectious period α is $e^{-\lambda\alpha}$. Hence the probability of the observed numbers, B and C, given $B + C$, is

$$\binom{B + C}{B} e^{-C\lambda\alpha}(1 - e^{-\lambda\alpha})^B. \tag{15.2}$$

Further, the distribution of the time-interval τ, from the beginning of the infectious period to the point at which infection of the second case actually takes place is evidently

$$f(\tau) = \lambda e^{-\lambda\tau}(1 - e^{-\lambda a})^{-1}, \quad 0 \leqslant \tau \leqslant \alpha. \tag{15.3}$$

Let distribution B arise from a variable $\zeta = \xi + \tau$, where, of course, ξ has the frequency function

$$f(\xi) = (2\pi\sigma^2)^{-\frac{1}{2}} \exp\{-(\xi - \mu)^2/(2\sigma^2)\}, \quad -\infty < \xi < \infty. \tag{15.4}$$

The frequency distribution of ζ is obtained by using (15.3) and (15.4) to write down the joint frequency distribution for ξ and τ, replacing ξ by $\zeta - \tau$, and integrating out τ. This gives

$$f(\zeta) = \frac{\lambda \exp\{-\lambda(\zeta - \mu - \frac{1}{2}\lambda\sigma^2)\}}{1 - \exp(-\lambda\alpha)} \int_{u'}^{u} \frac{1}{\sqrt{(2\pi)}} \exp(-\frac{1}{2}t^2)dt, \tag{15.5}$$

where $\quad u = \sigma^{-1}\{\zeta - (\mu + \lambda\sigma^2)\} \quad$ and $\quad u' = u - \alpha\sigma^{-1}. \tag{15.6}$

We shall also need the sample mean, $\bar{\zeta}$, and variance, v, of the B-distribution, together with the observed second moment about the origin, $V = \Sigma\omega^2/A$, for the A-distribution.

15.4   Estimation of parameters

Using the three frequency functions given in (15.1), (15.2) and 15.5) above, we can proceed in the usual way to derive maximum-likelihood scores and information functions for the parameters λ, α, μ and σ. In order to do this as concisely as possible let us first write

$$R(\zeta) \equiv \int_{u'}^{u} \frac{1}{\sqrt{(2\pi)}} \exp(-\frac{1}{2}t^2)dt, \tag{15.7}$$

and

$$T_\theta = \frac{1}{R}\frac{\partial R}{\partial\theta}, \quad \theta = \lambda, \alpha, \mu, \sigma. \tag{15.8}$$

Amalgamating the three contributions to each score then gives quite simply

$$\left.\begin{aligned}
S_\lambda &\equiv \partial L/\partial\lambda = B(\mu - \bar{\zeta} + \lambda^{-1} + \lambda\sigma^2) - C\alpha && + \sum_\zeta T_\lambda, \\
S_a &\equiv \partial L/\partial\alpha = && -C\lambda && + \sum_\zeta T_\alpha, \\
S_\mu &\equiv \partial L/\partial\mu = && B\lambda && + \sum_\zeta T_\mu, \\
S_\sigma &\equiv \partial L/\partial\sigma = A\sigma^{-1}(\frac{1}{2}V\sigma^{-2} - 1) && + B\lambda^2\sigma && + \sum_\zeta T_\sigma,
\end{aligned}\right\} \tag{15.9}$$

where L is as usual the log likelihood. The quantities T_θ are most easily calculated from the functions

$$Q(x) = \frac{1}{\sqrt{(2\pi)}} \exp\left(-\tfrac{1}{2}x^2\right), \quad P(x) = \int_{-x}^{x} Q(t)\,dt, \quad x \geqslant 0, \\
\left.\begin{array}{r} = -P(|x|), \quad x \leqslant 0, \end{array}\right\} \tag{15.10}$$

using the tables published by the New York W.P.A. (1942). We then have

$$\left.\begin{array}{ll}
R = \tfrac{1}{2}(P - P'), & \partial R/\partial\lambda = -\sigma(Q - Q'), \\[4pt]
\partial R/\partial\alpha = \sigma^{-1}Q', & \partial R/\partial\mu = -\sigma^{-1}(Q - Q'), \\[4pt]
\partial R/\partial\sigma = -\sigma^{-1}(uQ - u'Q') - 2\lambda(Q - Q'), \\[4pt]
\text{where} \quad P \equiv P(u), \quad P' \equiv P(u'), \quad Q \equiv Q(u), \quad Q' \equiv Q(u').
\end{array}\right\} \tag{15.11}$$

The T_θ are then obtained from (15.8), (15.10) and (15.11).

It should be noted that in the first edition of this book there was an error in the score S_σ in the fourth line of the old equation (7.9), where $B\lambda\sigma^2$ appeared instead of $B\lambda^2\sigma$. The correct form is given in (15.9) above.

The derivation of information functions also goes in a straightforward way. A minor point worth mentioning is that if we differentiate T_θ with respect to one of the parameters, say ϕ, we obtain

$$-T_\theta T_\phi + \frac{1}{R}\frac{\partial^2 R}{\partial\phi\,\partial\theta}.$$

The expectation of $R^{-1}\partial^2 R/\partial\phi\,\partial\theta$ is easily found since when multiplying by the frequency function in (15.5) the factors R in numerator and denominator cancel, and the integration with respect to ζ gives no special difficulty. With $T_\theta T_\phi$, on the other hand, the integrand involves a factor R^{-1}, and it seems best to leave these terms as observed quantities. In any case the individual values of T_θ and T_ϕ for each ζ have already been calculated in finding the scores. The information matrix, I, for the parameters λ, α, μ and σ, in that order, then turns out to be the symmetric array

$$\begin{bmatrix}
\begin{array}{l} \Sigma T_\lambda^2 \\ -\bar{B}(\lambda^2\sigma^4 + \sigma^2 - \lambda^{-2}), \end{array} & \begin{array}{l} \Sigma T_\lambda T_\alpha \\ +\dfrac{\bar{B}(1 + \lambda^2\sigma^2)}{e^{\lambda\alpha} - 1}, \end{array} & \begin{array}{l} \Sigma T_\lambda T_\mu \\ -\bar{B}(1 + \lambda^2\sigma^2), \end{array} & \begin{array}{l} \Sigma T_\lambda T_\sigma \\ -\bar{B}\lambda^3\sigma^3, \end{array} \\[20pt]
 & \begin{array}{l} \Sigma T_\alpha^2 \\ +\dfrac{\bar{B}\lambda^2}{e^{\lambda\alpha} - 1}, \end{array} & \begin{array}{l} \Sigma T_\alpha T_\mu \\ +\dfrac{\bar{B}\lambda^2}{e^{\lambda\alpha} - 1}, \end{array} & \begin{array}{l} \Sigma T_\alpha T_\sigma \\ +\dfrac{\bar{B}\lambda^3\sigma}{e^{\lambda\alpha} - 1}, \end{array} \\[20pt]
 & & \begin{array}{l} \Sigma T_\mu^2 \\ -\bar{B}\lambda^2, \end{array} & \begin{array}{l} \Sigma T_\mu T_\sigma \\ -\bar{B}\lambda^3\sigma, \end{array} \\[20pt]
 & & & \begin{array}{l} \Sigma T_\sigma^2 \\ -\bar{B}\lambda^4\sigma^2 + 2A\sigma^{-2} \end{array}
\end{bmatrix}$$

$$\tag{15.12}$$

where $$\bar{B} = (B + C)(1 - e^{-\lambda\alpha}),\tag{15.13}$$

and where the elements below the leading diagonal can be filled in by symmetry Writing $\mathbf{S}$ for the vector of scores calculated at trial values given by the vector $\boldsymbol{\theta}$, we calculate approximate maximum-likelihood values, $\boldsymbol{\theta}_1$, given by

$$\boldsymbol{\theta}_1 = \boldsymbol{\theta} + \boldsymbol{\Gamma}^{-1}\mathbf{S},\tag{15.14}$$

as is well known. The procedure is then repeated using $\boldsymbol{\theta}_1$ for the trial values until sufficient accuracy is obtained.

To obtain initial trial values it is convenient to use approximate estimates given by setting $V, C, \bar{\zeta}$ and v equal to their expectations. The first two of these are $2\sigma^2$ and $(B + C)e^{-\lambda\alpha}$, derived from (15.1) and (15.2), while the last two are given in (15.18) below. This leads to the values

$$\left.\begin{array}{l} \check{\lambda} = (1 - T)^{\frac{1}{2}}U^{-\frac{1}{2}}, \\[2mm] \check{\alpha} = \check{\lambda}^{-1}\log(1 + Y), \\[2mm] \check{\mu} = \bar{\zeta} - \check{\lambda}^{-1} + \check{\alpha}Y^{-1}, \\[2mm] \check{\sigma} = (\tfrac{1}{2}V)^{\frac{1}{2}}, \end{array}\right\}\tag{15.15}$$

where

$$\left.\begin{array}{l} T = Y^{-1}(1 + Y^{-1})\{\log(1 + Y)\}^2, \\[2mm] U = v - \tfrac{1}{2}V, \\[2mm] Y = B/C. \end{array}\right\}\tag{15.16}$$

Expressions for the large-sample variances of the estimates appearing in (15.15) are given in Bailey (1955), but as their precision seems on the whole to be rather low, it is recommended that they be used only as trial values to start the maximum-likelihood scoring procedure.

If it should happen that in any set of data A were small or zero then no satisfactory initial estimate of σ would be available from (15.15). However, it is still possible to obtain rough estimates by setting B equal to its expectation, leading to

$$\lambda\alpha = \log(1 + Y) \equiv F,\tag{15.17}$$

and by putting the first three sample cumulants, $\bar{\zeta}, v$ and m_3, in the B-distribution equal to their expectations, namely

$$\left.\begin{array}{ll} \kappa_1 \equiv \mu + \lambda^{-1} - \alpha(e^{\lambda\alpha} - 1)^{-1} & = \bar{\zeta}, \\[2mm] \kappa_2 \equiv \sigma^2 + \lambda^{-2} - \alpha^2 e^{\lambda\alpha}(e^{\lambda\alpha} - 1)^{-2} & = v, \\[2mm] \kappa_3 \equiv \quad 2\lambda^{-3} - \alpha^3 e^{\lambda\alpha}(e^{\lambda\alpha} + 1)(e^{\lambda\alpha} - 1)^{-3} & = m_3. \end{array}\right\}\tag{15.18}$$

Using (15.17) and (15.18), we can solve to the required estimates successively as follows.

$$
\left.
\begin{aligned}
\alpha^3 &= m_3\{2F^{-3} - Y^{-3}(1 + Y)(2 + Y)\}^{-1}, \\
\sigma^2 &= v - \alpha^2\{F^{-2} - Y^{-2}(1 + Y)\}, \\
\mu &= \bar{\xi} - \alpha(F^{-1} - Y^{-1}), \\
\lambda &= F\alpha^{-1}.
\end{aligned}
\right\}
\qquad (15.19)
$$

15.41   Application to measles data

Let us now apply the foregoing maximum-likelihood scoring procedure to Hope Simpson's measles data exhibited in Table 15.1. It has not been feasible to repeat the original calculations using the corrected form for S_σ, since these took several man-weeks on a desk computer. The following first-edition account has therefore been left unchanged for consistency of discussion. Actually, the errors involved are very small, as can be seen from the corrected results given in Section 15.7, which were obtained from a computerized method requiring only a few minutes of machine time.

Examination of the observed frequencies shows immediately that in attempting to fit any reasonably smooth curve to B we are likely to be troubled by an apparent excess of observations for days 7 and 14 (with corresponding deficits for adjacent days). This could be due to a small unconscious bias towards an integral number of weeks. A similar situation is not uncommon in other fields, e.g. interviewees may show a preference for ages ending in 0 or 5, and measurements of blood-pressure sometimes show a marked excess of readings which are even multiples of 10. One way of offsetting such bias is to pool the frequencies for, say, days 6, 7 and 8 in one group, and for 13, 14 and 15 in another group, when carrying out a goodness-of-fit test.

Preliminary estimates obtained from (15.15) are

$$
\left.
\begin{aligned}
\lambda &= 0.203, \\
\alpha &= 8.13 \text{ days}, \\
\mu &= 7.94 \text{ days}, \\
\sigma &= 1.32 \text{ days}.
\end{aligned}
\right\}
\qquad (15.20)
$$

Since these estimates are likely to be rather inefficient, we should not be surprised if the maximum-likelihood values are appreciably different. After one cycle of successive approximation the second set of estimates did in fact show large changes. When the third set of values was obtained the information matrix was recalculated, and convergence was then rapid. Stability was practically achieved with the fourth approximation—a final fifth stage gave only very small further corrections. The maximum-likelihood estimates found in this way are

$$\left.\begin{array}{l} \hat{\lambda} = 0\cdot256 \pm 0\cdot032, \\[6pt] \hat{\alpha} = 6\cdot57 \pm 0\cdot76 \text{ days}, \\[6pt] \hat{\mu} = 8\cdot58 \pm 0\cdot32 \text{ days}, \\[6pt] \hat{\sigma} = 1\cdot77 \pm 0\cdot13 \text{ days}. \end{array}\right\} \tag{15.21}$$

The average incubation period, given by $\hat{\alpha} + \hat{\mu}$, is thus $15\cdot15 \pm 0\cdot51$ days. (To obtain the latter standard error we must refer to the covariance matrix because we require the covariance of $\hat{\alpha}$ and $\hat{\mu}$ as well as their variances. It appears that these estimates have a strong negative correlation.)

When carrying out the usual goodness-of-fit test it is convenient to use the last approximation but one, if sufficiently accurate, since we need not then recalculate the $R(\zeta)$ in computing the function given by (15.5). In practice, of course, the data will normally be grouped in units of 1 day, as in Table 15.1. The fitted values for distribution B were obtained merely by calculating $f(\zeta)$ at the midpoint of each interval, as the small additional accuracy resulting from integration over the interval was not thought worth the extra labour of computation. On the other hand, integrated values for distribution A are immediately available from the tabulated values of $P(x)$ in (15.10). It can be seen from Table 15.1 that the agreement between observed and expected values is on the whole quite good. For the usual goodness-of-fit test the classes bracketed together have been pooled so as to avoid small expectations. There are sixteen classes for the combined A- and B-distribution, giving 15 d.f.; and two classes, giving 1 d.f., for the numbers B and C. From the total of 16 d.f. we must remove 4 to allow for the parameters estimated. We find an overall χ^2 of $20\cdot3$ on 12 d.f. As the 5 percent point is at $21\cdot0$, we can regard the fit as just adequate. Actually, we have already remarked the possibility of unconscious bias in the records producing local peaks at 7 and 14 days, and suggested that it could be minimized by amalgamating the frequencies for 6, 7 and 8 days in one group, and 13, 14 and 15 in another. When this is done we obtain a χ^2 of $12\cdot9$ on 8 d.f., which is entirely satisfactory since the 10 percent point is at $13\cdot4$.

It is also of some interest to see what would happen if certain portions of the data were missing. There may, for example, be no families with a double primary, i.e. $A = 0$. All we have to do is to remove the term $2A\sigma^{-2}$ from $I_{\sigma\sigma}$ in (15.12) before inverting the information matrix. Alternatively, there may be no record of C, the number of families with a single case only. No information about λ and α is then available from the frequency distribution in (15.2). Accordingly, we must remove from $I_{\lambda\lambda}$, $I_{\lambda\alpha}$ and $I_{\alpha\alpha}$ the contributions $W\alpha^2$, $W\alpha\lambda$ and $W\lambda^2$, respectively, where

$$W = (B + C)(e^{\lambda\alpha} - 1)^{-1}.$$

Again, both these items may be missing, and we may only have data on families with a primary and a secondary case. These results are summarized in Table 15.2, which shows the appropriate efficiencies derived by comparing the variances of the estimates in each case with the "best" values given by the squares of the standard errors appearing in (15.21). It is worth noticing that reasonably

Table 15.2 *Efficiencies (in percentages) of estimates with parts of data absent*

Data available	λ	α	μ	σ
All three sources present	100	100	100	100
No double primaries ($A = 0$)	79	70	77	60
No single cases ($C = 0$)	23	100	83	99
B-distribution only ($A = C = 0$)	22	70	68	59

efficient estimates of all four parameters can be obtained in the absence of double primary data, but that knowledge of the number of families with a single case is essential for an efficient determination of λ. Without the B-distribution, of course, little information of value would be forthcoming.

15.5 Various modifications

15.51 Effect of variation in chance of infection

As we saw above in Section 14.4, chain-binomials gave a satisfactory goodness-of-fit for the Providence measles data when analysed stage by stage only on the assumption that the chance of cross-infection, p, varied between households. In the notation of this chapter we have

$$p = 1 - e^{-\lambda\alpha}. \tag{15.22}$$

It follows that we ought in the present context to consider the possibility of variations in λ. We could hardly expect to make any precise estimate of parameters in the distribution of λ in households of two, but it is worth making a rough estimate of the likely consequences. We can do this by calculating the expectation, with respect to appropriate variations in λ, of the expected frequencies in the model. Now for the distribution of p given in (14.16), the mean and variance of p are

$$\left. \begin{array}{l} \bar{p} = 0 \cdot 81, \\[2mm] v_p = \dfrac{pqz}{1+z} = 0 \cdot 063, \end{array} \right\} \tag{15.23}$$

using the pooled estimates of p and z based on households of three and four, shown at the end of Section 14.42. Using the estimates of λ and α in (15.21), we see that the value of p given by (15.22) is about 0·81, the same as the estimate in (15.23) taken from the Providence data. If we now suppose p to vary about this mean value, the expected frequencies for the observations B

and C will remain unchanged. The A-distribution will also be the same since it involves only σ. However, the B-distribution given in (15.5) will be modified, and may be replaced, approximately, by

$$f(\zeta) + \frac{v_p}{2}\frac{\partial^2 f}{\partial p^2} = f(\zeta) + \frac{v_p e^{2\lambda\alpha}}{2\alpha^2}\left(\alpha\frac{\partial f}{\partial \lambda} + \frac{\partial^2 f}{\partial \lambda^2}\right), \qquad (15.24)$$

where we have simply expanded in powers of $\delta p = p - \bar{p}$ and have taken expectations, neglecting terms of third and higher order in δp. It may be noted that the additional quantities on the right-hand side of (15.24) are all easily calculated from those already available. It turns out that the net result is to flatten and displace slightly towards the origin the peak of the fitted curve. The χ^2 values are then a little higher. The data grouped so as to minimize the peaks at 7 and 14 days give a χ^2 of 14·3 on 8 d.f., which is still satisfactory. Without this adjustment we obtain 21·5 on 12 d.f., which is just significant at the 5 percent level. We conclude that the results would probably not be appreciably influenced by only moderate variations in the chance of infection.

15.52   Effect of variation in infectious period

A somewhat similar analysis can be undertaken in respect of variations in the length of the infectious period, α, but this is more complicated in that both the A- and B-distributions are affected, and each involves considering two independently variable infectious periods. Moreover, with measles at any rate, there is little scope for introducing any substantial variations of α into the present model. This can be seen from the fact that if the variance of α were v_α the expected second moment about the origin of the A-distribution would be $2\sigma^2 + 2v_\alpha$, and the observed value is only 3·48. However, it can be shown that even if v_α were, say, approximately unity, although the effect on the goodness-of-fit would be very small so far as the A-distribution is concerned, there would be an appreciable flattening of the B-curve. This is clearly a matter that requires further investigation.

15.53   Allowance for misclassification of chains

So far we have assumed that the basic chains of the mathematical model (almost trivial for households of two) can be correctly identified. For the class with only one case there is no possibility of error. When there are two cases, however, and the A- and B-distributions overlap, then there is a definite chance of misclassification. In the example discussed above, where the two distributions overlap only to a very small extent, the effect is likely to be only a minor one confined to a few borderline observations. With more substantial overlapping it is desirable to make proper allowance for it in the analysis. This can be done by introducing a new parameter, ψ, which is the prior probability that a family is of type A. Maximum-likelihood scoring for the five unknown parameters, λ, μ, α, σ and ψ, can then be carried through as before. It is, however, considerably more complicated than the case already discussed. For this reason an indication only of the modified procedure will be given. See Section 15.7 for a computerized method of handling.

First consider the information available from the number of families, C, with one case only. The expected proportion is clearly $(1 - \psi)e^{-\lambda\alpha}$ and this must now be referred to the whole sample N, and not merely to $B + C$ as before. The analogue of (15.2) is thus

$$\binom{N}{C}(1 - \psi)^C e^{-C\lambda\alpha}\{1 - (1 - \psi)e^{-\lambda\alpha}\}^{N-C}. \tag{15.25}$$

Next consider the $N - C$ families which are liable to misclassification with regard to the A- and B-distributions. If we write the frequency functions in (15.1) and (15.5) as f_1 and f_2, the contribution to the likelihood from any family with two cases separated by an interval of w days is

$$\frac{\psi f_1(w) + (1 - \psi)(1 - e^{-\lambda\alpha})f_2(w)}{1 - (1 - \psi)e^{-\lambda\alpha}}. \tag{15.26}$$

Combining the contributions from (15.25) and (15.26) gives for the log likelihood

$$L = C \log (1 - \psi) - C\lambda\alpha + \sum_w \log \{\psi f_1(w) + (1 - \psi)(1 - e^{-\lambda\alpha})f_2(w)\},$$

$$\tag{15.27}$$

where the summation is taken over the $N - C$ values of w.

Now suppose that there are A and B families that are almost certainly of types A and B, respectively, and D families of uncertain classification. Almost certain classification means that the value of w is such that one of the two frequencies $f_1(w)$ and $f_2(w)$ is negligibly small. In doubtful cases it may be safer to take $A = B = 0$. For the A and B almost certain families we therefore put $f_2 = 0$ and $f_1 = 0$, respectively. This leads to the modified expression

$$\begin{aligned} L = \; & A \log \psi + (B + C) \log (1 - \psi) - C\lambda\alpha \\ & + B \log (1 - e^{-\lambda\alpha}) \\ & + \sum_A \log f_1 + \sum_B \log f_2 \\ & + \sum_D \log \{\psi f_1 + (1 - \psi)(1 - e^{-\lambda\alpha})f_2\}. \end{aligned} \tag{15.28}$$

The expressions (15.27) or (15.28) can be used as a basis for the standard technique. Although the scores and information functions are now much more complicated, they contain certain components that are the same as in the simpler situation.

15.6 Extension to households of three

When we try to extend the ideas of the previous section to households of three we find that certain new features appear. The analysis is rather more complicated, though parts of it are very similar to that just described. As households of three are quite common, it is worth devoting some space to a discussion of the calculations required. Larger households can be dealt with in the same kind of way, but the procedure becomes rapidly more difficult, especially as misclassification of links in the chain develops into an item of major importance.

15.61 Classification of data

As shown above in Section 15.3, for households of two, the data, consisting of say a total of N households with at least one case, fall naturally into three parts. There are A households with two cases, both having been infected simultaneously by an outside contact. There are a further B households with two cases, where the second case is derived from the first by cross-infection within the household. We also know the time-interval between the two cases, ω for the first type and ζ for the second. As a first approximation we assume that these two types, which we can label $\{2\}$ and $\{1^2\}$ in chain-binomial notation, can be accurately distinguished. The third type of household, of which there are C, contains only a single case and is labelled $\{1\}$.

When dealing with households of three, the parts of the data involving one or two cases only can again be described as above and we shall use the same notation. But we also have in addition D households containing three cases, so that now $N = A + B + C + D$. These households are of four kinds, represented by the chain-binomial symbols $\{1^3\}$, $\{12\}$, $\{3\}$ and $\{21\}$, with actual numbers E, F, G and H, respectively, where $D = E + F + G + H$. This time there are two time-intervals to be recorded: u between the first and second cases, and v between the second and third cases. Assuming for the time being that the different types of chain can be correctly identified, we must consider the type of information they provide in some detail.

First, take the E households of type $\{1^3\}$, where the second case is derived from the first, and the third from the second, both by cross-infection within the household. The two intervals, u and v, are clearly each a "ζ-type" variable such as arises from the B households giving a $\{1^2\}$ pattern. Secondly, the F households of type $\{12\}$, where the second and third cases have been simultaneously infected by the first, also provide two ζ-type observations, but these are now given by u and $u + v$. We therefore have in all $J = B + 2(E + F)$ ζ-type observations which can be subjected to the analysis already presented in Section 15.3.

Next, we consider the G households of type $\{3\}$, where all three cases have been simultaneously infected by an outside contact. These must be examined separately as they cannot be put in terms of other types of data already discussed. The appropriate analysis is given in the next section.

The H households of type $\{21\}$, where the first two cases are derived from a simultaneous infection and the third by cross-infection, present a special difficulty. The first interval u is plainly an "ω-type" variable and can be taken in conjunction with the data for the A households of type $\{2\}$, giving $K = A + H$ households altogether. The second interval v has a very much more complicated distribution, since the third case could have been infected during either of the infectious periods of the first two cases. It seems better to ignore the small amount of information available from this source in order to avoid excessive complexity.

Table 15.3 *Distribution of time-interval for 15 households of three with two cases*

Time-interval in days	0	1	2	3	4		5	6	7	8	9	10	11	12	13	14
Number of families	.	2	.	1	1		.	2	1	1	.	.	3	1	2	1
Probable type of chain			$\{2\}$									$\{1^2\}$				
Total number			$A = 4$									$B = 11$				

Table 15.4 *Distribution of time-intervals (u, v) for 57 households of three with three cases*

Time (v) between second and third cases in days	Time (u) between first and second cases in days																	Total
	0	1	2	3	4	5	6	7	8	9	10	11	12	13	14	15	16	
0	.	1	1	.	.	.	.	.	.	6	1	3	1	1	.	.	.	14
1	2	1	.	.	.	.	1	.	.	.	3	3	1	.	.	.	1	12
2	1	.	.	.	.	.	1	1	.	2	2	3	.	.	2	.	.	12
3	.	.	1	.	.	.	.	.	1	1	.	1	.	.	.	.	.	4
4	.	.	.	.	.	.	.	2	.	.	.	.	.	.	.	.	.	2
5	.	.	.	.	.	.	1	.	2	.	.	.	.	.	.	.	.	3
6	.	.	.	1	.	.	.	.	.	.	.	.	.	.	.	.	.	1
7	.	.	.	.	.	.	.	.	.	.	.	.	.	.	.	.	.	.
8	.	.	.	.	.	.	.	.	.	.	.	.	.	1	.	.	.	1
9	1	.	.	.	.	.	.	.	.	.	.	.	.	.	1	.	.	2
10	.	.	1	.	.	.	.	.	.	.	.	.	.	.	.	.	.	1
11	.	1	.	.	.	.	.	.	.	.	.	.	.	.	.	.	.	1
12	1	1	.	.	.	.	.	.	.	.	.	.	.	.	.	.	.	2
13	.	.	.	.	.	.	.	.	.	.	.	.	.	.	.	1	.	1
14	1	.	.	.	.	.	.	.	.	.	.	.	.	.	.	.	.	1
Total	6	4	3	1	.	.	3	3	3	9	6	10	2	2	3	1	1	$57 = D$

Finally, we can analyse the data according to the numbers of households showing different types of chain, apart from the time-intervals involved. The main subdivision here depends on whether the disease is introduced by a single case or by two simultaneously infected cases. A triple introduction adds nothing further to what has already been mentioned in the last paragraph but one. When there are two initial cases, i.e. A of type $\{2\}$ or H of type $\{21\}$, the treatment is very similar to that given in Section 15.3 for the distribution of B, given $B + C$. When there is a single introduction we have types $\{1\}$, $\{1^2\}$, $\{1^3\}$ and $\{12\}$, with observed numbers C, B, E and F, where we write $M = B + C + E + F$.

A new point arises here in connexion with the possibility of variations in the chance of infection. As shown in Section 15.51, the ζ-type distribution is relatively insensitive to such variations, while the ω-type variables are quite unaffected. The mean frequencies of A and H will also be unchanged. Variation in the chance of infection is therefore ignored so far as those sections of the

Table 15.5   *Summary of Table 15.4 giving probable types of chain with observed numbers, based on a dividing line between 4 and 5 days*

$\{3\}$	$\{12\}$
$G = 7$	$F = 37$
$\{21\}$	$\{1^3\}$
$H = 7$	$E = 6$

Table 15.6   *Amalgamated frequencies for ω-distribution, with a total of $K = A + H$ observations (households of three)*

Time-interval in days	Observed number	Expected number
0	3 ⎱ 7	1·87 ⎱ 5·29
1	4 ⎰	3·42 ⎰
2	1 ⎱	2·61 ⎱
3	2 ⎰ 4	1·64 ⎰ 5·71
4	1 ⎰	0·88 ⎰
⩾5	·	0·58 ⎰
Total	11 = K	11·00

data are concerned. However, it has been shown in Section 14.4 that the chain-binomial analysis of households of three with a single initial case *is* considerably influenced by variations in the chance of infection. An additional parameter must therefore be introduced when this part of the data is analysed.

The last matter to be mentioned in this section is the question of correctly identifying the links of the chains involved. The distinction between $\{1^2\}$ and $\{2\}$ is accomplished in a similar manner to that described in Section 15.3.

Table 15.3 shows the distribution of 15 observations of this sort with an approximate dichotomy being made, as before, between 4 and 5 days. It is a little more difficult to separate the four groups of families with three cases and we now need to inspect a two-way table. The distribution of 57 observations is shown in Tables 15.4 and 15.5. Inspection of the marginal totals

Table 15.7 *Amalgamated frequencies for ζ-distribution, with a total of $J = B + 2(E + F)$ observations (households of three)*

Time-interval in days	Observed number	Expected number
0	⎫	⎫
1	⎪	⎪
2	⎪	0·01 ⎪
3	⎬ 8	0·04 ⎬ 4·32
4	⎪	0·24 ⎪
5	3	1·01 ⎪
6	5 ⎭	3·02 ⎭
7	5	6·64
8	6	10·97
9	17	14·16
10	7 ⎫ 31	15·00 ⎫ 28·80
11	24 ⎭	13·80 ⎭
12	10	11·55
13	10	8·87
14	5	6·03
15	1 ⎫	3·43 ⎫
16	3 ⎬ 5	1·54 ⎬ 5·66
17	1 ⎪	0·53 ⎪
≥18	⎭	0·16 ⎭
Total	97 = J	97·00

suggests that an appropriate division can again be made between 4 and 5 days, but there is now a somewhat greater possibility of overlap than appeared with households of two. The chance of misclassification can be allowed for by the introduction of additional parameters, but seems hardly worth embarking on at present. Tables 15.6 and 15.7 give the amalgamated expected and observed numbers for those parts of the data giving rise to ω- and ζ-type distributions, while analyses of the chains for households with two and three cases are presented in Table 15.8.

15.62 Derivation of scores and information functions

It will be remembered that we assume the latent period ξ to be normally distributed with mean μ and variance σ^2, and the ensuing infectious period to be of constant length α. Infection of further susceptibles during this time is taken to be a Poisson process such that the chance of a given susceptible contracting the disease in time dt is λdt. The five main aspects of the data that are fairly easily analysed will now be described in detail.

Table 15.8   *Analysis of chains for two and three cases (households of three)*

Type of introduction	Type of chain	Symbol	Observed number	Expected number
	$\{1\}$	C	6	8·62
	$\{1^2\}$	B	11	6·23
Single	$\{1^3\}$	E	6	9·81
	$\{12\}$	F	37	35·34
	Total	M	60	60·00
	$\{2\}$	A	4	3·05
Double	$\{21\}$	H	7	7·95
	Total	K	11	11·00

The ω- and ζ-type distributions arising from the data are easily dealt with according to the theory already described in Section 15.3, the only difference being that there all contributions to scores and information functions were amalgamated (see equations (15.9) and (15.12)), whereas here it is more convenient to have the individual contributions displayed separately.

ω-type distribution

There are K households giving ω-type observations, and the appropriate score and information function are

$$S_\sigma = K\sigma^{-1}(\tfrac{1}{2}V\sigma^{-2} - 1),\qquad(15.29)$$

$$I_{\sigma\sigma} = 2K\sigma^{-2},\qquad(15.30)$$

where, as before, V is the observed second moment of the distribution about the origin.

ζ-type distribution

Here we have J households in all, yielding ζ-type observations. The four scores are

$$S_\lambda = J\{\mu - \bar{\zeta} + \lambda^{-1} + \lambda\sigma^2 - \alpha(e^{\lambda\alpha} - 1)^{-1}\} + \sum_\zeta T_\lambda,$$

$$S_\alpha = \qquad\qquad -J\lambda(e^{\lambda\alpha} - 1)^{-1} + \sum_\zeta T_\alpha,$$

$$S_\mu = \qquad\qquad J\lambda \qquad\qquad + \sum_\zeta T_\mu,$$

$$S_\sigma = \qquad\qquad J\lambda^2\sigma \qquad\qquad + \sum_\zeta T_\sigma,$$

(15.31)

where $\bar{\zeta}$ and v are the mean and variance of the observed distribution, and T_θ is defined as in (15.8) and summed over the observed values of ζ. The corresponding information functions are

$$I_{\lambda\lambda} = \sum_\zeta T_\lambda^2 - J\{\lambda^2\sigma^4 + \sigma^2 - \lambda^{-2} + \alpha^2 e^{\lambda\alpha}(e^{\lambda\alpha} - 1)^{-2}\},$$

$$I_{\lambda\alpha} = \sum_\zeta T_\lambda T_\alpha + J\{(1 + \lambda^2\sigma^2)(e^{\lambda\alpha} - 1)^{-1} - \lambda\alpha e^{\lambda\alpha}(e^{\lambda\alpha} - 1)^{-2}\},$$

$$I_{\lambda\mu} = \sum_\zeta T_\lambda T_\mu - J(1 + \lambda^2\sigma^2),$$

$$I_{\lambda\sigma} = \sum_\zeta T_\lambda T_\sigma - J\lambda^3\sigma^3,$$

$$I_{\alpha\alpha} = \sum_\zeta T_\alpha^2 - J\lambda^2(e^{\lambda\alpha} - 1)^{-2},$$

$$I_{\alpha\mu} = \sum_\zeta T_\alpha T_\mu + J\lambda^2(e^{\lambda\alpha} - 1)^{-1},$$

$$I_{\alpha\sigma} = \sum_\zeta T_\alpha T_\sigma + J\lambda^3\sigma(e^{\lambda\alpha} - 1)^{-1},$$

$$I_{\mu\mu} = \sum_\zeta T_\mu^2 - J\lambda^2,$$

$$I_{\mu\sigma} = \sum_\zeta T_\mu T_\sigma - J\lambda^3\sigma,$$

$$I_{\sigma\sigma} = \sum_\zeta T_\sigma^2 - J\lambda^4\sigma.$$

(15.32)

Chains with double introductions

We now take the K households with a double introduction, i.e. A of type $\{2\}$ and H of type $\{21\}$. Using the Greenwood rather than the Reed–Frost formulation, the relative frequencies are $e^{-\lambda\alpha}$ and $1 - e^{-\lambda\alpha}$. Contributions to the scores and information functions are therefore

$$S_\lambda = H\alpha(e^{\lambda\alpha} - 1)^{-1} - A\alpha, \quad S_\alpha = \lambda\alpha^{-1}S_\lambda, \qquad (15.33)$$

and

$$I_{\lambda\lambda} = K\alpha^2(e^{\lambda\alpha} - 1)^{-1}, \quad I_{\lambda\alpha} = \lambda\alpha^{-1}I_{\lambda\lambda}, \quad I_{\alpha\alpha} = \lambda^2\alpha^{-2}I_{\lambda\lambda}. \quad (15.34)$$

There is no special difficulty in developing corresponding formulae for the Reed–Frost variant if required, though variation in the chance of infection must then be allowed for.

Chains with single introductions

As mentioned above, it is necessary to take into account the possibility of variations in the chance of infection when analysing the frequencies of the several chains starting with only a single introductory case. This has already been discussed at length in Section 14.4. The chief assumption made was that the chance of cross-infection, p, which when constant equals $1 - e^{-\lambda\alpha}$ in our present notation, followed the beta-distribution shown in (14.16). The appropriate scores and observed information functions for the two parameters p and z, previously given in (14.20) and (14.21), are repeated below using the present symbols for the observations, namely

$$\left.\begin{aligned} S'_p &= \frac{B+E+F}{p} - \frac{B+C+E}{q} + \frac{E+F}{p+z} - \frac{B+C}{q+z}, \\ S'_z &= -\frac{M}{1+z} - \frac{2(B+E)}{1+2z} + \frac{E+F}{p+z} + \frac{B+C}{q+z}, \end{aligned}\right\} \quad (15.35)$$

and

$$\left.\begin{aligned} I'_{pp} &= \frac{B+E+F}{p^2} + \frac{B+C+E}{q^2} + \frac{E+F}{(p+z)^2} + \frac{B+C}{(q+z)^2}, \\ I'_{pz} &= \qquad\qquad\qquad\qquad \frac{E+F}{(p+z)^2} - \frac{B+C}{(q+z)^2}, \\ I'_{zz} &= -\frac{M}{(1+z)^2} - \frac{4(B+E)}{(1+2z)^2} + \frac{E+F}{(p+z)^2} + \frac{B+C}{(q+z)^2}. \end{aligned}\right\} \quad (15.36)$$

Primes are used here to distinguish these *auxiliary* scores and information functions from those with which we shall be more immediately concerned.

Such a procedure entails using two parameters to specify the probability of infection. The parameter λ, which we are using in the present chapter to score data that are relatively insensitive to variations in the chance of infection, can be regarded as an average probability. We therefore need to introduce one additional parameter, and it is convenient to use the z referred to above. We now suppose the frequencies to have been written in terms of λ, α and z, instead of p and z. Use of the functional relation

$$p = 1 - e^{-\lambda\alpha} \quad (15.37)$$

then leads by the usual processes of differentiation to the scores and information functions appropriate to the present context. These can be conveniently written in terms of the auxiliary expressions appearing in (15.35) and (15.36) as follows:

$$S_\lambda = \alpha q S'_p, \quad S_\alpha = \lambda q S'_p, \quad S_z = S'_z, \quad (15.38)$$

and

$$I_{\lambda\lambda} = \alpha^2 q(qI'_{pp} + S'_p), \quad I_{\lambda\alpha} = \lambda\alpha^{-1}I_{\lambda\lambda} - qS'_p,$$

$$I_{\lambda z} = \alpha qI'_{pz}, \qquad\qquad I_{\alpha\alpha} = \lambda^2\alpha^{-2}I_{\lambda\lambda},$$

$$I_{\alpha z} = \lambda\alpha^{-1}I_{\lambda z}, \qquad\qquad I_{zz} = I'_{zz}. \qquad\qquad (15.39)$$

Time-interval distribution for triple introductions

The last item to be discussed is the extraction of information from the G households involving a triple introduction. Each basic observation is the number-pair (u, v), where $u \leqslant v$. Let the times at which symptoms occur in the three patients, measuring from the common point of infection as origin, be π_1, π_2 and π_3. Then these variables are normally and independently distributed with mean $\mu + \alpha$ and variance σ^2. The joint frequency distribution of the *ordered* trio (π_1, π_2, π_3) is

$$f(\pi_1 \leqslant \pi_2 \leqslant \pi_3)d\pi_1 d\pi_2 d\pi_3 = \frac{3!}{(2\pi\sigma^2)^{\frac{3}{2}}} \exp\left\{-\frac{1}{2\sigma^2} \sum_{i=1}^{3} (\pi_i - \mu - \alpha)^2\right\} d\pi_1 d\pi_2 d\pi_3.$$

$$(15.40)$$

If we now use the transformation

$$u = \pi_2 - \pi_1,$$

$$v = \pi_3 - \pi_2,$$

$$s = \pi_1 + \pi_2 + \pi_3, \qquad\qquad (15.41)$$

to write down the joint distribution of u, v and s, we can then integrate out s to give the required joint distribution of u and v only. This turns out to be

$$f(u, v)du\,dv = \frac{\sqrt{3}}{\pi\sigma^2} \exp\left\{-\frac{1}{3\sigma^2} (u^2 + uv + v^2)\right\} du\,dv. \qquad (15.42)$$

We can now derive a score and information function for σ in the usual way. If for a set of observed number-pairs

$$(u_i, v_i), \quad i = 1, ..., G,$$

we put

$$Z = \sum_{i=1}^{G} (u^2_i + u_i v_i + v^2_i), \qquad\qquad (15.43)$$

we obtain

$$S_\sigma = -2G\sigma^{-1} + \tfrac{2}{3}Z\sigma^{-3}, \quad I_{\sigma\sigma} = 4G\sigma^{-2}. \qquad (15.44)$$

These results are, moreover, not affected by variations in the chance of infection.

This now completes the derivation of all the various components of the scores and information functions required for obtaining maximum-likelihood estimates for the five parameters, λ, α, μ, σ and z. The only elements of the 5×5 information matrix which have not been mentioned explicitly are $I_{\mu z}$ and $I_{\sigma z}$, and these are easily seen to be identically zero. In analysing actual data we first classify them according to the five main aspects above. Next, we calculate in each case, for trial values of the parameters, the appropriate contributions to scores and information functions. Corresponding contributions are then added and the resultant vector of overall scores multiplied by the inverse of the complete information matrix to give first corrections to the trial values, as indicated by the general equation (15.14). The process is then repeated as usual until the desired accuracy is achieved.

15.63   Application to measles data

The foregoing maximum-likelihood scores and information functions can now be applied to Hope Simpson's data, the relevant aspects of which are exhibited in Tables 15.3 to 15.8. A preliminary inspection of the data shows that so far as the ζ-distribution in Table 15.7 goes, a really satisfactory fit is unlikely to be obtained on account of the apparent excess of observations at 11 days with a counterbalancing deficit at 10 days. In Section 15.3 a difficulty of this sort was encountered with households of two in the appearance of possibly spurious peaks at 7 and 14 days. This was thought to be due to an unconscious bias associated with integral multiples of a week. In the present case no very satisfactory explanation can be discerned. However, as the agreement between hypothesis and observation seems in other respects to be quite good, the best plan seems to be to pool the frequencies for 10 and 11 days when proceeding to test goodness-of-fit.

Preliminary estimates for λ, α, μ and σ can be taken from the final values previously obtained for households of two, while a trial value of z is available from the earlier analysis of data in Section 14.4. After carrying out the standard procedure of maximum-likelihood scoring, the final estimates turn out to be

$$\left.\begin{aligned}
\hat{\lambda} &= 0.180 \pm 0.039, \\
\hat{\alpha} &= 7.05 \pm 1.13 \text{ days}, \\
\hat{\mu} &= 7.63 \pm 0.50 \text{ days}, \\
\hat{\sigma} &= 1.59 \pm 0.26 \text{ days}, \\
\hat{z} &= 0.50 \pm 0.29.
\end{aligned}\right\} \qquad (15.45)$$

These estimates of λ, α, μ and σ are rather less precise than those given in equation (15.21) for households of two, but it may be noted that in no case are the two estimates of any parameter significantly different. The parameter z is not determined with much precision, although the estimate obtained does suggest a significant amount of variation in the chance of infection from household to household ($\hat{z}$ is significantly different from zero on a one-sided test).

In testing goodness-of-fit, based as before on the last set of estimates but one in the iteration, the classes bracketed together have been pooled to avoid small expectations. We have also amalgamated the frequencies for 10 and 11 days in the ζ-distribution as indicated above. The total number of degrees of freedom is 13, i.e. 1 from the ω-distribution in Table 15.6, 8 from the ζ-distribution in Table 15.7 and 4 in all from Table 15.8, while 5 must be removed to allow for the parameters estimated. We actually obtain an overall χ^2 of 14·6 on 8 degrees of freedom. As the 5 percent point is at 15·5 we can regard the fit as reasonably satisfactory, except of course for the anomalous behaviour of the frequencies in the 10- and 11-day classes of the ζ-distribution. Whether this is due to some bias in collecting the data, or whether it is of genuine biological significance is a matter which requires further investigation, and should be given special attention when new data of this type are collected.

Some consideration should be given at this point to the consequences of neglecting the effect of variations in λ on the form of the ζ-distribution. Using the method of Section 15.51, it can be shown that the fairly substantial variation envisaged there would in the present case actually improve the fit very slightly, reducing χ^2 by about 0·5.

15.7   Computerized applications

The basic model introduced in Section 15.3 is relatively simple in its essential features. Moreover, the results obtained from actual data, as for example in Sections 15.4 and 15.6, can be presented and interpreted in a quite straightforward fashion. Nevertheless the approach seems to have been used but rarely by practical epidemiologists (see, however, Owada, Sakamoto and Tanaka, 1971 for an application to 1022 families of three involving influenza). The main reasons for this are probably the complexity of the underlying mathematics as presented above, and the considerable labour involved in the computations, at least using a desk calculator. It must also be admitted that data of the right form are not very easy to come by, but increased efforts might be made if more streamlined methods of analysis were available.

It was only when Dr K. Petersen of the Gesundheitsbehörde, Hamburg, suggested that the writer might like to analyse some excellent data available on infectious hepatitis, that a real attempt was made to develop more accessible methods of analysis. This led to the paper by Bailey and Alff-Steinberger (1970), to which reference should be made for details additional to those set out below. The main epidemiological discussion is in Petersen (1970).

In principle, straightforward computerization of the maximum-likelihood scoring methods set out above would lead to a great saving of time and effort. But, as already pointed out in Chapter 4, once an electronic computer is available the simplest course is to maximize the log likelihood directly, using some standard maximization program, thus saving even more time.

For households of two, we can combine the frequency functions in (15.1), (15.2) and (15.5) to give a total log likelihood, ignoring an arbitrary constant, of

$$L = -A \log \sigma + B \log \lambda - C\lambda\alpha + B\lambda(\mu + \tfrac{1}{2}\lambda\sigma^2)$$

$$-\tfrac{1}{4}\sigma^{-2} \sum_{i=1}^{A} \omega_i^2 - \lambda \sum_{j=1}^{B} \zeta_j + \sum_{j=1}^{B} \log \left(\int_{b_j'}^{b_j} e^{-\frac{1}{2}t^2} dt \right), \qquad (15.46)$$

where ω_i and ζ_j are observed values of the variables ω and ζ, respectively, and

$$b_j = \sigma^{-1}\{\zeta_j - (\mu + \lambda\sigma^2)\}, \quad b_j' = b_j - \alpha\sigma^{-1}. \tag{15.47}$$

If we wish to make use of the suggestion in Section 15.53 for allowing for the misclassification of chains, then we can work directly with the expression in (15.27), which involves the additional parameter ψ. Little extra work is required beyond defining the log likelihood in the relevant programming language.

Thus (15.46) or (15.27) provide the functions to be maximized. Starting values of the parameters λ, α, μ and σ can be obtained from (15.15) or (15.19), as before. If we wish to use ψ as well, then A and B must be estimated empirically by inspecting the data. This will suffice in order to use (15.15). For ψ itself, a reasonable starting value is $\psi = A/N$.

The work is a little more complicated for households of three, but most of the heavy algebra is avoided. First of all, there is the contribution to the log likelihood arising from the three continuous types of variables given in (15.1), (15.5) and (15.42). This is

$$L_1 = \sum_{i=1}^{K} \log f(\omega_i) + \sum_{j=1}^{J} \log f(\zeta_j) + \sum_{k=1}^{G} \log f(u_k, v_k). \tag{15.48}$$

Some algebraic simplification is possible if we pick out exponential factors explicitly before taking logarithms.

Next, we consider the information arising from the numbers of different types of chains. Basically, we appeal to the approach of Section 14.4, introducing an additional parameter z. For the K double introductions, the contribution to the log likelihood on the Greenwood model is

$$L_2 = A \log q + H \log p, \tag{15.49}$$

while for the Reed–Frost formulation we have

$$L_2' = A \log q + H \log p + A \log (q + z) + H \log (q + z + 1) - K \log (z + 1). \tag{15.50}$$

This last expression for L_2' easily follows from applying the approach mentioned to the frequencies shown in Table 14.2 for double introductions.

For the M single introductions, frequencies are the same for both Greenwood and Reed–Frost models, and are shown in Table 14.12. The contribution to the log likelihood is evidently

$$L_3 = (B + E + F) \log p + (B + C + E) \log q + (E + F) \log (p + z)$$
$$+ (B + C) \log (q + z) - M \log (1 + z) - (B + E) \log (1 + 2z). \tag{15.51}$$

The required final expression for the log likelihood is therefore the sum of

L_1, L_2 or L_2', and L_3. We carry out the maximization for the parameters λ, α, μ, σ and z, making use of the fact that $p \; (= 1 - q)$ is expressible in terms of λ and α, as given by (15.37).

The problem of handling the situation where individual chains are not clearly distinguishable could perhaps be dealt with in households of three by introducing two further parameters, ψ_1 and ψ_2, which specify the probabilities that a household is introduced into the records by a single or double primary. There are, however, certain combinatorial aspects that have not as yet been fully resolved.

15.71   Application to measles data

The measles data already analysed in Sections 15.4 and 15.6 were reinvestigated by directly maximizing the log likelihood, using the expressions set out above. Bailey and Alff-Steinberger actually used the MINROS program originally written in the CERN version of FORTRAN. This is based on the Rosenbrock maximization technique, but involves calculating all second-order partial differential coefficients at the final stage of the iterations, followed by inversion of what is in fact the matrix of observed information functions. Standard errors of the maximum-likelihood estimates are thus provided automatically. The formulae proposed in (15.15) and (15.19) for starting values, and appropriate χ^2 goodness-of-fit tests were also incorporated in the overall program. The latter was then used to obtain the results shown in Table 15.9. Only a few minutes of computer time on an IBM 360 Model 40 were required to obtain any single column of results, as compared with several man-weeks previously needed using a desk calculating machine.

Table 15.9   *Results of computerized analysis of measles data*

Parameter	Households of two		Households of three	
	(1)	(2)	Greenwood	Reed–Frost
λ	0.257 ± 0.043	0.281 ± 0.057	0.181 ± 0.038	0.173 ± 0.037
α (days)	$6.58 \;\; \pm 1.05$	$5.96 \;\; \pm 1.25$	$7.02 \;\; \pm 1.20$	$7.06 \;\; \pm 1.21$
μ (days)	$8.59 \;\; \pm 0.38$	$8.90 \;\; \pm 0.45$	$7.63 \;\; \pm 0.56$	$7.60 \;\; \pm 0.58$
σ (days)	$1.81 \;\; \pm 0.19$	$1.87 \;\; \pm 0.22$	$1.62 \;\; \pm 0.24$	$1.62 \;\; \pm 0.24$
ψ	–	0.122 ± 0.021	–	–
z	–	–	$0.50 \;\; \pm 0.27$	$0.63 \;\; \pm 0.30$
χ^2	21.3 (14.0)	20.4 (12.6)	14.0	14.0
Degrees of freedom	12 (8)	12 (7)	8	7
5% point	21.0 (15.5)	21.0 (14.1)	15.5	14.1

Column (1) of Table 15.9, under "Households of two", is to be compared with (15.21) above. Differences in values of the estimates, which are slight except for σ, must be due to the error in the score for σ already noted in Section 15.41. The goodness-of-fit figures shown in parentheses refer to the results obtained when adjustments are made for the peaks observed in the data at 7 and 14 days. When allowance is made, as in column (2), for the misclassification parameter ψ, there are some changes in the estimates, though these are not large in comparison with the standard errors involved.

With households of three, the new estimates are virtually indistinguishable from the earlier ones in (15.45), using the Greenwood model for double introductions. When the Reed—Frost model is adopted for this part of the data, some changes occur in the estimates, but they are small compared with the standard errors.

15.72 Application to infectious hepatitis data

After so much detailed analysis of measles data it was refreshing to have the opportunity to try out the model under discussion with a different disease. Dr Petersen's Hamburg material, already referred to, relates to infectious hepatitis outbreaks in 224 households of three children under the age of 16, during the years 1959—67. No parents were affected, and they were assumed not to be epidemiologically involved. Accepting that there are always difficulties in the clinical diagnosis of infectious hepatitis, all patients were admitted to hospital and subjected to extensive clinical and laboratory investigations. The resultant data should therefore show considerable freedom from major inaccuracies.

Of the $N = 224$ households, there were $C = 157$ with one case only, 41 with two cases and 26 with three cases. Table 15.10 gives the serial interval distribution for the 41 households with two cases, while Table 15.11 shows the joint distribution of the 26 pairs of successive serial intervals when there were three cases. The best choice of a suitable cut-off point to separate out the various sub-distributions was not altogether clear. To begin with, a point between 12 and 13 days was assumed. In Table 15.10 this means $A = 11$ households of type $\{2\}$, and $B = 30$ households of type $\{1^2\}$.

In Table 15.11 we obtain the values shown for E, F, H and G, a small refinement having been used in comparison with the method of subdivision previously used in Table 15.4 for the measles data. Suppose that the arbitrarily chosen cut-off point is at d days. Then for group $\{3\}$ we should expect all the data to lie above and to the left of a line $u + v = d$. This is because $u + v$ is in fact approximately an ω-type variable, and so we should have $u + v < d$. For groups $\{12\}$ and $\{1^3\}$ the dividing lines should be drawn as before.

We can now identify the three types of continuous variables as follows. There are $K = A + H = 14$ households producing intervals of ω-type, whose distribution is shown in Table 15.12. And there are $J = B + 2(E + F) = 72$ households yielding ζ-type variables, the distribution appearing in Table 15.13. Finally the $G = 2$ households giving (u, v) pairs can be found in the last line of Table 15.11.

Routine computer analysis then gave the figures shown in Table 15.14.

Table 15.10 *Distribution of time-interval for 41 households of three with two cases*

Interval (days)	0	1	2	3	4	5	6	7	8	9	10	11	12	13
Freq.	2	1	2	.	2	1	1	.	.	.	1	.	1	.
Interval (days)	14	15	16	17	18	19	20	21	22	23	24	25	26	27
Freq.	2	1	.	1	1	.	.	1	1	.	2	4	2	.
Interval (days)	28	29	30	31	32	33	34	35	36	37	38	39	40	41	42
Freq.	1	.	1	2	3	.	1	1	1	2	1	.	1	.	1

Table 15.11 *Distribution of 26 time-interval pairs (u, v) for households of three cases, measured in days*

Type of chain	Number of households observed	(u, v) intervals observed
$\{1^3\}$	$E = 8$	(16, 15) (22, 37) (25, 36) (28, 31) (32, 33) (34, 14) (36, 21) (36, 30)
$\{12\}$	$F = 13$	(13, 1) (16, 0) (16, 6) (19, 9) (21, 5) (23, 3) (23, 11) (24, 1) (25, 2) (25, 5) (27, 1) (28, 3) (34, 2)
$\{21\}$	$H = 3$	(1, 24) (7, 22) (9, 18)
$\{3\}$	$G = 2$	(1, 0) (1, 2)

Table 15.12 *Amalgamated frequencies for the ω distribution based on $K = A + H = 14$ observations*

Interval (days)	0	1	2	3	4	5	6	7	8	9	10	11	12
Freq.	2	2	2	.	2	1	1	1	.	1	1	.	1

Table 15.13 *Amalgamated frequencies for the ζ distribution based on $J = B + 2(E + F) = 72$ observations*

Interval (days)	13	14	15	16	17	18	19	20	21	22
Freq.	1	4	2	4	1	1	1	.	3	3
Interval (days)	23	24	25	26	27	28	29	30	31	32
Freq.	2	3	8	4	2	5	.	3	4	4
Interval (days)	33	34	35	36	37	38	39	40	41	42
Freq.	1	4	1	5	3	1	.	1	.	1

Table 15.14   *Results of computerized analysis of infectious hepatitis data*

Parameter	Estimate
λ	0.0073 ± 0.0013
α	21.73 ± 2.54 days
μ	15.62 ± 1.53 days
σ	3.95 ± 0.57 days
z	0.33 ± 0.13
χ^2	11.2
Degrees of freedom	11
5% point	19.7

The overall conclusion of this analysis may be stated quite simply as follows. A good description of the data is obtained by assuming a latent period of about $15\frac{1}{2}$ days, with a standard deviation of about 4 days, followed by an infectious period of $21\frac{1}{2}$ days. This makes an incubation period of 37 days with a standard deviation of 4 days. It must be admitted that the range of variation appropriate to the incubation period is here somewhat smaller than is sometimes suggested in the literature. The figures given above imply that about 95 percent of incubation periods should lie between 29 and 45 days. Nevertheless, these are the best estimates currently available from the Hamburg data. It may be that there is some epidemiological peculiarity here that is revealed by the type of quantitative analysis undertaken.

15.8   Extension to larger groups

The general procedure described here for households of three can clearly be extended to larger households. By picking out contributions to ω- and ζ-type distributions we could use the scores and information functions given in (15.29) to (15.32) directly. When analysing the different kinds of chain allowing for a variable chance of infection the formulae given above in (15.37) to (15.39) would have to be applied to the extensions of (15.35) and (15.36). Double and triple introductions can also be dealt with as above. Other multiple introductions require the obvious extensions of (15.40) to (15.44). We have in the present discussion neglected to make use of the distribution of v-intervals in chains of type {21} because of undue complexity. With larger households there would be further relatively intractable items of this sort. Another point of importance is that with small households the errors introduced by neglecting to make allowance for the probability of chains being misclassified are likely to be small, while in large households this source of error would be much more pronounced because of the greater opportunity for the distributions of different kinds of chains to overlap. If sufficient data of this kind are forthcoming, the difficulty could be tackled along the lines suggested in Section 15.53.

The difficulties of analysis stem from the fact that the processes entailed are non-Markovian in character, and the resultant complexities are not readily handled in terms of smaller components. An associated Markov process can be constructed by the inclusion of supplementary variables such as unelapsed latent and infectious periods. Unfortunately, this does not seem to lead to a computationally feasible method of parameter estimation. Further research on this topic could prove extremely useful, especially if one could learn to handle the more general situation of several interacting groups such as exist in a community consisting of many households.

Bailey and Alff-Steinberger (1972, unpublished; quoted in Bailey, 1973a) have attempted a form of analysis of the observed interremoval times, without trying to identify any specific patterns of case-to-case transmission. The idea is that one computes, on the basis of the model already used in the present chapter, the probability of each observed interval *given* the previously observed pattern. The product of all such conditional probabilities then supplies the likelihood of the observed data for the parameter set used. As before, a computerized method is used to choose the parameter set that maximizes the likelihood.

The difficulty of this approach is that the removal, next after any given set of consecutive removals starting with the first one, is possibly only the first of several removals of individuals who have already become infected at an earlier stage. If we ignore the influence of the latter individuals, then it is possible easily to construct a formal expression for the probability that the next removal occurs when it does, since all the infectious intervals during which infection might have occurred are known. However, because of the doubts attaching to the method it is hardly worth giving more precise details.

Bailey and Alff-Steinberger applied the above procedure in a heuristic way to the Abakaliki smallpox data already presented in Section 6.8. In the latter it was used to illustrate a mathematically exact form of analysis based on the general stochastic epidemic. The estimates obtained by the present method were

$$\left.\begin{aligned}
\hat{\lambda} &= 0\cdot010 \pm 0\cdot004, \\
\hat{\alpha} &= 1\cdot0 \quad \pm 0\cdot4 \text{ days}, \\
\hat{\mu} &= 9\cdot8 \quad \pm 2\cdot2 \text{ days}, \\
\hat{\sigma} &= 4\cdot2 \quad \pm 1\cdot0 \text{ days}.
\end{aligned}\right\} \qquad (15.52)$$

Even if these estimates are unlikely to be mathematically very respectable, we can still ask how intrinsically reliable are they as a matter of empirical fact. One way of answering this question is as follows.

For a given set of parametric values, those in (15.52) for example, we construct a large number of simulated sets of data based on the model in question. For each simulated data set we use the proposed method of analysis, and then see how the series of computed estimates compare with the "true" values used to build the simulations. Thus fifty simulated epidemics for groups of size 120 (the value for Abakaliki) were prepared using the estimates in (15.52) as the "true" parametric values. The means of the fifty independent computed values of each parameter turned out to be

$$\left.\begin{aligned}
\bar{\lambda} &= \ 0\cdot013, \\
\bar{\alpha} &= \ 0\cdot81 \ \text{days}, \\
\bar{\mu} &= 10\cdot4 \ \text{days}, \\
\bar{\sigma} &= \ 3\cdot7 \ \text{days}.
\end{aligned}\right\} \tag{15.53}$$

The differences between the mean computed values of (15.53) and the assumed "true" values in (15.52) are not unduly large compared with the standard errors of the latter based on a single real epidemic. This is an encouraging result, indicating that the approach does perhaps deserve further investigation, especially in the context of larger samples containing more information.

It should also be mentioned that it can be shown that the estimates in (15.53) are in fact significantly different from the "true" values, showing the existence of bias. In principle, we should be able to adjust the original estimates of (15.52) so as to remove the biases and obtain more accurate estimates. Again, investigations were made into the series of computed standard errors, but on the whole it was felt that samples were rather too small for reliable and consistent results to be expected.

In any case the Abakaliki data were not very extensive, entailing only a single smallpox epidemic of 30 cases in a community of 120 people, so that the results should be treated with caution. The estimated average incubation period of about 11 days agrees quite well with the commonly accepted figure of 12 days. The estimated standard deviation of approximately 4 days for the latent period or incubation period seems rather high, but a range between 7 and 17 days is commonly accepted. The estimate of one day for the length of the infectious period is a rather small value for smallpox by ordinary epidemiological standards. It must not be forgotten, however, that we are measuring from the end of the latent period to the moment at which the case is removed from circulation. In this model we are not concerned with infectiousness that may well exist after isolation. As a final comment, we mention that there are some general epidemiological reasons for thinking that the Abakaliki outbreak was somewhat atypical.

16

Simple multistate models

16.1 Introduction

The applications of the previous two chapters have been concerned with attempts to fit specific stochastic models to relatively small bodies of data, but with a major emphasis on parameter estimation and goodness-of-fit testing. The results of such work can have an important bearing both on epidemiological theory and on public health control mechanisms. In the present chapter we shall look at some simplified, and deterministic, models that have come to be used in recent years to evaluate the possible consequences of various alternative public health interventions. These models have been especially useful in the area of bacterial diseases such as tuberculosis, typhoid fever, cerebrospinal meningitis, cholera, tetanus, etc.

With such diseases there is often a considerable amount of clinical, biological and epidemiological knowledge, including forms of treatment, immunization or vaccination leading to possible control measures. What is needed to evaluate alternative control strategies in any given community is a fairly realistic and broadly based model that incorporates all the categories of individuals that are considered to be of epidemiological importance for the disease in question, together with an account of the mechanisms, or at least the transfer-rates, according to which individuals pass from one category to another. Great mathematical rigour or epidemiological predictive accuracy are in general probably unnecessary, though there is no reason to avoid them if they can be included without undue labour.

In previously discussed models we have usually confined ourselves to a small number of categories such as "susceptible", "infected but uninfectious" (implying a latent period), "infected and infectious", "removed" (i.e. isolated, dead, or recovered and immune), etc. But with diseases like tuberculosis or typhoid even the simplest models seem to require nine or ten categories, with a much higher number of transfer-rates between categories. Although, when constructed, such a model may seem to be rather complex, it may in fact be very simple since it consists of a number of elementary components, each of which can be described in an uncomplicated, straightforward manner.

We shall give below, in Section 16.2, an example of the construction and use of such multistate, or multicompartment, models in the specific area of tuberculosis control. Pioneer work has been done in this area in recent years by a variety of authors who have helped to develop underlying epidemiological models, on the basis of which associated optimization and control models could be evolved. As a result, considerably improved insight into the principles of control has been obtained.

In Section 16.3 we shall briefly review similar applications that have been made to a range of other diseases.

16.2   Tuberculosis models

Tuberculosis is a chronic bacterial disease that still represents a serious world problem. There is a total of some 15-20 million cases of infectious tuberculosis in the world, more than three-quarters of these being in developing countries. The case-fatality rate per year is of the order of 5-10 percent, and about 2-3 million new infectious cases occur each year. Effective disease control depends on a combination of BCG vaccination for susceptibles and chemotherapeutic treatment for actual cases. Many alternative control strategies exist, and a major problem in resource allocation is to be able to evaluate the effectiveness of these alternatives in advance of putting any actual program into operation. There are many important problems in tuberculosis control whose solutions are relatively insensitive to the underlying epidemiological assumptions (e.g. Feldstein, Piot and Sundaresan, 1973).

Nevertheless, it is desirable in general to base such investigations on descriptive models which represent the epidemiological dynamics in a reasonably satisfactory way. This enables subsequent criticism to be handled more effectively, and often allows unforeseen problems and difficulties to be answered without having to reformulate the whole model.

The first effective modelling of the epidemiological dynamics of tuberculosis appears to be that of Waaler, Geser and Andersen (1962). These authors used an essentially three-category model, involving noninfected individuals, infected non-cases, and infected cases, to compare the future consequences of existing trends in three different situations, namely, with no control, with adequate treatment of two-thirds of the active cases, and with BCG vaccination.

A more complex extension of this model was later developed by Brøgger (1967), in which there were six distinct epidemiological categories each divided into 15 one-year age groups for ages 0-14 years, and 15 five-year age groups for ages 15-89 years. Several other important studies, with the main emphasis on operational research and systems aspects, including cost—benefit analyses, have been carried out by Mahler and Piot (1966a,b), Waaler (1968a,b), Waaler and Piot (1969, 1970), ReVelle and Male (1970), and Feldstein, Piot and Sundaresan (1973).

Most of these investigations make use in one way or another of an underlying epidemiological model. However, they all assume that the number of new infections occurring in any time-interval Δt is jointly proportional only to Δt and to the number of actively infectious cases. This is equivalent to assuming that the total number of susceptibles remains effectively constant. For epidemic processes in which the number of susceptibles is subjected only to relatively small variations, the assumption is a reasonable and valid approximation. But if we need a model that will handle wider ranges of variation in the numbers of both infected individuals and susceptibles, then we ought to make the number of new cases in Δt jointly proportional to Δt, the number of infectives, *and* the number of susceptibles, in accordance with the ideas generally adopted throughout this book.

This more general specification of the rate of spread of infection in tuberculosis modelling was, with a certain important modification described below, first introduced by ReVelle (1967), and was also incorporated in the work of ReVelle, Lynn and Feldmann (1967). For purposes of illustration we shall describe in some detail the model developed by the latter authors. A somewhat more comprehensive model, based on consensus views obtained at a workshop on model methodology, has been reported briefly by Lynn and ReVelle (1968).

The essential structure of the ReVelle, Lynn and Feldmann model is shown in Fig. 16.1. This is almost self-explanatory, but it is worth describing the various components in some detail so as to indicate some of the thinking that has gone into the construction of the model, and to make more explicit the various assumptions involved. It should be remembered that in applications to a specific disease we expect to do more than merely indicate a few salient features of the dynamic process entailed: we hope to be able to achieve a degree of realism sufficient for us to discriminate between the predicted consequences of different control strategies.

It is supposed, first of all, that the population consists of two broad groups: susceptibles, who have never been infected, and cases who have been infected at some time or other. There are no individuals who can be categorized as "removed", in the sense of the definition previously used in Chapter 6, for example. Secondly, the cases can be divided into those who are active and those who are inactive. So far, this classification is virtually identical with that of Waaler, Geser and Andersen (1962) mentioned above. However, the present model introduces further subclassifications of both susceptible and inactive categories.

There is a major distinction between susceptibles who have and those who have not been subjected to BCG vaccination. This creates two parallel subsystems, though it is convenient to distinguish only one category of active

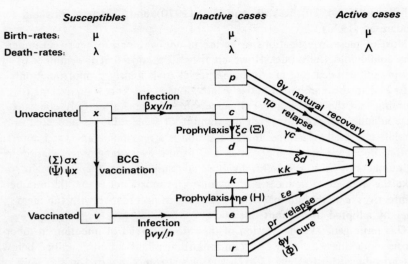

Fig. 16.1   A model of tuberculosis control by vaccination, prophylaxis and treatment. Arrows show directions of transfer, and associated symbols indicate actual rates of transfer per unit time. Symbols in boxes show actual numbers at a given time. (Based on ReVelle, Lynn and Feldmann, 1967)

cases, on the assumption that all active cases are, at least approximately, equally infectious, independently of their previous path through the system.

Unvaccinated susceptibles, x in number, at time t are considered to give rise to new, but initially inactive, cases at rate $\beta xy/n$, where y is the total number of active cases, β is the infection-rate, and n is the total population size. If n is constant it can be absorbed into the parameter β, and the infection-rate is identical with that of Chapter 6. But if n is variable, use of the quantity $\beta xy/n$ is equivalent to assuming a restriction of homogeneous mixing, as previously employed in the host-vector and venereal disease models of Chapter 11. Thus we can interpret β as the rate at which any specified individual achieves contacts that are sufficiently close to transmit infection if one individual is susceptible and the other is an active case. It follows that y active cases will make a total of $\beta y \Delta t$ contacts in time Δt. Of these contacts, only a proportion x/n will be with susceptibles and so give rise to new cases. The actual number of new cases will therefore be $\beta xy \, \Delta t/n$ in Δt, giving the rate of occurrence of new (inactive) cases as $\beta xy/n$.

Let the number of inactive cases at time t that have been derived directly from the unvaccinated susceptible category by infection be $\check{c}$. These inactive cases are assumed to become active at a rate γ. They are also detected and given prophylactic treatment, with say isoniazid, at a rate ξ. The number of inactive cases receiving prophylaxis is d, and these become active at rate δ. If the prophylaxis is helpful, δ will be less than γ and it has in one study been estimated to be about one-half of γ.

The use of BCG vaccination transfers susceptibles from the unvaccinated category to the vaccinated category, for which the actual number is v. It is convenient to distinguish two kinds of vaccinations: those who are vaccinated routinely soon after birth at rate σ, and those who are vaccinated in mass campaigns at rate ψ. We might suppose σ to be relatively constant, while ψ will be nonzero only during rather restricted campaign periods. More will be said about time-dependence aspects below.

Vaccinated susceptibles undergo transfers to inactive categories by infection, with possible subsequent prophylaxis, in a similar manner to the unvaccinated susceptibles. The rate of occurrence of new (inactive) cases will clearly be $\beta vy/n$, using the same reasoning as before, assuming that a vaccinated individual's resistance to infection is no different from that of an unvaccinated susceptible.

Let the number of inactive cases that have been derived in this way from the vaccinated susceptible category be e. The latter inactive cases are assumed to become active at rate ϵ. They are also detected and given prophylactic treatment at rate η. The number of inactive cases receiving prophylaxis is k, and these become active at rate κ. It is expected that effect of the vaccination, while not changing the resistance to infection in the first place, will have some effect on the tendency to develop into an active case. Some studies have estimated ϵ to be as low as one-fifth of γ. The use of prophylaxis should lower the risk of activation still further.

As mentioned above, this model uses only a single category of active cases. These may recover naturally without treatment at rate θ, transferring to an inactive status. The actual number of the latter category is p. Relapses back to active status occur at rate π. Active cases can also be treated by isoniazid and supporting drugs, resulting in a certain proportion of "cures", that is, patients who revert, at rate ϕ say, to inactive status. The number in the latter category is designated by r, and the relapse rate for these individuals is indicated by ρ. In general, we expect ρ to be less than π.

Since treatment is one of the forms of control, it may be convenient to distinguish the arbitrary rate of treatment, ζ say, and the rate ω at which treated patients recover sufficiently to become inactive. Thus $\phi = \zeta\omega$.

In addition to the above transfer rates the model also allows for birth and death. The assumptions made are that all groups have the same birth-rate μ, every newborn individual being susceptible, but that susceptibles and inactive cases have a death-rate λ, while active cases have a higher death-rate Λ. Less restrictive assumptions could be adopted if this were thought to be useful.

We have now defined the dynamic flows within the total system in sufficient detail to describe the latter's behaviour over a specified period of time by nine ordinary differential equations, namely

$$\frac{dx}{dt} = -\frac{\beta xy}{n} + \mu n - (\lambda + \sigma + \psi)x,$$

$$\frac{dv}{dt} = -\frac{\beta vy}{n} - \lambda v + (\sigma + \psi)x,$$

$$\frac{dc}{dt} = \frac{\beta xy}{n} - (\lambda + \gamma + \xi)c,$$

$$\frac{dd}{dt} = -(\lambda + \delta)d + \xi c,$$

$$\frac{de}{dt} = \frac{\beta vy}{n} - (\lambda + \epsilon + \eta)e, \qquad (16.1)$$

$$\frac{dk}{dt} = -(\lambda + \kappa)k + \eta e,$$

$$\frac{dp}{dt} = -(\lambda + \pi)p + \theta y,$$

$$\frac{dr}{dt} = -(\lambda + \rho)r + \phi y,$$

$$\frac{dy}{dt} = -(\Lambda + \theta + \phi)y + \pi p + \gamma c + \delta d + \kappa k + \epsilon e + \rho r.$$

We also have an equation for the total population size n, which may be written down directly, or obtained by adding all nine equations in (16.1), i.e.

$$\frac{dn}{dt} = \mu n - \lambda(n - y) - \Lambda y. \qquad (16.2)$$

Now the parameters β, μ, λ, Λ, θ, π, γ, δ, κ, ϵ and ρ may be regarded as constants for a given population within a specified social and physical environment. But σ, ψ, ξ, η and ϕ, relating to BCG vaccination, prophylaxis and treatment, are to a greater or less extent under direct control and may therefore vary with time according to the control strategy adopted and the amount of effort expended.

One method of proceeding is to work with a succession of time-intervals, each of which might for convenience be one year in length. Equations (16.1) would then hold for the ith year, say, but with the controllable parameters having a suffix i attached, namely σ_i, ψ_i, ξ_i, η_i and ϕ_i. For any given set of "natural" parameters β, μ, λ, etc., the consequences of a particular control strategy may be evaluated by solving the sets of equations (16.1) over the relevant range of i. The initial values of the state variables x, v, p, etc. for any interval are of course simply the final values for the previous interval.

In fact, ReVelle, Lynn and Feldmann (1967) use a version of (16.1) in which the actual numbers of *controllable* transfers are held constant in any given time-period. Thus for the ith year they define, in effect, the control variables given by

$$\sigma_i x = \Sigma_i, \quad \psi_i x = \Psi_i, \quad \xi_i c = \Xi_i, \quad \eta_i e = H_i, \quad \phi_i y = \Phi_i. \quad (16.3)$$

This leads to certain simplifications, especially in using the model for optimization purposes. It might in some cases be even more realistic, but difficulties could arise such as negative numbers of individuals sometimes occurring in certain categories. Additional assumptions would then be required to avoid such problems. These would be easy to handle in computerized numerical studies.

In general, the sets of nonlinear differential equations do not admit of explicit analytical solutions. But for practical purposes we can use computerized forms of numerical integration to make the required time-projections. However, it must not be forgotten that a mathematical examination of the properties of such systems might reveal unexpected features, help to avoid computational pitfalls, and suggest new forms of control.

It is not our purpose here to review in detail the numerical results obtained by various authors, notable ReVelle, Lynn and Feldmann (1967), which the reader should consult for further particulars. However, there are certain broad aspects that are worth mentioning. The first is that in order to obtain guidance for the control of tuberculosis in any given community we need estimates of all the parameters for *that* specific community. To get started, it may not be necessary to have highly accurate estimates. In any case subsequent computation may be able to show whether important results are sensitive to changes in certain parameters. When this occurs, special steps may have to be taken to obtain more accurate information.

Some parameters, like birth- and death-rates or relapse- and recovery-rates, may be directly derivable from appropriate demographic or epidemiological data. Others, like β, may have to be based on a certain amount of guesswork. In principle, it should be possible to obtain some parameters by an appropriate statistical estimation procedure such as least squares or maximum likelihood. This aspect seems to have received insufficient attention so far. Further developments along these lines might necessitate the examination of stochastic models, as opposed to the purely deterministic version introduced above.

Actually ReVelle, Lynn and Feldmann (1967) do not study a specific tuberculosis situation, but draw on the literature to construct a hypothetical model, the parameters of which might be considered broadly representative of some developing countries, and from which certain general conclusions can be drawn.

Another aspect which must be considered in any public health context is the question of cost, especially the problem of the optimal allocation of resources. Since fairly realistic estimates can be made of the cost of vaccination, prophylaxis and chemotherapeutic treatment, it is clear that we should be able to use the basic dynamic population model (or some variant of it) already introduced above to determine what combination of controls will achieve a specific result most efficiently.

A special application of the foregoing model was developed by ReVelle (1967) (see also ReVelle, Feldmann and Lynn, 1969) in order to make use of linear programming techniques. Although equations (16.1) are not linear as they stand, a workable linearizing approximation can be derived as follows.

It is supposed that the number y of active cases can be reduced in any year by an appropriate use of controls. The special device used is to specify the value of y we intend to achieve at the end of the year, and then ask what combinations of vaccination, prophylaxis and treatment will enable us to reach the objective. Given the costs of these various measures, we look for an optimal combination. Since y is now fixed at the beginning and end of the interval, we take the average $\bar{y}$ of these two values and use it throughout the interval. Equations (16.1) then become

$$\frac{dx}{dt} = -\left(\frac{\beta\bar{y}}{n} + \lambda\right)x + \mu n - \Sigma - \Psi,$$

$$\frac{dv}{dt} = -\left(\frac{\beta\bar{y}}{n} + \lambda\right)v + \Sigma + \Psi,$$

$$\frac{dc}{dt} = \frac{\beta\bar{y}}{n}x - (\lambda + \gamma)c - \Xi,$$

$$\frac{dd}{dt} = -(\lambda + \delta)d + \Xi,$$

$$\frac{de}{dt} = \frac{\beta\bar{y}}{n}v - (\lambda + \epsilon)e - H,$$

$$\frac{dk}{dt} = -(\lambda + \kappa)k + H,$$ (16.4)

$$\frac{dp}{dt} = -(\lambda + \pi)p + \theta\bar{y},$$

$$\frac{dr}{dt} = -(\lambda + \rho)r + \Phi,$$

$$\frac{dy}{dt} = -(\Lambda + \theta + \phi)\bar{y} + \pi p + \gamma c + \delta d + \kappa k + \epsilon e + \rho r,$$

where we have used the form with constant control variables defined as in (16.3), and have dropped all suffixes i for convenience. Equations (16.4) are all linear in form and can be solved in sequence by elementary means using integrating factors though the algebraic expressions so obtained are somewhat unwieldy. Numerical-integration has been used to show that at least in certain circumstances quite good approximate solutions can be obtained.

It is not appropriate here to discuss all the technical details of the linear programming formulation. The interested reader should consult ReVelle, Feldmann and Lynn (1969) for further particulars. Suffice it to say that development along the lines indicated above leads, for any given year, to a system of eight linear equations in twelve unknowns, the latter comprising seven final conditions and the values of the five control variables. An extension to the more practical situation of an appreciable planning period, involving say a 20-year time horizon, is achieved by determining in advance some alternative patterns of active case reduction. For any one pattern, the y-values are given for the beginning and end of each year. For every year we have a set of linear relationships as described above. We next combine these sets over all years to form a single large set of linear relationships in a larger number of variables. Optimization then selects the forms of control that achieve the specified reduction program at lowest cost.

Consider, for example, an illustration given in detail by ReVelle *et al.* (1969). The initial condition involved 22 000 active cases. Four schedules of active case reduction were considered. Schedule 1 provided a slow but steady reduction to 14 400 active cases in 12 years, followed by a sharp decrease to 2000 cases at the end of 20 years. Schedule 4, on the other hand, envisaged a fast initial decrease to 7200 in six years, after which there was a slow decline to the same end point of 2000 cases. Schedules 3 and 4 were intermediate alternatives. Each schedule was subjected to the optimizing process outlined above, so as to determine the cheapest program of operation, given appropriate values of the underlying parameters.

A typical result, assuming BCG vaccination to be 70 percent efficient, was the following. The overall cost of Schedule 1 was $7.8 million, involving a total of 284 000 man-years of tuberculosis experience. Schedule 4, at the other end of the range, entailed 162 000 man-years of tuberculosis experience, but cost $11.4 million. The balance between human morbidity and dollar costs for the various schedules could thus be exhibited in a single table. Similar comparisons were presented for the alternative assumptions that BCG was only 30 percent efficient, and that it was not used at all.

Although this illustration is hypothetical, it does show very clearly how a sound mathematical model can be used as a basis for providing a public health decision-maker with an explicit set of forecasts for each of a range of strategies within his power of choice.

There are many additional technical complications in the full discussion, but it is obvious that ReVelle has devised a very useful technique for circumventing the difficulties arising from the nonlinear character of the basic epidemiological model. Further elaboration of the public health applications of tuberculosis modelling may be found in the recent book by Grundy and Reinke (1973, p.187).

16.3   Other applications

The kind of studies first successfully developed in detail for the control of tuberculosis, reviewed in the previous section, have in recent years come to be applied to a number of other bacterial diseases.

For example, Cvjetanović, Grab and Uemura (1971) have constructed a deterministic multistate model for endemic typhoid fever involving ten distinct categories. The purpose of this was to show how the endemic level was related to controllable factors such as vaccination and sanitation. A hypothetical model was established using parametric values derived from a variety of special studies in different countries. The basic equations characterizing the process were established in finite difference form, and numerical computations were carried out using a basic time-interval of one day.

The results of the extensive calculations carried out suggested that in general a single mass vaccination reduces the disease incidence very considerably, but that this gain largely disappears in a few years. Repeated vaccination, at say 5-year intervals, is an improvement, but there is a diminishing returns effect. On the other hand, improved sanitation has a long-lasting effect and in this respect is more effective than vaccination. The model can be used not only for predicting the consequences of specific preventive measures, but also as a basis for cost—benefit studies and general planning. In particular, certain demographic and epidemiological indices typical of Western Samoa and some other Pacific islands were incorporated in the calculations so as to provide conclusions that might well be of direct practical importance in this area.

A somewhat similar model involving nine categories has also been developed for tetanus by Cvjetanović, Grab, Uemura and Bytchenko (1972). There are a number of special features here. In particular, tetanus is one of the few infections diseases that are not transmitted directly from individual to individual. Again, it is desirable to make an explicit distinction between tetanus of the newborn and tetanus in the remaining population. Vaccination is the only effective and rapid method of control available, and so particular importance attaches to the study of alternative vaccination programs. A variety of computerized calculations were carried out, using parametric values typical of many developing countries. In particular, certain cost—effectiveness and cost—benefit analyses were undertaken. One important result was the demonstration of the advantages of continuously immunizing pregnant women in order to control tetanus of the newborn, both from the point of view of effectiveness and economic benefit.

A subsequent publication by Cvjetanović, Uemura, Grab and Sundaresan (1973) not only reviews the above work on typhoid and tetanus, but also introduces a brief account of the modelling of cholera. The latter is of special importance for areas like Bengal where cholera is endemic. Further details are given in Sundaresan, Grab, Uemura and Cvjetanović (1974). The cholera model includes certain additional features of practical importance such as epidemic outbreaks and seasonal variations. In general it is clear that improving sanitation is a more effective and cheaper measure than immunization, though in communities with a low incidence, treatment may be preferable from a cost—benefit point of view.

Again, a start has been made by Lechat (1971) in developing a simple multistate model for planning and evaluating leprosy control activities.

It seems probable that such studies as the above will be extended to many other diseases in the next few years. To begin with fairly simple deterministic models can be quite effective in supplying a quantitative framework for discussion of any infectious disease for which a certain amount of biological and epidemiological knowledge is available. These models have already been used to sharpen discussion of planning preventive measures and of optimizing resource allocation. However, further refinements will obviously be called for as more applications are made to specific communities, involving all the statistical problems of estimating the parameters relevant to those communities, and testing the adequacy of the models to describe available data with sufficient accuracy.

Additional discussion of the more specifically public health aspects of the application of multistate models to the control of typhoid, tuberculosis and cholera can be found in Grundy and Reinke (1973, Ch.5).

17
Parasitic diseases

17.1 Introduction

In Chapter 11 we dealt in a rather broad way with a theoretical approach to some host-vector and venereal disease models. Such models involving two populations are inevitably more complicated than situations in which a disease is, to all intents and purposes, transferred directly from one person to another. Moreover, when we come to look in a detailed way at individual diseases, there are liable to be a large number of special features which it is difficult to ignore or push into the background without incurring the charge that the proposed applications are hopelessly unrealistic. Malaria is a case in point, on which we shall concentrate attention in the present chapter. A mathematical approach to the study of malaria goes back to the work of Ronald Ross in 1911. Later (Ross, 1915, 1916, 1917; Ross and Hudson, 1917) he extended his ideas in developing a rather general theory of population disease processes under the name of "*a priori* pathometry". There has been a considerable amount of controversy ever since about the value of mathematical modelling in the practical control of malaria. Writers such as Martini (1921), Moshkovskii (1950) and Macdonald (1957) have certainly been enthusiastic supporters of attempts to unravel the quantitative complexities of malaria dynamics by means of mathematical techniques. From the standpoint of the present book, the generalities of Chapter 11 can be regarded as providing no more than a broad quantitative background. For practical applications we need investigations that are more specific and detailed.

In conformity with an emphasis on malaria, we shall give a brief overview of the chief aspects of the latter's epidemiology in Section 17.2. The basic deterministic model of Ross (1911), together with certain conclusions of Lotka (1923b), are introduced in Section 17.3. A more developed model is reviewed in Section 17.4, being based largely on the work of Macdonald (1950 and later) but including some additional discussion of the implications of the phenomenon of superinfection. Recent developments in malaria modelling, due to Dietz (1971) and Dietz, Molineaux and Thomas (1974), are outlined in

Section 17.5. Finally, Section 17.6 contains a brief commentary on the gradual
growth of applications to other parasitic diseases, notably to schistosomiasis
(bilharziasis) as exemplified in the recent work by Nåsell (1972) and Nåsell
and Hirsch (1971, 1972, 1973a, b).

17.2 Epidemiology of malaria

It is not proposed here to attempt to describe the epidemiology of malaria
in great depth. Brief references to some of the major features were made at
the end of Chapter 3, as well as in Sections 11.1 and 11.2. However, for the
more detailed and specific applications of the present chapter, it is necessary
to provide a somewhat more structured picture than we have used hitherto.
For an extensive discussion of the whole epidemiological scene, the reader
should refer to the now classical work by Macdonald (1957, 1973).

Malaria in man is due to infection by one of four organisms belonging to
the genus *Plasmodium*, namely *P. falciparum*, *P. vivax*, *P. malariae* or *P. ovale*.
These different species have similar life histories, but there are quite a number
of differences of detail. A human host is infected through being bitten by a
female mosquito whose salivary glands have been invaded by sporozoite forms
of the parasite. These sporozoites find their way to the liver of the host, where
they multiply further in an asexual manner. There is a subsequent liberation
of trophozoite forms into the blood-stream where they invade and settle in
the red blood-cells. In due course the red cells rupture and release merozoite
forms. The latter can invade new red cells, the cycle being repeated several
times. At a certain point some of the merozoites give rise to gametocytes,
which are sexual forms of the parasite.

The blood of an infected person may thus contain a number of different
forms of the parasite, and we may find it convenient to distinguish, for example, between the gametocyte-rate for a population (i.e. the proportion of the
population with detectable levels of gametocytes in their blood-streams), the
trophozoite-rate, and the overall parasite-rate (including all forms).

Now it is the gametocytes that infect biting female mosquitoes when they
take the blood meal that is necessary to the development of the eggs. The
latter are laid on water every two or three days. They hatch out into larvae
which change into pupae, from which emerge the adult mosquitoes.

In the meantime, male and female gametocytes mate in the mosquito's
stomach to form zygotes, which penetrate the stomach wall and form oöcysts,
which in turn rupture to liberate large numbers of sporozoites. Some of these
make their way to the mosquito's salivary glands and the whole cycle repeats
itself. In the mosquito population the sporozoite-rate (i.e. the proportion of
the population with detectable levels of sporozoites in their salivary glands) is
an important index of infectiousness.

It will be realized that the foregoing description is in broad qualitative
terms only. Quantitative details will vary not only from one species of parasite

to another, but also between different mosquito populations, and between different human populations. Moreover, all of these biological processes will involve a considerable amount of natural statistical variation.

To begin with at any rate, most of these aspects can be dealt with in a deterministic way using average values of the various rates and measurements involved. There are, of course, many additional complications that need to be thought about, such as the relationship between infectiousness and gametocyte densities in persons found to be positive.

Again, there are problems of changing immunity. When a human host is subjected to repeated infection with malaria a certain amount of resistance or immunity is built up. This leads to lower parasite densities in the blood. More sophisticated models can take account of different immunity classes in man.

The extent to which demographic, climatological, epidemiological, parasitological, entomological, and immunological details, to mention only some aspects, need to be incorporated in applied models is a matter for empirical investigation. As usual, we try to start with the simplest models incorporating obvious major features, progressively introducing additional factors as required for the understanding of actual data and the control of real-life processes in the field.

17.3   Basic deterministic model of malaria

A basic deterministic formulation of the essentials of the population dynamics of malaria was given by Ronald Ross as long ago as 1911. Although to some extent paralleling the more abstract discussion of Section 11.2, it is convenient to exhibit here the development of Ross's original differential equations in the more explicit context of malaria itself, bearing in mind the epidemiological picture outlined above in Section 17.2.

Using t to represent the time variable, we define the following parameters (with some minor modifications to Ross's own notation) for the human population:

    n : total population size at a given time;

    y : total number of infected individuals;

    f : proportion of infected individuals who are also infectious;

    γ : recovery-rate;

    μ : birth-rate;

    ν : death-rate.

A similar set of definitions, employing the same symbols with primes, i.e. n', y', f', γ', μ' and ν', can be applied to the mosquito population.

As described in Section 11.2, we adopt the concept of a restricted form of homogeneous mixing, based on the assumption that the mosquitoes have a man-biting rate b'. So that in time Δt we see that y' infected mosquitoes make $b'f'y' \, \Delta t$ infectious bites, of which a proportion $(n - y)/n$ are on susceptible humans. Thus, the number of new human infections in Δt is $b'f'y'(n-y)\Delta t/n$.

Taking into account the recovery- and death-rates, it follows immediately that the differential equation describing the rate of growth of the human infected population is

$$\frac{dy}{dt} = \frac{b'f'y'(n-y)}{n} - (\gamma + \nu)y. \tag{17.1}$$

An exactly analogous argument *vis-à-vis* the infected mosquito population leads to

$$\frac{dy'}{dt} = \frac{b'fy(n'-y')}{n} - (\gamma' + \nu')y'. \tag{17.2}$$

Notice that the two equations (17.1) and (17.2) are not exactly symmetrical with regard to the presence and absence of primes. The transmission of disease from a mosquito to man, or vice versa, is in each case controlled by the man-biting habit of the mosquitoes. Thus, only b' exists: there is no corresponding quantity b, since man does not bite mosquitoes.

The above formulation assumes incidentally that no new births are infected: all newborns are taken to be susceptible. In addition, Ross concluded that in man ν was negligible compared with γ, and that in the mosquito, conversely, γ' was negligible compared with ν'. Moreover, if attention was confined to populations in which the birth- and death-rates exactly balanced each other, ν' could be replaced by μ'. Using these approximations, we can rewrite (17.1) and (17.2) approximately as

$$\left.\begin{array}{l} \dfrac{dy}{dt} = \dfrac{b'f'y'(n-y)}{n} - \gamma y, \\[3mm] \dfrac{dy'}{dt} = \dfrac{b'fy(n'-y')}{n} - \mu'y'. \end{array}\right\} \tag{17.3}$$

and

In these equations, given by Ross, the possible effects of migration are ignored.

Rewriting (17.3) in terms of the malaria-rate in man, defined by $m = y/n$, and the density of infected mosquitoes per head of human population, given by $u = y'/n$, leads to

$$\left.\begin{array}{l} \dfrac{dm}{dt} = b'f'u(1-m) - \gamma m, \\[3mm] \dfrac{du}{dt} = b'fm(a-u) - \mu'u, \end{array}\right\} \tag{17.4}$$

and

where we have written $a = n'/n$, the overall mosquito density per human.

These nonlinear equations were studied in some detail by Lotka (1923b). There are two equilibrium points to be obtained by putting $dm/dt = 0 = du/dt$ in (17.4). One solution is obviously given by

$$m = u = 0. \tag{17.5}$$

The other can be obtained by dividing through the equations

$$b'f'u(1-m)-\gamma m = 0,$$

and
$$b'fm(a-u)-\mu'u = 0,$$
(17.6)

by mu, and solving the resulting simultaneous equations which are linear in m^{-1} and u^{-1}. The required solution is easily found to be

$$n = \frac{ab'^2 ff' - \gamma\mu'}{b'f(\gamma + ab'f')}, \quad u = \frac{ab'^2 ff' - \gamma\mu'}{b'f'(\mu' + b'f)}.$$
(17.7)

Lotka investigated approximate time-dependent solutions near these equilibria. For any given set of parametric values, only one solution can be achieved in practice. Thus, the first point in (17.5) is stable if

$$\frac{ab'^2 ff'}{\gamma\mu'} \leqslant 1.$$
(17.8)

This means that, when (17.8) holds, a few malaria cases introduced into a malaria-free population will not give rise to any epidemic or endemic process, and the disease soon disappears again.

On the other hand, if

$$\frac{ab'^2 ff'}{\gamma\mu'} > 1,$$
(17.9)

the introduction of a small amount of disease will cause the prevalence to rise to an endemic level given by the second equilibrium in (17.7).

Ross (1911) also set up another, single, differential equation of first order to represent the course of malaria in an infected community. Obviously, this could be at best only an approximation to the theory indicated above, which involves a system of two differential equations equivalent to a pair of two separate equations of second order, one in y and t, the other in y' and t. For an extensive mathematical discussion of the comparison and implications of Ross's malaria models the reader should consult Lotka (1923b).

It is convenient to designate the left-hand sides of the inequalities in (17.8) and (17.9) by the single quantity

$$z_0 = \frac{ab'^2 ff'}{\gamma\nu'},$$
(17.10)

where we have used our assumption that $\mu' = \nu'$. This quantity z_0 is essentially what Macdonald (1952b, 1957) later called the *basic reproduction rate*. It can be interpreted as the average number of secondary cases arising from a single primary case in a very large population of susceptibles. An immediate heuristic derivation can be derived as follows.

Take a single primary case. With a recovery-rate of γ, the average time spent in an infected state is $1/\gamma$. During this time, the average number of mosquito bites received from a susceptible mosquitoes each with a biting rate of b' is ab'/γ. Of these bites a proportion f are actually infectious. We thus have a total of approximately $ab'f/\gamma$ mosquitoes infected by the primary human case. Each of these mosquitoes survives for an average time of $1/\nu'$, largely on susceptible humans, a total of $b'f/\nu'$ infectious bites. The total number of secondary cases is thus $(ab'f/\gamma).(b'f/\nu') = ab'^2 ff'/\gamma\nu'$.

The control of malaria therefore depends, at least from the present standpoint, on reducing the basic reproduction rate to a value below unity. It is evident that intervention measures, such as antimalarial drugs, mosquito nets, insecticides and larvicides, all tend to reduce z_0. However, in any actual epidemic or endemic malaria situation it may be difficult to determine what is likely to be an effective practical combination of strategies. There are many statistical problems of parameter estimation to be faced, and these will be discussed further in the next section, where a more structured model is developed.

17.4 An extended malaria model

The discussion of the previous section is still in a somewhat theoretical form, although we have already modified the general approach of Chapter 11 so as to refer it specifically to malaria. We continue to be some way from the practical problems of identifying and interpreting actual field observations. Moreover, some of the factors introduced so far are hard to disentangle from one another as the relevant parameters tend to occur only in certain functional combinations.

It is, accordingly, necessary to describe the biological processes involved in a little more quantitative detail. There is a good deal of epidemiological controversy in these matters about which formulae appearing in the literature are valid, and which interpretations are appropriate. Nevertheless, the main lines of development seem clear enough. These are in the direction of specifying models that clarify existing biological concepts and which, with a minimum of complexity, are capable of explaining major observable phenomena, so as to lead on to the public health control or eradication of the disease.

Now one of the biological aspects, about which it is important to be clear, is the phenomenon of *superinfection*. This refers to the fact that there may be, not just a single class of infected humans, but several distinct classes, depending on how many broods of organisms, derived from different infectious mosquito bites, are flourishing in their human host side by side.

Thus, Ross (1916) had already used the following form of analysis, writing x for the proportion of people affected, h for the proportion of the population receiving infected bites per unit time, and r for the recovery-rate. Superinfection is ignored, or at any rate additional infections are supposed to be lost if they occur. It follows that, in time-interval Δt, the affected proportion of the population x is reduced by an amount $rx \Delta t$ due to recovery, and increased by $h(1 - x)\Delta t$ due to infection of the susceptible proportion $1 - x$. Hence we have

$$\frac{dx}{dt} = h(1-x) - rx = h - (r+h)x. \qquad (17.11)$$

On the assumption that h could be regarded as constant, and not varying with, for example, the changing incidence of disease, the solution of (17.11) is

$$x = \frac{h}{r+h} - \left(\frac{h}{r+h} - x_0\right) e^{-(r+h)t}, \qquad (17.12)$$

where x_0 is the initial value of x.

If we concentrate on a cohort of newborn susceptibles we can take $x_0 = 0$. Equation (17.12) then becomes

$$x = \frac{h}{r+h}(1 - e^{-(r+h)t}). \qquad (17.13)$$

Now Macdonald (1950a) pointed out that the analysis of observed data on parasite-rates by age-groups, based on the above result of Ross, leads to difficulties. Curves can be fitted reasonably well, but the estimated recovery-rates are far below what could normally be regarded as acceptable. Macdonald therefore proposed to look more closely at the phenomenon of superinfection, and to make appropriate allowances for it in the description of the basic model. Unfortunately, the modified form of (17.11) proposed by Macdonald, namely

$$\left. \begin{aligned} \frac{dx}{dt} &= h - rx, \quad h \leqslant r, \\ &= h(1-x), \quad h \geqslant r, \end{aligned} \right\} \qquad (17.14)$$

does not adequately represent the implications of the proposed extension. It is in fact necessary to consider explicitly the proportion of infected individuals harbouring any given number of broods of parasites.

Suppose, for example, that the population contains a proportion of persons f_j with exactly j broods, $j \geqslant 1$. When $j = 0$, we have the proportion of susceptibles f_0 ($\equiv 1 - x$, in the foregoing notation). Thus,

$$\sum_{j=0}^{\infty} f_j = 1. \qquad (17.15)$$

If h is the inoculation-rate, irrespective of how many broods an individual already has, and if r is the elimination-rate for any given brood, then consideration of the rate of change of the proportion of the population with exactly j broods leads immediately to the differential equation

$$\frac{df_j}{dt} = hf_{j-1} - (h+jr)f_j + r(j+1)f_{j+1}, \quad j \geqslant 0, \qquad (17.16)$$

this single formula holding for all $j \geqslant 0$, provided we take $f_{-1} \equiv 0$.

For equilibrium conditions we put all $df_j/dt = 0$, to give

$$hf_{j-1} - (h+jr)f_j + r(j+1)f_{j+1} = 0,$$

which can be rearranged in the form

$$hf_{j-1} - rjf_j = hf_j - r(j+1)f_{j+1}, \quad j \geqslant 0. \tag{17.17}$$

Using (17.17) recursively, we see that

$$rjf_j = hf_{j-1}, \quad j \geqslant 1.$$

Hence

$$f_j = \frac{(h/r)^j}{j!} f_0, \quad j \geqslant 1. \tag{17.18}$$

It now follows from (17.15) that

$$f_0 = e^{-h/r},$$

and so

$$f_j = \frac{e^{-h/r}(h/r)^j}{j!}, \quad j \geqslant 0. \tag{17.19}$$

The proportion of individuals harbouring different numbers of broods therefore follows a Poisson distribution with parameter h/r.

The corresponding time-dependent distribution can also be derived quite straightforwardly from (17.16). Defining the generating function

$$F(w, t) = \sum_{j=0}^{\infty} w^j f_j, \tag{17.20}$$

we multiply (17.16) by w^j and sum over all j. In an obvious way we readily obtain

$$\frac{\partial F}{\partial t} = h(w-1)F - r(w-1)\frac{\partial F}{\partial w}, \tag{17.21}$$

subject to the initial condition, relevant to studying the progress of a susceptible group of newborns, given by

$$F(w, 0) = 1. \tag{17.22}$$

Now (17.21) is a linear partial differential equation with subsidiary equations

$$\frac{dt}{1} = \frac{dw}{r(w-1)} = \frac{dF}{h(w-1)F}. \tag{17.23}$$

Two intermediate integrals are easily found, e.g.

$$(w-1)e^{-rt} = \text{const.}, \qquad Fe^{-hw/r} = \text{const.} \tag{17.24}$$

We can thus write the general solution in the form

$$F = e^{hw/r}\Phi\{(w-1)e^{-rt}\}, \tag{17.25}$$

where Φ is an arbitrary function.

Putting $t = 0$ in (17.25) and using (17.22) shows that

$$1 = e^{hw/r}\Phi(w-1).$$

Hence, writing $v = w - 1$, we obtain Φ explicitly as

$$\Phi(v) = e^{-h(v+1)/r}. \tag{17.26}$$

Combining (17.25) and (17.26) now gives the complete solution as

$$F(w, t) = e^{hw/r} \exp\left[-\frac{h}{r}\{1 + (w - 1)e^{-rt}\}\right]$$
$$= \exp\left\{\frac{h}{r}(w - 1)(1 - e^{-rt})\right\}. \tag{17.27}$$

The distribution is thus again of Poisson form, this time with parameter $(h/r)(1 - e^{-rt})$. This time-dependent result was first mentioned to me by Dr Klaus Dietz (personal communication), who derived it as a special interpretation of an appropriately defined homogeneous stochastic immigration–death process.

The proportion of individuals infected with at least one brood is $1 - f_0$. Putting $w = 0$ in (17.27) immediately yields $f_0(t)$. Hence, for this superinfection model, we can write

$$x(t) \equiv 1 - f_0(t) = 1 - \exp\left\{-\frac{h}{r}(1 - e^{-rt})\right\}, \tag{17.28}$$

the corresponding equilibrium value being

$$x = 1 - e^{-h/r}. \tag{17.29}$$

Equations (17.28) or (17.29) thus supply information about the parameters h and r jointly, in terms of the observed human prevalence–rate. Whether one works in terms of the gametocyte-rate or the overall parasite-rate is a matter of convenience, though it is of course essential to be consistent.

Let us now turn to consideration of the mosquito population. Instead of trying to develop a symbolism entirely consistent with our previous treatments, we shall use the notation adopted in the detailed investigations of Macdonald (1950a and later), Armitage (1953), and Macdonald, Cuellar and Foll (1968), since this has been widely referred to in the literature on malaria.

We continue to use the foregoing definitions of h, r and x. But in addition we need:

m : the mosquito density per human;

a : the average number of humans bitten per day by any one mosquito;

s : the proportion of mosquitoes with sporozoites in their salivary glands;

b : the proportion of mosquitoes, having sporozoites in their salivary glands, that are actually infectious;

n : the time taken for the extrinsic parasite cycle in the mosquito;

p : the probability of a mosquito surviving over any given day.

First, it follows from general biological considerations that the inoculation rate h must be given by $\qquad\qquad h = mabs.$ $\qquad\qquad\qquad$ (17.30)

Secondly, let the mosquito death-rate be ν', as in the previous section. The proportion of insects living for more than t days is $e^{-\nu' t}$, on the assumption of a negative exponential survival curve. The proportion of a stationary population between ages t and $t + \Delta t$ is then $\nu' e^{-\nu' t} \Delta t$. Suppose we now take into account the length, n, of the extrinsic cycle, that is the time elapsing between a mosquito's receiving infection in the form of gametocytes after biting an infected human to the invasion of its salivary glands by sporozoites. Mosquitoes of age less than n have not had time to become infectious. We consider therefore only those of ages $t > n$. There will have been an interval of length $t - n$ such that any infection acquired during it will have had time to develop and make the mosquito infectious at least by age t.

We continue to assume, as with Ross in the previous section, that the removal-rate in mosquitoes is negligible compared with the death-rate. Thus, once infectious, the mosquito remains so during the rest of its lifetime. During the interval $t - n$ the distribution of adequate contacts with infected humans can be taken to be Poisson, with parameter $ax(t - n)$. The chance of at least one such contact is $1 - \exp\{-ax(t - n)\}$. It follows that the proportion of infected mosquitoes in the population must be given by

$$s = \int_n^\infty [1 - \exp\{-ax(t - n)\}] \nu' e^{-\nu' t} dt$$
$$= \frac{ax\, e^{-\nu' n}}{ax + \nu'}. \qquad\qquad (17.31)$$

With a death-rate of ν', the probability p of a mosquito surviving for one day is

$$p = e^{-\nu'}. \qquad\qquad (17.32)$$

Substitution in (17.31) gives Macdonald's formula

$$s = \frac{axp^n}{ax - \log p} \qquad\qquad (17.33)$$

for the sporozoite-rate. This can of course be measured in practice and gives further help in estimating unknown parameters.

Information on the parameters m, a, n and p is derivable more or less directly from appropriate biological observations, though these have often been obtained in practice in rather artificial experimental situations which do not necessarily reproduce actual field conditions in a realistic way. In addition, the parameter b is a little more elusive, though it can be expressed in terms of h, a, m and s, via (17.30).

The above discussion introduces the basic implications of Macdonald's pioneer work on malaria modelling. A fuller account of the detailed conclusions that can be drawn in relation to various types of observable data is given in the mathematical statement in Appendix I to Macdonald's (1957) book. It is not worth while to discuss these various ramifications here, though the interested reader should consult the reference given. In fact, there are a number of difficulties about Macdonald's work which suggest that practical applications require further development of certain aspects.

First of all, there is the problem of handling the possibility of superinfection, already discussed above, in an adequate and consistent manner. Next, there is the major aspect of the development of immunity in response to repeated infection. This is discussed verbally by Macdonald, but not included in his mathematical treatment. Another substantial factor which needs incorporation is the fact of the enormous seasonal variations that frequently occur in mosquito populations. It is quite unrealistic to try to work with values that are averaged out over twelve months. Again, in order to pursue the implications of his modelling, Macdonald draws on parameter estimates derived from a range of relevant, but often heterogeneous, sources of data. This tends to produce a quantitative picture which may be typical, but not specific to any actual situation anywhere. To achieve the latter demands that, so far as possible, all parameter estimates be derived from the population under study. This is a general problem that has already been noted in trying to apply, for example, the multistate models of Chapter 16.

These comments are not intended to be in any sense destructive of Macdonald's work, which has constituted a major advance. Nevertheless, part of its very success has consisted in clarifying what is needed for the next steps towards constructing models that can represent actual field situations in a realistic fashion. Any models which are to be used in support of public health interventions must undergo careful fitting to data and be subjected to proper statistical validation. It is not sufficient, as is sometimes done, merely to extract from the work of Macdonald or others certain formulae which appear to be convenient, and then to use them in contexts to which they may not apply. Recent attempts to develop and apply a more integrated approach are described in the next section.

17.5   Recent developments in malaria modelling

In conformity with the remarks made at the end of the previous section, recent developments in malaria modelling have been directed towards the handling of specific field situations, especially with regard to parameter estimation and goodness-of-fit testing. This implies, of course, that such models must include major factors influencing the population dynamics of the disease, such as the development of immunity or seasonal variations in the mosquito population density. From the point of view of general *eradication* theory it may be unnecessary to introduce certain aspects like the effect of immunity on transmission. But for *control* theory such features may be crucial, since here we are concerned with the possibility of achieving a new balance between host and parasite populations within some specified period of time.

Thus the model described in Dietz (1971) was developed in close cooperation with epidemiologists, entomologists and immunologists in connection with a field project involving specific villages in Northern Nigeria. Data were in process of collection, and were expected to provide a basis for testing the model. The latter assumed that superinfection had no influence on the chance of recovery in the human population, but the notion of several immunity classes was included. Thus both infected and uninfected individuals were divided into K immunity classes. The infected classes differed from each other in respect of both infectivity and recovery-rates, while the susceptible classes varied with regard to susceptibility. Similarly, the mosquitoes were divided into K classes differing in infectivity, depending on the immunity class of humans from which they were infected. Allowance was also made for the presence of several different species of mosquitoes.

So long as an individual was infected, he could pass from one immunity class to the next class with a higher level of immunity. Similarly, a recovered individual could pass from one immunity class to the next with a lower level of immunity. Births and deaths were also included, newborns entering the class with lowest immunity.

A description of the mosquito population dynamics was also developed using several parameters of entomological importance.

Mathematical details (for these, see Dietz, 1971) are not given here as the model was later superseded (Dietz, Molineaux and Thomas, 1974). The latter

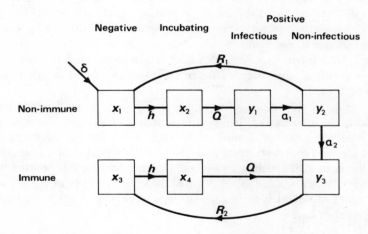

Fig. 17.1 Epidemiological model of malaria. Arrows show directions of transfer. Associated symbols are relevant transfer-rates (see text for definitions). Symbols in boxes indicate population proportions at a given time. All classes also have a death-rate δ (Based on Dietz, Molineaux and Thomas, 1974.)

authors noted that the earlier model gave a good fit to the yearly average age-distribution of malaria prevalence, but could not reproduce in a satisfactory manner the seasonal fluctuations later observed in two places chosen for testing. Appropriate modifications of the model were therefore indicated. Super-infection was reintroduced, and the immunity structure was made simpler and at the same time rather more specific.

For the human population, Fig. 17.1 shows the essence of the model adopted. The symbols x_i and y_i, defined in detail below, refer to the *proportions* of the human population in the relevant epidemiological classes. In this scheme individuals are called *positive* (y_1, y_2 and y_3) only if they have parasites in the blood. Those with parasites in the liver only (x_2 and x_4) are said to be *incubating*, while those with no parasites in the body at all are *negative* (x_1 and x_3). Of the positive persons, a distinction is made between those that are *infectious* (y_1) and those that are *non-infectious* (y_2 and y_3).

It is assumed that newborns enter the class of "non-immune negatives", having a proportion x_1, at constant rate δ. The death-rate from all classes is also δ. The inoculation-rate h defines the rate of transfer to an "incubating" class with proportion x_2, followed after a fixed incubation period of length N by conversion to the class of "infectious positives", having proportion y_1, at a rate Q to be defined below. Infectivity is then lost at a constant rate α_1, and individuals transfer to the class of "non-infectious positives", having proportion y_2. From here they may lose their immunity, recover, and go back directly to the "non-immune negatives" at rate R_1 (defined below). Alternatively, they may pass to another class of "non-infectious positives", having proportion y_3, at a constant rate α_2. These individuals retain their immunity and transfer to the class of "immune negatives", with proportion x_3, at rate R_2 (defined below). They also keep a high recovery-rate from any reinfections that occur. The latter take place at rate h, and result in individuals moving to the class of "incubating immunes", with proportion x_4, at rate h. A return to the class of "non-infectious positives" then occurs after an incubation period of length N, at rate Q (defined below).

With the above definitions we can immediately write down the equations determining the dynamics of the human population. There are, however, two further points to be borne in mind at this stage. First, the assumption of a constant incubation period of length N leads to the inclusion of a time-lag in Q, and the associated variables x_1 and x_3. The time variable t is omitted below, except where a lagged value of $t - N$ is required. Secondly, from a computational point of view it is more convenient to work with a difference equation format. We thus have

$$\Delta x_1 = \delta + R_1 y_2 - (h + \delta)x_1,$$
$$\Delta x_2 = hx_1 - Qx_1(t - N) - \delta x_2,$$
$$\Delta x_3 = R_2 y_3 - (h + \delta)x_3,$$
$$\Delta x_4 = hx_3 - Qx_3(t - N) - \delta x_4,$$
$$\Delta y_1 = Qx_1(t - N) - (\alpha_1 + \delta)y_1,$$
$$\Delta y_2 = \alpha_1 y_1 - (\alpha_2 + R_1 + \delta)y_2,$$
$$\Delta y_3 = \alpha_2 y_2 + Qx_3(t - N) - (R_2 + \delta)y_3,$$

$$(17.34)$$

where the quantities Q, R_1 and R_2 have to be defined more explicitly. Note also that all the variables x_i and y_i, and all parameters except for δ, α_1 and α_2, are taken to be time-dependent.

Consider now the transfers from the x_2 group to the y_1 group. These are individuals who were infected at time $t - N$ when in the "non-immune negative" group, with proportion $x_1(t - N)$ and inoculation-rate $h(t - N)$. With a death-rate of δ, the proportion of newly infected individuals who survive the incubation period of N days is approximately $(1 - \delta)^N$. Hence the quantity transferring to the "non-infectious positive" class in unit time is

$$(1 - \delta)^N h(t - N)x_1(t - N), \quad \text{i.e.}$$
$$Q = (1 - \delta)^N h(t - N). \qquad (17.35)$$

Next we have to derive R_1 and R_2 on the basis of the occurrence of super-infection. In general, ignoring suffixes for the moment, we adopt the basic assumptions of the detailed discussion of superinfection in Section 17.4. Thus, h is the inoculation-rate, irrespective of how many broods an individual already has, and r is the elimination-rate for any given brood. Let us assume that h varies sufficiently slowly with time for the equilibrium results of (17.19) to apply. For present purposes we want an expression for the average rate at which positive individuals become negative. In fact, transfers of this type occur only from the class with one brood to the class of susceptibles. In time Δt the proportion of the population so transferred is $rf_1 \Delta t$, but the total proportion of positives is $1 - f_0$. Hence the required transfer-rate R from positive to negative status is given by

$$R = \frac{rf_1}{1 - f_0}$$
$$= \frac{h}{e^{h/r} - 1}, \qquad (17.36)$$

using (17.19). Thus for R_1 and R_2 we can write

$$R_1 = \frac{h}{e^{h/r_1} - 1}, \qquad R_2 = \frac{h}{e^{h/r_2} - 1}. \qquad (17.37)$$

The parameters r_1 and r_2 may be regarded as fixed, though they will need to be estimated. On the other hand, in the context of equations (17.34) we must consider the inoculation-rate to be a function of time, i.e. $h(t)$. This will depend to a very marked degree on the behaviour of the mosquito population, which may easily undergo drastic seasonal fluctuations. Fortunately, most of the relevant information about the mosquito population can be combined into a single variable $C(t)$ called the *vectorial capacity* (Garrett-Jones, 1964; Garrett-Jones and Shidrawi, 1969). This index can be defined as follows. Consider a single individual who is bitten on day t by a certain number of mosquitoes. Then the vectorial capacity $C(t)$ is the total number of bites distributed by those mosquitoes that survive beyond the extrinsic cycle of duration n.

In terms of Macdonald's notation in Section 17.4, the average number of bites per individual per day is ma. The proportion of these mosquities surviving for n days is p^n. And those that survive have an average expectation of life of $(-\log p)^{-1}$, using the value of $(\nu')^{-1}$ given by (17.32). Since these survivors distribute bites at rate a, it follows that

$$C(t) = (ma) \cdot p^n \cdot (-\log p)^{-1} \cdot a$$

$$= \frac{ma^2 p^n}{(-\log p)}. \tag{17.38}$$

Thus C depends on entomological parameters and the length of the extrinsic cycle, but not on the parasite-rate or sporozoite-rate.

Next we derive an approximate expression for the inoculation-rate. It is clear from the definition of $C(t)$ that the average number of potentially successful contacts, which the infectious positives existing on day $t - n$ make on day t and thereafter, is $C(t-n)y_1(t-n)$. For a fairly short-lived vector it is not unreasonable to assume that all the latter bites occur on day t itself. If we further suppose that these bites have a Poisson distribution, the probability that any given susceptible receives at least one infectious bite is

$$1 - \exp\{-C(t-n)y_1(t-n)\}.$$

We now postulate a susceptibility parameter g, so that

$$h(t) = g[1 - \exp\{-C(t-n)y_1(t-n)\}]. \tag{17.39}$$

This formulation entails a strongly density-dependent aspect. While $h(t)$ is linearly related to C for small values of the latter, high vectorial capacities cause the inoculation-rate to reach a saturation level.

Thus, given the average annual pattern of the vectorial capacity $C(t)$ (which may in fact vary appreciably from year to year), we can use equations (17.34) to simulate the transmission dynamics of malaria in a given population.

As a refinement, Dietz, Molineaux and Thomas (*loc. cit.*) introduce the notion of the detectability of parasites in the blood of a positive individual, according to the class to which he belongs. Probabilities q_i are associated with y_i, $i = 1, 2, 3$, where it can be assumed that $q_1 = q_2 > q_3$.

After an initial period of operation to allow the attainment of equilibrium, the computer program used will produce a representation of the seasonal variations in any variable of interest. Of special importance are the daily inoculation-rate $h(t)$, the observed proportion of positives,

$$z = \sum_{i=1}^{3} q_i y_i,$$

the true proportion of positives,

$$y = \sum_{i=1}^{3} y_i,$$

the proportion of positives that are actually infectious, i.e. y_1/y; etc.

Dietz, Molineaux and Thomas also use the following ingenious device to compute the age-specific values of any variables investigated, assuming that the chosen pattern of vectorial capacity goes on repeating itself periodically. After equilibrium is achieved for the whole population as described above, the yearly pattern for the inoculation-rate is applied to a cohort of newborns, conveniently represented by an initial $x_1 = 1$. The time parameter can now be interpreted as the age of the cohort. Moreover, the inoculation-rate in this application is given, so the vectorial capacity is not involved as an input parameter. Finally, the parameter δ is put equal to zero, since the cohort is by definition not augmented by birth, and age-specific rates of the type mentioned above are unaffected by death.

The above theoretical approach was applied to field data collected from a total of 16 villages (totalling approximately 5000 individuals) involved in a WHO malarial research project in the African savannah in Kano State, Northern Nigeria. The most complete entomological, parasitological and epidemiological observations were collected from 8 of the villages in five surveys at ten week intervals during 1971, and extensive studies of this baseline material have been made. However, the paper of Dietz, Molineaux and Thomas (*loc. cit.*) is only an interim report dealing with the possibility of fitting a model to the baseline data in order to try to predict the prevalence and incidence of the parasite (primarily *Plasmodium falciparum* in this case) from the entomological observations. Subsequent investigations will deal with the control phase of the project, involving intervention measures such as the use of larvicides, adulticides or drugs, alone or in combination.

For a detailed statistical discussion the reader is referred to the paper quoted. In the present account we shall merely give a broad indication of the results obtained. Two villages were selected on the basis of showing the most extreme values of vectorial densities. They were used to examine whether the two epidemiological situations could be adequately simulated assuming the same model and the same parameters, the only difference being the two widely different levels of vectorial capacity.

In order to make the estimation problem more manageable, at least to begin with, the number of parameters to be estimated was reduced by assuming reasonable values for some of them, namely:

δ = 0·0001 per day per person. This corresponds to annual birth- and death-rates of 36·5 per thousand, with an expectation of life of about 27 years.

r_2/r_1 = 10. This ratio of elimination was regarded as reasonable, leaving only one of the parameters to be estimated, r, say.

q_1, q_2 = 1; q_3 = 0·7. Only the class of non-infectious positives retaining their immunity was considered to have a probability of detection less than unity.

n = 10 days. This is the approximate length of the extrinsic cycle, i.e. the incubation period in the mosquito.

N = 15 days. The approximate incubation period in humans.

α_1 = 0·002 per day. The rate at which infectivity is considered to be lost in the group of infectious positives.

These assumptions leave α_2, g and r_1, to be estimated from the parasitological data, given the values of $C(t)$ drawn from the entomological observations. A minimum-χ^2 technique was adopted, using the CERN computer program MINROS. Because of the large-sample equivalence of the minimum-χ^2 and maximum-likelihood approaches, this computerized method also yields the relevant standard errors. The estimates obtained were

$$\left.\begin{aligned}
\hat{\alpha}_2 &= 0·000\,19 \pm 0·000\,01, \\
\hat{g} &= 0·097 \pm 0·017, \\
\hat{r}_1 &= 0·0023 \pm 0·0005.
\end{aligned}\right\} \quad (17.40)$$

These results were derived from a total of 52 data points, the actual minimum value of χ^2 being 53·5. Since three parameters have been estimated, the number of degrees of freedom is 49. Thus, so far as the investigation has gone, the goodness-of-fit is entirely satisfactory. However, more searching analyses by the authors in question are to be expected later.

An important means of evaluating the general malaria situation in any given community is to determine the critical vectorial capacity C^*, below which the disease cannot maintain itself at an endemic level. This quantity C^* can be calculated from the relationship that holds when the basic reproduction rate $z_0 = 1$. Formula (17.10) defined z_0 in terms of the parameters used in the models of Section 17.3. In the present context we can obtain the average number of secondary cases generated from a single primary infectious case as follows. The average period during which a case is infectious is $(\alpha_1 + \delta)^{-1}$. During this time, for small vectorial capacities, (17.39) gives the approximate number of successful contacts per unit of time as gC, of which $gC(1-\delta)^N$ survive to the end of the incubation period. Hence

$$C^* = (\alpha_1 + \delta)/\{g(1-\delta)^N\}. \qquad (17.41)$$

For the parametric values assumed or estimated in the above application, we obtain 0·021 contacts per day as the critical vectorial capacity.

In order to obtain a broad qualitative impression of the intensity of effort required to achieve some degree of malaria control, the model can be used to compute the yearly average crude parasite-rate as a function of the yearly average vectorial capacity. The village with the highest vectorial capacities showed average values of about 0·2 during the dry season, and anything up to 30 during the wet season. The yearly average was 8. It could be shown that the latter value would have to be reduced by a factor of more than 170 in order to lower the yearly average crude parasite-rate to half its original value.

An investigation of data from the subsequent control phase of the project can be expected to show to what extent such qualitative forecasts are approximately valid, and able to be used as a planning guide. It is obvious that this work is at an exciting stage of development. Further studies will be required to see if the existing model is adequate for practical purposes, or whether additional modifications may be required.

17.6 Other parasitic diseases

Although there are many serious parasitic diseases in the world, malaria is pre-eminent in the degree to which it has been possible to develop the underlying mathematical theory to the point where the latter is both realistic and useful. For this reason we have concentrated on outlining the various stages through which this theory has evolved. Progress has been slow but continuous, though it is worth emphasizing that some 65 years have passed since Ross's initial work on the subject.

In more recent times attention has begun to turn towards some of the other diseases, especially schistosomiasis (bilharziasis). This is a disease caused by flatworms from the genus *Schistosoma*. There are a number of biological complications that tend to preclude any very simple mathematical treatment. To begin with, we may consider Man as the definitive host for the parasite, while certain species of snails act as intermediate hosts. Humans acquire the infection by contact with the free-swimming form of the parasite, called a cercaria. The latter occurs in water and may be male or female. The cercariae penetrate the skin and in due course mating takes place within the body of the definitive host. Eggs of the adult schistosomes are discharged from the body of the host, and if they find suitable water will develop into a free-swimming larva, or miracidium. If this reaches a snail of an appropriate species an asexual phase of reproduction may be initiated within the body of the snail. This is followed by

the production of the cercariae with which we started the description of the
whole cycle.

Human disease is caused by an accumulation of adult parasites through
repeated infections like the superinfection already discussed in Section 17.4 in
relation to malaria. Severity of disease and level of infectivity both depend on
the number of parasites present. This aspect therefore has to be taken into
account quite explicitly. We are accordingly committed to dealing with the
population dynamics of at least three species: the human host, the intermediate
host, and the parasite.

Schistosomiasis produces a variety of serious morbid symptoms. It not only
leads to the possibility of death directly, but also predisposes the sufferers to
attack from other diseases. A variety of control measures are available, including
reduction of snail populations and direct attacks on the parasite at various stages
of its life cycle. Limitations occur in connexion with most of these methods, so
that important questions arise as to the most effective and economical combinations of intervention procedures.

The whole situation is exacerbated by the fact that other supposedly bene-
ficial social developments may increase the incidence of the disease. A case in
point is the construction of dams and the formation of artificial lakes for irri-
gation purposes. The advantages of the latter may be offset by the provision of
new breeding grounds for the snails that act as intermediate hosts for the
schistosomiasis parasites.

The first big step forward in the quantitative modelling of schistosomiasis
appears to be the preliminary biometrical investigations of Hairston (1962).
This was followed by further studies by the same author (Hairston, 1965a, b).
Additional mathematical details were added by Macdonald (1965a). Since then
several writers have contributed to the development of a more structured mathematical analysis. Leyton (1968) dealt with sexual mating functions, while
Linhart (1968) investigated stochastic models to account for age prevalence
curves. The population dynamics of the parasites has been studied stochastically
by Tallis and Leyton (1969), and deterministically by Goffman and Warren
(1970).

Considerable developments of a somewhat intricate nature have recently
been made by Nåsell (1972), and Nåsell and Hirsch (1971; 1972; 1973a, b).
Although much of this work is highly theoretical in form it does appear to
have appreciable practical relevance, and is therefore referred to here rather
than in the "general theory" of Chapter 11. It is evident that a realistic model
of any given parasitic disease will tend to be rather specific to that disease,
because of the unique biological peculiarities that have been incorporated.
Nevertheless, it may well be that the theoretical work of Nåsell and Hirsch
could be adapted to deal with other diseases that have the same broad features
as schistosomiasis, e.g. the existence of an intermediate host, the multiplication
of parasites outside the definitive and intermediate hosts, the accumulation of

parasites in man causing disease of varying severity and infectivity, etc.

It is clear that this work is still in the opening stages of development. An excellent start has been made, but much more needs to be done before models of the type evolved for malaria can be used in a practical way for schistosomiasis to facilitate the choice between alternative intervention strategies. Moreover, we may hope that in due course the approach, already established for malaria and now being developed for schistosomiasis, will be extended to other major parasitic diseases such as filariasis, onchocerciasis, and trypanosomiasis.

18

Interference models

18.1 Introduction

Many communicable diseases, especially in developing countries, occur not as population processes to be studied in isolation, but as part of a more complicated pattern of spread involving two or more competing and interfering infective agents. Relatively little theoretical work has been done so far in this area which appears to have considerable public health importance. In any multi-disease situation, interventions aimed at one disease may well have consequences for the other coexisting diseases, especially if some kind of interference is present.

Specific examples, with sufficiently detailed data for mathematical analysis, are hard to come by. However, the apparent acceleration of the 1957 New Guinea yaws epidemic by a concomitant outbreak of chickenpox is a case in point. A suitable deterministic model due to Gart (1968) is described in Section 18.2, and a more sophisticated stochastic model of Reed—Frost type (also due to Gart, 1971, 1972) is developed in Section 18.3. The latter approach is particularly useful where appreciable statistical variation is present, and it also permits the ready estimation of parameters and the testing of various alternative hypotheses. Applications of all these methods to the yaws and chickenpox data of de Vries (Gart and de Vries, 1966) are described in Section 18.4.

In addition to these theoretically based mathematical and statistical investigations, a very important series of empirical studies based on computer simulations has been developed in recent years by Lila Elveback (1964 and onwards) and her co-workers. A series of six fundamental models of increasing complexity are described in Section 18.5. These have been developed in the context of the public health control of poliomyelitis by means of live polio vaccine, the operative mechanism being a degree of interference and competition between the two viral agents. The effects of different intervention strategies can be studied. In addition, the more advanced models deal with more than two infective agents, for example, where the effect of the vaccine on the naturally occurring virus is inhibited by a third enterovirus infection.

Although the Elveback models do not as yet have a highly developed theoretical basis, their practical importance should not be underestimated. They portray the interference mechanisms more realistically than the Gart models, though the latter's work points the way to a sound statistical analysis of real data.

18.2 Deterministic model

Let us first consider the deterministic analysis of a model with two kinds of susceptibles that can be used to gauge the possible interaction between two diseases. We shall follow the theoretical discussion of Gart (1968) in this section, reserving an examination of a practical application to de Vries' data on yaws and chickenpox in Section 18.4.

The essential feature of this model is that the population contains two kinds of susceptibles whose numbers initially at $t = 0$ are n_1 and n_2, where $n_1 + n_2 = n$. The number of infectives introduced into the population at the start of the outbreak is a. We now assume that the disease in question spreads according to a straightforward extension of the simple deterministic epidemic of Section 5.2. There are thus no removals of any kind. Suppose that at time t the n_1 susceptibles of the first group have given rise to y_1 infectives, with x_1 susceptibles still remaining. The corresponding quantities for the second group of n_2 individuals are y_2 and x_2, respectively. Thus, so far, we have

$$x_1 + y_1 = n_1, \quad x_2 + y_2 = n_2, \quad n = n_1 + n_2. \tag{18.1}$$

It is also convenient to distinguish the total number of infectives y, where

$$y = a + y_1 + y_2, \tag{18.2}$$

and the total number of susceptibles x, where

$$x = x_1 + x_2. \tag{18.3}$$

We shall assume that the numbers of new infections in the two groups in the time-interval Δt are $\beta_1 x_1 y \, \Delta t$ and $\beta_2 x_2 y \, \Delta t$, where β_1 and β_2 are the relevant infection-rates of susceptibles in the two groups. Homogeneous mixing is thus assumed, but the chance of disease developing in a susceptible depends on the group to which he belongs. The infectives are all considered to be equally infectious, whether they are initial cases or are derived from the first or second groups of susceptibles.

With these assumptions, the epidemic process will be described by an obvious extension of (5.1) or (5.6) in t-time, namely

$$\frac{dx_1}{dt} = -\beta_1 x_1 y = -\beta_1 x_1 (n - x + a), \tag{18.4}$$

and

$$\frac{dx_2}{dt} = -\beta_2 x_2 y = -\beta_2 x_2 (n - x + a), \tag{18.5}$$

with initial conditions

$$x_1 = n_1, \quad y_1 = 0; \quad x_2 = n_2, \quad y_2 = 0; \quad t = 0. \tag{18.6}$$

From (18.4) and (18.5), we obtain by division

$$\frac{dx_1}{dx_2} = \frac{\beta_1 x_1}{\beta_2 x_2} = \lambda \frac{x_1}{x_2}, \tag{18.7}$$

where $\lambda = \beta_1 / \beta_2$ is the relative infection-rate in the first group as compared with the second. Equation (18.7) can be solved immediately, subject to (18.6), by elementary means to give

$$\log(x_1/n_1) = \lambda \log(x_2/n_2). \tag{18.8}$$

An exact formal solution follows from writing (18.8) as

$$x_1 = n_1 n_2^{-\lambda} x_2^{\lambda} \tag{18.9}$$

and substituting for x_1 on the right of (18.5) to yield

$$\frac{dx_2}{dt} = -\beta_2 x_2 (n + a - x_2 - n_1 n_2^{-\lambda} x_2^{\lambda}). \tag{18.10}$$

An implicit solution for x_2 is therefore given by

$$\int_{x_2}^{n_2} \frac{du}{u(n + a - u - n_1 n_2^{-\lambda} u^{\lambda})} = \beta_2 t. \tag{18.11}$$

In a similar way x_1 can be found as the implicit solution of

$$\int_{x_1}^{n_1} \frac{du}{u(n + a - u - n_2 n_1^{-1/\lambda} u^{1/\lambda})} = \beta_1 t. \tag{18.12}$$

However, it is not clear how one would use (18.11) and (18.12) to estimate the infection-rates β_1 and β_2. An approximate solution turns out to be more useful. We first add (18.4) and (18.5) to obtain

$$\frac{dx}{dt} = -(\beta_1 x_1 + \beta_2 x_2) y. \tag{18.13}$$

Since $y = n + a - x$ and $x_1 = n + a - y - x_2$, we can substitute in (18.13) to give

$$\frac{dy}{dt} = \beta_1 y \{n + a - y - (1 - \lambda^{-1}) x_2\}. \tag{18.14}$$

Let us observe the epidemic up to some fixed time $t = T$. (This could be the point at which the whole situation is changed by the intervention of treatment.) Furthermore, we shall be particularly interested in processes for which $\lambda \gg 1$, i.e. where the first group of susceptibles have a much higher infection-rate than the second group. Since $x_2 \leqslant n_2$ and $\lambda > 1$, it follows from (18.14) that

$$\frac{dy}{dt} \geqslant \beta_1 y\{n + a - n_2(1 - \lambda^{-1}) - y\}$$

$$= \beta_1 y(a + n_1 + n_2\lambda^{-1} - y), \tag{18.15}$$

the equality holding at $t = 0$ when $y = a$.

Solving (18.15) then gives

$$y \geqslant \frac{a(a + n_1 + n_2/\lambda)}{a + (n_1 + n_2/\lambda) \exp\{-(a + n_1 + n_2/\lambda)\beta_1 t\}}. \tag{18.16}$$

If the total number of infectives in the second group is small, $x_2(T) \sim n_2$. The right-hand side of (18.16) is then a reasonable approximation to y. It corresponds exactly to the solution of the simple deterministic epidemic given in (5.8) (with $x = n + a - y$), provided that we now interpret the population size as $a + n_1 + n_2/\lambda$. We shall call the latter the *effective population size*.

An upper bound on y can also be obtained from (18.14) by using the fact that $x_2(t) \geqslant x_2(T)$. Arguing in a manner similar to the previous derivation leads to

$$y \leqslant \frac{a\{a + n - (1 - \lambda^{-1})x_2(T)\}}{a + \{n - (1 - \lambda^{-1})x_2(T)\} \exp\left[-\{a + n - (1 - \lambda^{-1})x_2(T)\}\beta_1 t\right]}, \tag{18.17}$$

where this time the quantity corresponding to the effective population size is $a + n - (1 - \lambda^{-1})x_2(T)$.

In at least one special case the effective population size as defined above is very close to the actual population size of relevance to the model in question. Suppose, for example, that the first group is a homogeneous collection of susceptibles, while the second really consists of a mixture of immunes and susceptibles. We want to know the size v of this latter sub-group of susceptibles, but cannot observe it directly. Now it is reasonable to assume that the total *proportion* of susceptibles infected by time T in the first group is the same as in the second sub-group, i.e.

$$\frac{y_1(T)}{n_1} = \frac{y_2(T)}{v}. \tag{18.18}$$

Thus

$$v = n_1 y_2(T)/y_1(T), \tag{18.19}$$

and the *actual* total population of susceptibles and infectives is therefore

$$a + n_1 + v = a + n_1 + n_1 y_2(T)/y_1(T). \tag{18.20}$$

On the other hand, if we put $t = T$ in (18.8), we can write

$$\lambda = \frac{\log\{x_1(T)/n_1\}}{\log\{x_2(T)/n_2\}}$$

$$= \frac{\log\{1 - y_1(T)/n_1\}}{\log\{1 - y_2(T)/n_2\}}$$

$$\doteqdot \frac{n_2}{y_2(T)}\left\{\frac{y_1(T)}{n_1} + \frac{\{y_1(T)\}^2}{2n_1^2} + ...\right\}, \qquad (18.21)$$

expanding the logs in the second line and using the previous assumption that $y_2(T)/n_2$ is small. From (18.21) it follows that the effective population size is approximately given by

$$a + n_1 + n_2/\lambda \doteqdot a + n_1 + \frac{n_1 y_2(T)}{y_1(T)}\left\{1 + \frac{y_1(T)}{2n_1} + ...\right\}^{-1}. \qquad (18.22)$$

For $y_1(T) \ll 2n_1$, the result on the right of (18.22) is approximately the same as that in (18.20).

The implications of the foregoing analysis to actual data will, as already mentioned, be reviewed in Section 18.4.

18.3 Generalized chain-binomial model

While the deterministic treatment of the previous section can be quite useful in practice, a more searching analysis is needed if we are to handle satisfactorily the problems that arise from data involving an appreciable degree of statistical variability. Some kind of stochastic model is required. One possibility would be to use a continuous-time stochastic analogue of the previous deterministic model, as was done by Severo (1969c) (see also Section 5.10). An alternative approach developed by Gart (1971, 1972) is to employ a discrete-time analogue of the chain-binomial type. This certainly seems to be approximately applicable to the yaws and chickenpox situation discussed in Section 18.4, and it readily permits the estimation of the relevant parameters and the testing of various hypotheses.

The general theory of the chain-binomial approach has already been discussed in Chapter 8, and the statistical problems of practical applications have been extensively reviewed in Chapter 14. In this section we shall confine ourselves to formulating Gart's model and indicating how various statistical tests of interest can be carried out. A numerical illustration appears in the following section.

We suppose first that the time-scale is chosen so as to make the incubation period of unit length. We shall, accordingly, be concerned to characterize the process at the series of discrete-time points given by $t = 0, 1, 2, ..., T$. The susceptibles in the population are divided into k different kinds, the actual numbers at time t being specified by the random variables $X_i(t)$, $i = 1, 2, ..., k$.

The corresponding numbers of infectives that have arisen from the several kinds of susceptibles are indicated by $Y_i(t)$. So far as the spread of disease is concerned, only the total number of infectives $Y(t)$ is of importance. It follows that the number of new infectives arising from the ith kind of susceptible at time t is

$$\Delta Y_i(t) = X_i(t-1) - X_i(t). \tag{18.23}$$

If, therefore, infectives are removed from circulation immediately after the very short period of infectiousness that completes the incubation period, we have

$$Y(t) = \sum_{i=1}^{k} \Delta Y_i(t). \tag{18.24}$$

But if no removal occurs, then

$$Y(t) = Y(0) + \sum_{s=1}^{t} \sum_{i=1}^{k} \Delta Y_i(s), \tag{18.25}$$

where $Y(0)$ is the initial number of infectives.

Let us consider the case of no removals in more detail. The simple deterministic model involving only one kind of susceptible, and with infection-rate β_1, is, as shown in Section 5.2, characterized by the differential equation

$$\frac{dx}{dt} = -\beta xy,$$

or, alternatively, $\qquad\qquad \dfrac{dy}{dt} = \beta xy. \tag{18.26}$

An obvious stochastic, discrete-time analogue of Reed—Frost type (see Chapters 8 and 14), but with no removal, gives rise to the probability distribution

$$\Pr\{\Delta Y(t)|t\} = \binom{X(t-1)}{\Delta Y(t)} \{P(t)\}^{\Delta Y(t)} \{1-P(t)\}^{X(t-1)-\Delta Y(t)}, \tag{18.27}$$

where $\qquad\qquad P(t) = 1 - q^{Y(t-1)} \tag{18.28}$

$p = 1 - q$ being the chance of adequate contact.

Now assume that p is small. Heuristically we may argue as follows. The mean value of $\Delta Y(t)$ is

$$m(t) = X(t-1)P(t)$$
$$= X(t-1)(1 - a^{Y(t-1)}),$$

whence

$$\log q = \frac{\log\left(1 - \dfrac{m(t)}{X(t-1)}\right)}{Y(t-1)}$$

$$\sim -\frac{m(t)}{X(t)Y(t)},$$

provided that $m(t)/X(t-1)$ is small, and where we also assume that $X(t-1) \sim X(t)$, $Y(t-1) \sim Y(t)$. It follows that

$$m(t) \sim (-\log q)\, X(t)Y(t). \tag{18.29}$$

The expression on the right of (18.29) corresponds closely with the deterministic form in (18.26) if $\beta = -\log q$, i.e. if $p = 1 - e^{-\beta}$. With this relationship between the parameters, the deterministic and stochastic forms of the model have the kind of correspondence we should expect.

We can now generalize the simple model, whose probability distribution is shown in (18.27), to the case of k types of susceptibles and time-dependent contact-rates. Then the likelihood of the whole set of observed $X_i(t)$ and $Y_i(t)$ can be written as

$$e^L \propto \prod_{i=1}^{k} \prod_{t=1}^{T} \{P_i(t)\}^{\Delta Y_i(t)} \{1 - P_i(t)\}^{X_i(t-1) - \Delta Y_i(t)}, \tag{18.30}$$

where

$$P_i(t) = 1 - \{q_i(t)\}^{Y(t-1)}, \quad p_i(t) = 1 - q_i(t), \tag{18.31}$$

and L is the log likelihood. We assume, in conformity with the deterministic model, that the initial number of infectives is $Y(0) = a$.

There are three main types of models that are worth special consideration, namely:

(i) Time-homogeneous models:

$$p_i(t) = p_i, \quad t = 1, 2, ..., T; \quad i = 1, 2, ..., k.$$

(ii) Time-dependent models:

$$p_i(t) = p_i, \text{ all } t \neq s; \quad i = 1, 2, ..., k;$$

$$p_i(s) = p'_i, \quad i = 1, 2, ..., k.$$

(iii) Time-dependent and group-dependent models:

$$p_i(t) = p_i, \text{ all } t \neq s; \quad i = 1, 2, ..., k;$$

$$p_i(s) = p_i, \quad i = 1, ..., h,$$

$$= p'_i, \quad i = h+1, ..., k.$$

The above classification is by no means exhaustive, and specific variants may be required for individual problems. It is assumed, moreover, that all the p_i and p'_i are to be estimated from the data, and are not given *a priori*.

It follows from (18.30) that the log likelihood L can be expressed as

$$L = \text{const.} + \sum_{i=1}^{k} \sum_{t=1}^{T} \Delta Y_i(t) \log P_i(t)$$
$$+ \sum_{i=1}^{k} \sum_{t=1}^{T} \{X_i(t-1) - \Delta Y_i(t)\} \log\{1 - P_i(t)\}. \qquad (18.32)$$

We can now conveniently estimate the relevant parameters, taking into account the restrictions specified by the model in question, using the usual technique of maximum likelihood.

Thus for the time-homogeneous model (i), differentiation with respect to p_i gives, after a little rearrangement, the equation for the maximum-likelihood estimate $\hat{p}_i$ as

$$\frac{\partial L}{\partial p_i} \equiv q_i^{-1} \sum_{t=1}^{T} \left\{ \frac{\Delta Y_i(t) Y(t-1)}{P_i(t)} - X_i(t-1) Y(t-1) \right\} = 0. \qquad (18.33)$$

On differentiating a second time, we obtain the observed amount of information as

$$I(p_i) \equiv -\frac{\partial^2 L}{\partial p_i^2} = -q_i^{-2} \sum_{t=1}^{T} \left\{ \frac{\Delta Y_i(t) Y(t-1)}{P_i(t)} - X_i(t-1) Y(t-1) \right\}$$
$$+ q_i^{-1} \sum_{t=1}^{T} \frac{\Delta Y_i(t) Y^2(t-1) q_i^{Y(t-1)-1}}{P_i^2(t)}.$$

The first term on the right vanishes in virtue of (18.33), and the second can be simplified using $q_i^{Y(t-1)} = 1 - P_i(t)$ from (18.31). Thus

$$I(p_i) = q_i^{-2} \sum_{t=1}^{T} \frac{\Delta Y_i(t) Y^2(t-1)\{1 - P_i(t)\}}{P_i^2(t)}. \qquad (18.34)$$

Since the differential coefficients $\partial^2 L/\partial p_i \partial p_j$, $i \neq j$, all vanish, the information matrix is diagonal in form. It follows that, in large samples,

$$\text{var}(\hat{p}_i) \doteqdot \{I(\hat{p}_i)\}^{-1}, \qquad (18.35)$$

where $\hat{p}_i$ is the solution of (18.33), and $I(p_i)$ is given by (18.34).

Equation (18.33) can be solved iteratively using the maximum-likelihood scoring technique (e.g. as in Chapters 6, 14 and 15). Alternatively, since only one parameter is involved in each equation to be solved, it may be simpler to proceed by a process of inverse interpolation, as in Section 6.8. This latter method readily gives numerical estimates of both $\hat{p}_i$ and its variance var $(\hat{p}_i)$ without recourse to (18.34).

A similar approach can also be used for that part of model (ii) for which the parameters are time-homogeneous, restricting the summations to those values of t for which the parameters are to be considered constant. For the parameters $p_i(s) = p'_j$ in model (ii), explicit estimates can be found. Thus in place of (18.33) we obtain

$$q_i^{-1}(s) \left\{ \frac{\Delta y_i(s) Y(s-1)}{P_i(s)} - X_i(s-1) Y(s-1) \right\} = 0,$$

i.e. $$\Delta Y_i(s) = X_i(s-1) P_i(s), \qquad (18.36)$$

from which we readily deduce the required estimate

$$\hat{p}_i(s) = 1 - \left\{ 1 - \frac{\Delta Y_i(s)}{X_i(s-1)} \right\}^{\frac{1}{Y(s-1)}} \qquad (18.37)$$

The variance of $\hat{p}_i(s)$ can be derived from (18.35), retaining only the term for $t = s$ in the expression for $I(p_i)$ in (18.34). Thus it quickly follows that

$$\text{var} \{\hat{p}_i(s)\} \doteq \frac{P_i(s)}{X_i(s-1) Y^2(s-1) \{1 - P_i(s)\}^{1-(2/Y(s-1))}}, \qquad (18.38)$$

using (18.31), and substituting for $\Delta Y_i(s)$ from (18.36).

For model (iii), we have obvious extensions of the foregoing approach. No special difficulties are entailed. However, generally speaking, most models involve nonlinear maximum-likelihood equations which do not have explicit solutions. The part of model (ii) to which the explicit form in (18.37) applies is an exception. Thus, when electronic computing facilities are available, we are better off to use the approach of Chapter 4 (already adopted, for example, in Sections 6.8 and 15.7) and simply maximize the log likelihood directly, choosing a computerized maximization programme that will automatically supply standard errors of the final estimates as well.

Whatever method we choose for maximizing the likelihood, it is helpful to have rough starting values for the computations. A convenient procedure for the time-homogeneous model (i) or the time-homogeneous component of model (ii) is to form time-dependent estimates of the type shown in (18.37) for each relevant point of time, and then take a weighted average. We thus obtain a starting value p_{i0} for the ith group given by

$$p_{i0} = \frac{\sum\limits_{u} X_i(u-1) \hat{p}_i(u)}{\sum\limits_{u} X_i(u-1)}, \qquad (18.39)$$

where $\hat{p}_i(u)$ is obtained from (18.37), and the summation is over all values of u for which the parameters are really taken to be constant. Alternatively, we could use analogous estimates based on the deterministic model of Section 18.2 (see applications to data in Section 18.4).

An important aspect of examining alternative models is the question of how to choose between them. Elsewhere, e.g. in Chapter 14, we have made extensive use of χ^2 goodness-of-fit tests for discriminating between different models.

However, as pointed out by Gart (1972), there are advantages in exploiting a likelihood approach as well, and the latter will perhaps be more widely used in the future.

Suppose we define the vector $p \equiv (p_1, p_2, ..., p_k)$. Then, when considering two hypotheses H_i, and H_j, the "odds" in favour of H_i are $\Pr\{\hat{p}|H_i\}/\Pr\{\hat{p}|H_j\}$. When the parameter space of H_i is a proper subset of the parameter space of H_j, the hypothesis H_i may be tested against H_j by using the likelihood-ratio chi-square statistic

$$\chi_r^2 = -2 \log \left[\Pr\{\hat{p}|H_i\}/\Pr\{\hat{p}|H_j\} \right]$$

$$= -2 \{ L(\hat{p}|H_i) - L(\hat{p}|H_j) \}, \tag{18.40}$$

where r is the difference between the dimensions of the two parameter spaces (see Billingsley, 1961). If, however, the hypotheses are not nested in this manner, the approaches of Cox (1962) or Atkinson (1970) might be used, though the validity of these techniques has not yet been rigorously proved for applications to Markov processes. Generally speaking, it is probably wise in practice to use a judicious combination of χ^2 goodness-of-fit tests together with an evaluation based on likelihood ratios.

18.4 Applications to yaws and chickenpox

The foregoing deterministic and stochastic models have a direct application to the data collected by deVries (Gart and deVries, 1966) in 1957 in a village of New Guinea (now West Irian) on an epidemic of yaws. Yaws is a disease caused by the spirochete *Treponema pertenue*, and the outbreak in question occurred about a year and a half after a control survey involving total mass treatment had been carried out. Moreover, the spread of the disease was faster than normally observed, a particularly large increase in the number of cases occurring during the month following a concomitant outbreak of chickenpox. Elucidation of a possible interaction between the two diseases was considered to be of some importance for the planning of long-term surveillance and eventual public health control of yaws.

Basic data on the yaws epidemic are shown in Table 18.1, where the suffix 1 refers to a negative history of yaws, and suffix 2 to a positive history. This outbreak occurred between August 1956 and February 1957 in children of 10 years of age and younger. During October 1956 there was also an epidemic of chickenpox in the same population. Inspection of Table 18.1 certainly suggestes quite clearly that the yaws epidemic made a big advance in November. A more detailed statistical analysis of the basic data (see Gart and deVries, 1966) reveals that there were 48 children, presumed susceptible to yaws in November, and who had chickenpox in October. Of these 12 contracted yaws in November, giving an incidence rate of 25 percent. On the other hand, only one of the 49 susceptibles in the non-chickenpox group contracted yaws in November. This difference is highly significant. Later, in January and February, the trend appeared to be reversed, but not quite significantly so.

Table 18.1 *Numbers of infectives and susceptibles in yaws epidemic analysed according to previous yaws exposure*

		Negative history of yaws			Positive history of yaws			Total infectives
t	Deterministic model	$x_1(t)$	$y_1(t)$	–	$x_2(t)$	$y_2(t)$	–	$y(t)$
	Stochastic model	$X_1(t)$	$Y_1(t)$	$\Delta Y_1(t)$	$X_2(t)$	$Y_2(t)$	$\Delta Y_2(t)$	$Y(t)$
0	Aug. 1956	54	0	–	48	0	–	1*
1	Sept. 1956	53	1	1	48	0	0	2
2	Oct. 1956	53	1	0	48	0	0	2
3	Nov. 1956	42	12	11	46	2	2	15
4	Dec. 1956	39	15	3	46	2	0	18
5	Jan. 1957	35	19	4	44	4	2	24
6	Feb. 1957	26	28	9	41	7	3	36

* This was the initial case; thus $y(0) = Y(0) = a = 1$.

A strong short-term association between yaws and chickenpox appears to be indicated. There is some medical support for this view, since (1) the incubation period of yaws is usually assumed to be 20-30 days, (2) the spirochete causing yaws could gain entry more easily through the skin eruptions of chickenpox, and (3) infection with chickenpox is thought to increase susceptibility to yaws, due to stimulation of steroid production.

Further investigation of the presumed association can be pursued by the use of appropriate models. First, the hypothesis that the distribution of new cases of yaws could be explained by a random Poisson process was shown by Gart and deVries to be untenable. The data of Table 18.1 show two high points in the monthly incidence of yaws, one in November 1956 and one in February 1957. The latter seems to have resulted from a gradual epidemic build-up, after which the epidemic was brought to an end by mass treatment with long-acting penicillin. The former peak in November is clearly exceptional and requires special investigation.

Let us examine first the implications of the deterministic model of Section 18.2. With equation (18.8) in mind, we can use the data of Table 18.1 to graph $\log \{x_1(t)/n_1\}$ against $\log \{x_2(t)/n_2\}$ for $t = 1, ..., 6$. Even including November ($t = 3$), there is an approximately linear relationship including the origin, which agrees with the assumptions of the model.

Alternatively, estimates of λ can be made for each month using

$$\hat{\lambda}(t) = \frac{\log \{x_1(t)/n_1\}}{\log \{x_2(t)/n_2\}}, \tag{18.41}$$

as derived in an obvious way from (18.8) For the data available we can use (18.41) only for $t = 3, 4, 5, 6$, since division by zero is inadmissible. Calculating, on intuitive general principles, the least-squares estimate which is the weighted mean with weights proportional to $\{\log x_2(t)/n_2\}^2$, gives the value $\lambda_0 = 5\cdot28$.

The effective population size $a + n_1 + n_2/\lambda$ is thus approximately 64. Substitution in (18.16) gives, approximately,

$$y \doteqdot \frac{64}{1 + 63 \exp(-64\beta_1 t)}. \tag{18.42}$$

Hence

$$\beta_1 t = \frac{1}{64} \log \frac{63y(t)}{64 - y(t)} \equiv l(t), \tag{18.43}$$

where $l(t)$ represents the logit transformation.

Thus β_1 can be estimated from observed adjacent values of y. It turns out that the average estimated $\hat{\beta}_1$ for the two months before November is $5 \cdot 54 \times 10^{-3}$, and for the three months after November is $7 \cdot 47 \times 10^{-3}$. The figure for November itself is $35 \cdot 16 \times 10^{-3}$, about five times the average of the other months. A similar though less pronounced effect can be found in the available $\hat{\beta}_2$'s, using $\hat{\beta}_2 = \hat{\beta}_1/\lambda_0$.

This brief outline of the statistical analysis based on a deterministic model (see Gart, 1968, for a more detailed description) underlines the previous conclusion that the month of November was an exceptional point in the epidemic. And on general epidemiological grounds this seems quite likely to have been due to the action of the chickenpox outbreak in accelerating the transmission of yaws.

A more searching analysis can be made using the stochastic modified chain-binomial approach described in Section 18.3. This is especially useful from the point of view of hypothesis testing.

Since the incubation period of yaws is of the order of one month, it is perhaps permissible to adopt the assumption made in Section 18.3 of a Reed–Frost type of chain-binomial model, but without removal, using a basic discrete-time interval of one month.

It is now possible to review a series of alternative hypotheses. To start with, we could consider

$$H_1 : p_i(t) = p; \quad t = 1, ..., 6; \quad i = 1;$$

where no distinction is made between different kinds of susceptibles, and time-homogeneity is assumed; or

$$H_2 : p_i(t) = p_i; \quad t = 1, ..., 6; \quad i = 1, 2; \tag{18.44}$$

i.e. model (i) of Section 18.3, involving two kinds of susceptibles depending on their previous exposure to yaws. Both of these hypotheses can be dismissed fairly quickly, since when the parameters are estimated using the techniques of Section 18.3 a significant goodness-of-fit χ^2 is obtained each time.

The next hypothesis to try is the time-dependent model (ii), defined in the present context by

$$H_3 \ : \ p_i(t) = p_i; \quad t \neq 3; \quad i = 1, 2;$$
$$p_i(3) = p_i'; \quad i = 1, 2.$$
$$(18.45)$$

The maximum-likelihood estimates turn out to be

$$\hat{p}_1 = 0.0078 \pm 0.0019; \quad \hat{p}_2 = 0.0019 \pm 0.0008;$$
$$\hat{p}_1' = 0.110 \ \pm 0.031 \ ; \quad \hat{p}_2' = 0.021 \ \pm 0.015.$$
$$(18.46)$$

Thus $\hat{p}_1'$ is significantly greater than $\hat{p}_1$, while $\hat{p}_2'$ is greater than $\hat{p}_2$ but not significantly so. The χ^2 goodness-of-fit can be shown to be non-significant, and the log likelihood is $L(\hat{p}) = -107.6$. So far, there is clear evidence in favour of H_3.

A more diversified model of some interest is given by assuming all the $p_i(t)$ to be different, e.g.

$$H_4 \ : \ p_i(t) = p_{it}; \quad t = 1, ..., 6; \quad i = 1, 2. \qquad (18.47)$$

The two estimates for $t = 3$ turn out to be by far the largest, the overall log likelihood being increased to $L(\hat{p}) = -103.2$. The test statistic in (18.40) is thus $\chi_8^2 = 8.8$, the number of degrees of freedom being eight since that is the number of additional parameters fitted in a nested way. However, this improvement is clearly non-significant.

Further light can be shed on the role of the chickenpox factor by enunciating another hypothesis. Suppose we consider the fourfold classification of susceptibles at $t = 2$ given by distinguishing not only those with and without a history of yaws, but also those who contracted chickenpox at that time and those who did not. We assume that those who did not contract chickenpox in $t = 2$ had the same probability of developing yaws in $t = 3$, depending of course on their yaws history, as in other time-periods. On the other hand, those who did contract chickenpox in $t = 2$ are taken to have a greater probability of yaws in $t = 3$, but the same probability in other time-periods, again depending only on their yaws history.

This analysis requires a somewhat finer breakdown of the data in Table 18.1, at least for the time-periods $t = 2, 3$. Let us retain the suffixes 1 and 2 to indicate negative and positive histories of yaws in those who did not contract chickenpox, introducing the additional suffixes 3 and 4 for those with negative and positive histories of yaws, who did contract chickenpox. The relevant numerical data are in fact

$$X_1(2) = 30, \Delta Y_1(3) = 1; \quad X_2(2) = 23, \Delta Y_2(3) = 0;$$
$$X_3(2) = 23, \Delta Y_3(3) = 10; \quad X_4(2) = 25, \Delta Y_4(3) = 2.$$
$$(18.48)$$

Note that the additional groups are needed for susceptibles in $t = 2$ and for new cases in $t = 3$.

Formally, the hypothesis may be expressed as

$$H_5 \; : \; p_i(t) \; = \; p_i; \quad t \; = \; 1, ..., 6; \quad i \; = \; 1, 2; \\ p_3(3) = p', \; p_4(3) = p''. \tag{18.49}$$

The maximum-likelihood estimates come out to be

$$\hat{p}_1 \; = \; 0\cdot0081 \pm 0\cdot0019; \quad \hat{p}_2 \; = \; 0\cdot0018 \pm 0\cdot0008; \\ \hat{p}' \; = \; 0\cdot248 \;\; \pm 0\cdot069; \quad \hat{p}'' \; = \; 0\cdot041 \;\; \pm 0\cdot028. \tag{18.50}$$

Clearly $\hat{p}'$ exceeds $\hat{p}_1$ at a very high level of significance, though $\hat{p}''$ is not significantly greater than $\hat{p}_2$. The log likelihood is now increased to $L(\hat{\mathbf{p}}) = -99\cdot6$, and the goodness-of-fit χ^2 is non-significant. This analysis appears to implicate the chickenpox outbreak even more clearly, though the previous likelihood-ratio test cannot be used since H_5 is not nested in H_3 or H_4. However, it is of interest to note that the formal odds in favour of H_5 compared with H_3 are $e^8 \doteq 3000 : 1$.

In conclusion is may be remarked that further extensions of this kind of chain-binomial modelling could easily be made and would present no special difficulties in handling. The mathematics is not particularly elegant, but it does supply powerful analytical tools capable of producing results of epidemiological importance.

18.5 Simulation studies

The theoretical modelling exemplified in the three previous sections is in principle extremely powerful, but unfortunately very few data have so far become available for pursuing the process of parameter estimation and hypothesis testing. No doubt this deficiency will be made good in due course. In the meantime considerable progress has been made in recent years by Lila Elveback and her co-workers (see Elveback et al., 1964, 1965, 1968, 1971; Elveback, 1971; Ewy, 1971; Gatewood et al., 1971; Ewy et al., 1972) in developing a series of modifications and extensions of the basic Reed—Frost concepts. These have been used for the investigation by simulation of the behaviour of competing and interfering viruses in highly structured communities.

Although no major theoretical principles are involved, this work is obviously of considerable relevance to many practical problems of great importance in epidemiology and the public health control of communicable disease. It is therefore worth presenting the main types of models examined and the chief areas to which they are applicable. One might hope that further research would establish additional links between the detailed analytical investigations of Gart (1971, 1972), as described theoretically in Section 18.3 and applied in Section 18.4, and the simulation studies indicated below.

The latter have in fact been classified by Elveback et al., under six main headings, referred to as Models I-VI (at least, this is as far as the series goes at the time of writing). Model I is essentially the Reed–Frost model already discussed at length in Chapters 8 and 14, a further generalization being introduced in Section 18.3. As we have seen, each individual in the population is in one of three states: susceptible, infectious, and immune. There is a fixed latent period, followed by a very short infectious period (ideally reduced to a single point of time), after which symptoms appear. The patient is recognized as such and isolated. When he recovers he is considered to be immune. In many applications it is unnecessary to make a special distinction between the isolated and recovered individuals. They are then classified together under the single heading of "immune". Each individual has a fixed probability p of having adequate contact with any other specified individual. Thus, if there are r_t susceptibles just prior to time t, and s_t infected persons just prior to time t who will become infectious at time t, then $1 - q^{s_t}$ is the probability that a given susceptible will have adequate contact with at least one infective. Hence we can deduce the binomial probability distribution, already given in (8.3) and (14.1), for the number of new cases developing at time t. Moreover, because of the fixed latent period and very short infectious period, any outbreak consists of a series of discrete crops of cases, the distribution of the crop at each stage being an appropriate binomial distribution. This model is clearly very much of a first approximation, but modifications and extensions can be made to achieve greater realism.

In the present context of competing disease agents we first consider the formulation of Model II (Elveback *et al.*, 1964). This involves the assumption that there are two antigenically unrelated viral agents A and B. These two agents are supposed to interfere with each other in the following sense. Suppose that a person who is susceptible to both viruses becomes infected with A at time t_1. He becomes infectious for A at time t_2 and continues to be infectious until time t_3, after which he is immune to A. At some period during (t_1, t_3) his susceptibility to B is reduced. When this period of reduced susceptibility to B is over, the original degree of susceptibility is restored. In order to get started, a simplified version of this model can be used in which the interference is "total" or "complete", i.e. in the presence of A the probability of infection by B is reduced to zero over the whole period (t_1, t_3).

The ideas lead quite naturally to a model based on the eight mutually exclusive states shown in Table 18.2. We can suppose that the two-agent epidemic process develops in an obvious extension of the Reed–Frost Model I process, with fixed latent periods of unit length and infectious periods all contracted to single points of time.

Let us suppose, as a further simplification, that the probabilities of adequate contact for the two agents, p_A and p_B, are in fact both equal to p. Also let p_{ij} be the probability that an individual in state i at time t transfers to state j at time $(t + 1)$. It is evident from the definitions made above that $p_{44} = p_{53} = p_{64} = p_{72} = p_{84} = 1$.

Table 18.2 *Classification of states for Model II*

No. of state i	Description of state to which an individual may belong at any time t	States, j, to which individual may transfer at time $t+1$	Probability of transfer p_{ij}
1	Susceptible to both A and B	1, 5, 7	⎫
2	Susceptible to A, immune to B	2, 6	⎪ see text
3	Susceptible to B, immune to A	3, 8	⎭
4	Immune to both A and B	4	1
5	Infective for A, temporarily insusceptible to B	3	1
6	Infective for A, immune to B	4	1
7	Infective for B, temporarily insusceptible to A	2	1
8	Infective for B, immune to A	4	1

Next, write n_i for the number of persons in state i (at time t say), and put $n_A = n_5 + n_6$ and $n_B = n_7 + n_8$ for the total numbers of A and B infectives, respectively. Now it follows from the nature of the system summarized in Table 18.2 that there are just 12 non-zero transfer probabilities p_{ij}.

The probability of an individual in State I escaping infection by both A and B is $q^{n_A} \cdot q^{n_B} = q^{n_A + n_B}$. Hence $p_{11} = q^{n_A + n_B}$. The balance of probability, $1 - q^{n_A + n_B}$, must be allotted to infection by either A or B, but not both. It is intuitively obvious in the present case, with $p_A = p_B$, that we must have

$$p_{15} = \frac{n_A}{n_A + n_B}(1 - q^{n_A + n_B}), \qquad p_{17} = \frac{n_B}{n_A + n_B}(1 - q^{n_A + n_B}).$$

Again it is easily seen that $p_{22} = q^{n_A}$, $p_{26} = 1 - q^{n_A}$, $p_{33} = q^{n_B}$ and $p_{38} = 1 - q^{n_B}$. All other p_{ij} not mentioned so far are identically zero. When $p_A \neq p_B$ a little more care is needed over the expressions for p_{15} and p_{17}. Elveback *et al.* (1964) give results based on the idea of the infection processes actually taking place in continuous time over each interval. This raises complications that are not entirely in accord with the basic assumption of the Reed–Frost model that infectiousness is virtually confined to a single point of time. It seems that further work should be done on a more precise specification of the infection process in this general case of $p_A \neq p_B$.

It is evident that the foregoing definition of Model II is sufficient for carrying out computer simulations. Elveback *et al.* (1964) showed that, under typical assumptions, the distribution of the total number of cases due to one disease agent operating alone was practically unchanged by the presence of a competing and totally interfering agent. The value of these results for practical purposes was somewhat limited, but a basis had been laid for further more realistic developments.

Extensions of the above ideas were accordingly made in Model III (Elveback
et al., 1968). Allowance was made for the possibility of different agents having
different lengths of infectious periods by maintaining the infectiousness of any
individual over several basic time-intervals. The length of the infectious period
can easily be represented as a discrete random variable. A similar extension can
also be made to the period during which the interference operates. Model III
exhibited sufficient structure to study the possibility of using mass vaccinations
with a live vaccine to reduce, by interference, the epidemic potential of some
naturally occurring agent. Specific reference was made to the control of
Coxsackie B virus by means of the Sabin live-virus poliomyelitis vaccine. Simulation studies showed, for example, that the optimal vaccination schedule was
one which reduced the supply of susceptibles to the naturally occurring virus
below the appropriate threshold, and which held the supply at a sub-threshold
level until the original cases died out. It was further demonstrated that 100
percent vaccination on one weekend was less effective than other schedules
which spread the vaccination over two weekends. The latter schemes in fact
assured that the supply of Coxsackie susceptibles remained low for a longer
period of time.

Additional developments to take account of certain aspects of sociological
structure were incorporated in Model IV (Elveback *et al.*, 1971). Each individual
was regarded as belonging to three or four different mixing groups such as families, preschool play group, grade school, neighbourhood cluster of families, and
total community, depending on which of three major age-groups the individual
had been assigned to. The relative effects of various control measures such as
vaccination and the closing of schools were studied in relation to the distribution of initial cases.

A three-agent situation was also investigated by Elveback *et al.* (1971) in
Model V. Here studies were made of the effectiveness of the mass use of live
poliovirus vaccine in controlling an epidemic of wild poliomyelitis in a typical
developing country situation, where vaccination failures could be expected
because of interference from widespread enterovirus infections. The effectiveness of using the vaccine to reduce epidemic size, under certain specified conditions, was demonstrated.

An even more sophisticated development was Model VI (Ewy *et al.*, 1972).
This permitted the use of a more complex sociological stratification of the
community. It also analysed the chance of adequate contact into three components which depended on (1) the probability of physical contact, as a function of sociological behaviour, (2) the level of infectivity, a time-dependent
property of an infective, and (3) the level of susceptibility, a time-dependent
characteristic of a susceptible. Stochastic patterns of infectivity and susceptibility were incorporated as well. Both single-agent and multi-agent versions of
Model VI were described.

Obviously such a model can be structurally more realistic than the simple

Models I and II, though there may be difficulties in practical applications due to the large number of parameters involved. Nevertheless, as pointed out by Ewy *et al.*, Model VI should facilitate a number of sensitivity studies of great practical relevance. There are many questions affecting possible public health interventions that could be investigated, such as the effect of changing contact probabilities or the lengths of infectious periods by means of appropriate vaccination or immunization campaigns. Again, sensitivity analyses of model structure could produce estimates of the rewards and penalties of increasing the complexity of the model.

Finally, it should be repeated that although this work has so far achieved very little in the way of basic theoretical results, it does offer an extremely useful tool for analysing the probable consequences of alternative public health intervention strategies; and as such it is deserving of closer attention by those who are interested in the practical applications of the mathematical theory.

19
Geographical spread

19.1 Introduction

Some of the theoretical problems involved in the geographical distribution of infectious diseases have been discussed in Chapter 9, where we looked at both deterministic and stochastic models that explicitly incorporated a spatial element. The notion of several interacting groups of individuals had already been introduced in Sections 5.10 and 6.9, but these extensions of the single population models did not entail a direct use of two-dimensional distributions in space as such.

Nevertheless, the spread of a disease in space as well as time can be a matter of considerable practical importance. Several advances have been made in recent years in the USSR in the development of methods to predict the spread of influenza from one big city to another. The standpoint adopted there is intermediate between the two kinds of modelling mentioned above. Thus in the multigroup models of Sections 5.10 and 6.9 continuous interactions are envisaged between the different groups, although there is no explicit spatial structure, while in the genuinely spatial models of Chapter 9 assumptions are made that are mathematically appealing, though difficult to handle except under rather simplified conditions. The models developed in the USSR, on the other hand, describe the spread of disease within any given city in terms of restricted homogeneous mixing (as in Chapter 11, 16 and 17), but handle contacts between cities on a migration basis, the latter being derived empirically from the records of the transportation system. This simplification not only strikes a note of realism, but also leads to verifiable predictions derived from a computerized analysis.

Some of the general ideas involved in modelling the contact between groups in terms of migration rather than some form of random mixing are introduced in Section 19.2, and the specific approach adopted in the USSR for dealing with the spread of influenza between major cities is described in Section 19.3.

350

19.2   Migration models

Let us look first at the simplest possible way of describing a multigroup model in which the spread of disease within a group follows the general deterministic formulation of Section 6.2, but the contacts between groups are achieved by actual migration from one group to another. We now have to be rather more explicit about the different categories of individuals since it is unreasonable to suppose that those who are ill and isolated will be subject to migration. Let us therefore distinguish, in the ith group at time t, x_i susceptibles, y_i circulating infectives, u_i ill and isolated individuals, and z_i recovered and immune persons. If an appreciable number of people die we should have to introduce an additional category, but we shall ignore this complication for the time being. Let the total group size be n_i, there being G groups in all, so that

$$x_i + y_i + u_i + z_i = n_i, \quad i = 1, ..., G. \tag{19.1}$$

We can use a general infection-rate β, applicable to all groups, and a removal-rate γ, as before. So that the number of new infections within the ith group in time Δt is $\beta x_i y_i \Delta t$, and the number of removals is $\gamma y_i \Delta t$. The latter removals are of course observed new cases, as previously. However, they now join the ill and isolated category, for which we may assume a recovery-rate ω. Thus in time Δt there are $\omega u_i \Delta t$ individuals who transfer to the recovered and immune class. In addition, let us employ a migration-rate μ_{ij} which characterizes the rate of emigration of individuals from group i to group j, and which applies to all individuals except those who are ill and isolated.

The basic equations for group i are therefore

$$\left.\begin{aligned}
\frac{dx_i}{dt} &= -\beta x_i y_i + \sum_{j=1}^{G} (\mu_{ji} x_j - \mu_{ij} x_i), \\[2mm]
\frac{dy_i}{dt} &= \beta x_i y_i + \sum_{j=1}^{G} (u_{ji} y_j - \mu_{ij} y_i) - \gamma y_i, \\[2mm]
\frac{du_i}{dt} &= \gamma y_i - \omega u_i, \\[2mm]
\frac{dz_i}{dt} &= \omega u_i + \sum_{j=1}^{G} (\mu_{ji} z_j - \mu_{ij} z_i).
\end{aligned}\right\} \tag{19.2}$$

It will be noticed that, in this formulation, n_i is in general a variable quantity. But if

$$\sum_{i=1}^{G} n_i = N, \tag{19.3}$$

then N is the total number of individuals in all groups and is of course constant.

In equations (19.2) we have two kinds of parameters, first, the intrinsic epidemiological parameters β, γ and ω; and, secondly, the migration parameters μ_{ij}. The problem of estimation, using normally available data, presents some difficulties even in the present deterministic model. The recovery-rate ω can clearly be determined more or less directly from the observation of ill people. Again, it may be possible to estimate the μ_{ij} directly from observation, using data from the transportation network if these are available. The parameters β and γ are, as usual, more difficult since we only observe removals and not infections. However, for the purpose of initial explorations in specific instances it might be possible to set approximate *a priori* values on β and γ. (A more tractable modification of this model, approximately valid for the special case of influenza, is discussed in Section 19.3.)

Let us suppose that we can actually measure the rates of migration between all pairs of groups, σ_{ij} being the rate of transfer from group i to group j. Thus σ_{ij} is the rate for the whole group, while μ_{ij} as defined above is the rate per individual. Since the latter applies to all those who are not ill and isolated, it follows that

$$\sigma_{ij} = \mu_{ij}(n_i - u_i). \tag{19.4}$$

Thus if s_{ij} is the observed rate of transfer over some short interval of time, we can estimate μ_{ij} as

$$\overset{\smile}{\mu}_{ij} = \frac{s_{ij}}{n_i - u_i}. \tag{19.5}$$

If the data are not very abundant, we may have to combine data from different short intervals of time. This would give us the opportunity to test whether μ_{ij} appeared to vary with time or not. Obviously many practical statistical problems may arise in any specific context. These can be dealt with *ad hoc* by standard statistical methods, and we shall not pursue this aspect here.

Another matter to be examined is the validity of the assumption of homogeneous mixing so far as the spread of infection is concerned. We have already discussed some restrictions of this concept in Chapters 11, 16 and 17 in relation to malaria, venereal disease and tuberculosis. Suppose we imagine two cities, one k times as large in population as the other, and consider the contacts made in each by a given infectious individual. We can ask whether it is reasonable to assume that the rate at which the infective contacts other individuals in the larger of the two cities is really k times the rate obtaining in the smaller of the two cities. In many situations it seems more reasonable to assume for each individual a constant rate β of making contacts, irrespective of the total population size. However, this is a point which needs careful consideration whenever we are studying a particular disease in a specific community. For the moment, let us make this assumption. As we have seen in the previous discussions (Chapters 11, 16 and 17), this implies that the parameter β in (19.2) must be replaced by β/n_i.

With this restricted form of homogeneous mixing in mind, let us rewrite equations (19.2), using also (19.4) to replace the μ_{ij} by the σ_{ij}. We now have

$$\frac{dx_i}{dt} = -\frac{\beta x_i y_i}{n_i} + \sum_{j=1}^{G} \left(\frac{\sigma_{ji} x_j}{n_j - u_j} - \frac{\sigma_{ij} x_i}{n_i - u_i} \right),$$

$$\frac{dy_i}{dt} = \frac{\beta x_i y_i}{n_i} + \sum_{j=1}^{G} \left(\frac{\sigma_{ji} y_j}{n_j - u_j} - \frac{\sigma_{ij} y_i}{n_i - u_i} \right) - \gamma y_i,$$

$$\frac{du_i}{dt} = \gamma y_i - \omega u_i,$$

$$\frac{dz_i}{dt} = \omega u_i + \sum_{j=1}^{G} \left(\frac{\sigma_{ji} z_j}{n_j - u_j} - \frac{\sigma_{ij} z_i}{n_i - u_i} \right).$$

$$(19.6)$$

The models characterized by (19.2) and (19.6) have been introduced here largely on *a priori* grounds for the purpose of illustrating how the notion of migration, especially in relation to an observable transportation network, can be employed to set up a moderately realistic representation of the spread of a communicable disease over a large geographical area. They can be particularly useful in the case where the infection is initially introduced into a single group, subsequently spreading to other groups. A modified form of this approach, adopted in the USSR for studying the propagation of influenza throughout the country, is described in the following section. So far, no purely theoretical investigations have yet been carried out on the models of the present section, though it might in fact be quite useful to supplement specific, computerized applications with a deeper understanding of the structure of the processes involved.

19.3 The spread of influenza

The idea of describing the diffusion of a disease throughout a whole country, using the type of migration model introduced in the previous section, originated in the work of Baroyan and Rvachev (1967). This idea was subsequently developed and applied to the study of the spread of influenza in the USSR by Rvachev (1968b); Baroyan and Rvachev (1968); Baroyan, Genchikov, Rvachev and Shashkov (1969); Baroyan, Basilevsky, Ermakov, Frank, Rvachev and Shashkov (1970); Baroyan, Rvachev, Basilevsky, Ermakov, Frank, Rvachev and Shashkov (1971); Rvachev (1971, 1972); and Baroyan, Zhdanov, Soloviev, Zakstelskaya, Rvachev, Urbakh, Ermakov and Antonova (1972). Several of these papers exist only in the original Russian, but a useful coverage is provided by the English language communications of Baroyan *et al.* (1969, 1970, 1971). Two other papers by Rvachev (1967, 1968a) relate infectious processes in the organism to the structure of epidemics.

For the purposes of investigating influenza, Baroyan *et al.* used a somewhat simplified and modified version of the model presented in the previous section. Thus the *i*th group was considered to consist of n_i individuals, of whom x_i were susceptibles, y_i were circulating infectives who were all more or less ill but not sufficiently so to be isolated, and z_i were immunes, the class of ill and isolated persons being absent. One consequence of this formulation is that, at least in principle, it should be possible to observe y_i directly. In practice of course it has to be admitted that public health records are often far from complete, even when a disease is notifiable.

The groups themselves were identified with whole cities, and in the studies described 128 of the largest cities were chosen for convenience, i.e. $G = 128$ (this involved practically all cities with over 100 000 population).

In the earlier models infection-rates $\beta_i(t)$ were used, where there was dependence on both the individual group and the time. Thus the infection-rate might be related to population density, and it could also vary during the course of an epidemic owing to the susceptibles gradually building up a partial immunity through the wide circulation in the community of small doses of virus. However, in later versions of the model the assumption of a constant β was considered a reasonable first approximation.

So far, the above assumptions would lead to the simplified version of (19.6) given by

$$\left. \begin{aligned}
\frac{dx_i}{dt} &= -\frac{\beta x_i y_i}{n_i} + \sum_{j=1}^{G} \left(\frac{\sigma_{ji} x_j}{n_j} - \frac{\sigma_{ij} x_i}{n_i} \right), \\
\frac{dy_i}{dt} &= \frac{\beta x_i y_i}{n_i} + \sum_{j=1}^{G} \left(\frac{\sigma_{ji} y_j}{n_j} - \frac{\sigma_{ij} y_i}{n_i} \right) - \gamma y_i, \\
\frac{dz_i}{dt} &= \gamma y_i + \sum_{j=1}^{G} \left(\frac{\sigma_{ji} z_j}{n_j} - \frac{\sigma_{ij} z_i}{n_i} \right).
\end{aligned} \right\} \qquad (19.7)$$

If the disease starts in a single city, either by introduction from outside the country or from a virus mutation within the community, it should be possible to estimate the parameter β from statistical data on the initial stages of the local epidemic, while γ could be estimated from observed rates of recovery of sick persons. As indicated in the previous section, the migration coefficients σ_{ij} could also, hopefully, be derived from observations on the transportation system. We should then have enough information to make projections of the course of the epidemic over the whole country, given appropriate initial conditions, and to compare the projections with the events actually observed.

The assumption, in (19.7), of a constant removal-rate γ implies that the size of any given group of infectives decays in an exponential manner. However, the model of Baroyan et al. is formulated in a slightly more sophisticated fashion to allow for an age-dependent chance of recovery. Thus a distribution function $F(\tau)$ is defined for the duration of the illness, so that $F(\tau)$ is the proportion of newly infected persons who are ill for up to a period of τ time units. Further, is is convenient to define an auxiliary variable $\phi_i(t, l)$, where the number of individuals in group i at time t who fell sick in the time-interval $(l, l + \Delta l)$ is $\phi_i(t, l)\Delta l$ (for $l \leqslant t$), whether these individuals have recovered by time t or not. It follows from elementary considerations that

$$x_i(t) = x_i(0) - \int_0^t \phi_i(t, l)dl, \qquad (19.8)$$

and

$$y_i(t) = \int_0^\infty \phi_i(t, t - \tau)\{1 - F(\tau)\}d\tau, \qquad (19.9)$$

where (19.8) simply says that the number of susceptibles remaining at time t is equal to the initial number minus all the infections that have taken place, and (19.9) describes the fact that the number of infectives at time t is given by the total number of infections that have taken place at earlier times but have not yet recovered by time t. In practice it may be convenient to assume a maximum duration of illness T. In this case, $F(\tau) \equiv 1$ for $\tau \geqslant T$, and the upper limit of integration in (19.9) is T instead of ∞.

It is also evident that the number of infections taking place in group i in time-interval $(t, t + \Delta t)$ is $\phi_i(t, t)\Delta t$.

Thus

$$\phi_i(t, t) = \frac{\beta x_i y_i}{n_i} = \frac{\beta x_i(t)}{n_i} \int_0^\infty \phi_i(t, t - \tau)\{1 - F(\tau)\}d\tau, \qquad (19.10)$$

and the first equation of (19.7) can then be written

$$\frac{dx_i(t)}{dt} = \sum_{j=1}^G \left(\frac{\sigma_{ji} x_j(t)}{n_j} - \frac{\sigma_{ij} x_i(t)}{n_i} \right) - \phi_i(t, t). \qquad (19.11)$$

In addition, we consider how $\phi_i(t, l)$ may change with changes in t. The number of individuals $\phi_i(t, l)\Delta l$ is clearly affected only by migration. Hence

$$\frac{\partial \phi_i(t, l)}{\partial t} = \sum_{j=1}^G \left(\frac{\sigma_{ji} \phi_j(t, l)}{n_j} - \frac{\sigma_{ij} \phi_i(t, l)}{n_i} \right). \qquad (19.12)$$

Equations (19.10), (19.11) and (19.12), for $i = 1, ..., G$, are sufficient to determine the behaviour of the system as a whole for suitable initial conditions. The function $F(t)$ was estimated approximately from available epidemiological data on the duration of influenza. Estimation of the migration parameters σ_{ij} presented some difficulties. To begin with, an empirical approximation was used, given by $\sigma_{ij} = kn_i n_j$, where $k \doteq 2^{-32}$. This was derived from official transportation figures for traffic between Moscow and certain other cities in October 1966. Later it became possible to use more broadly based estimates obtained from a more extensive analysis of the reports of the traffic agencies.

This modified model was applied in 1967 by Baroyan et al. to the 1965 influenza epidemic, which was introduced first into Leningrad in January from Western Europe and which spread subsequently throughout the USSR. Statistics on the prevalence of influenza were available on a daily basis over the whole period of the local epidemic in Moscow, but only for the first few days in Leningrad. It was assumed as an approximation that the initial proportion of susceptibles was the same in all cities, i.e. $x_i(0) = Cn_i$, where C was a constant to be determined. Data from the initial period of the Moscow epidemic were used to determine estimates of β and C.

After these preliminary calculations, equations (19.10), (19.11) and (19.12) were used to compute the expected course of the epidemic over the whole network of 128 cities, *using only the initial epidemic data from Leningrad*, and assuming that the further introduction of influenza cases from outside the USSR was negligible. Detailed observations of subsequent outbreaks in other cities were originally available only for Moscow. It is remarkable that good qualitative predictions for the latter were obtained, relating to size, time of onset, and maximum point of the outbreak. Considering the extent and nature of the assumptions made in order to achieve these computerized predictions, the results were highly encouraging. Unfortunately, no use could be made at the time, i.e. 1967, of the predictions for the other 127 cities.

However, three years later in 1970, epidemiological data were collected by V. V. Ermakov showing the daily incidence of influenza in many other cities of the USSR over the previous ten years. Appropriate extracts from these records could then be compared with some of the computer predictions which had happily been preserved for all 128 cities in a thesis of Rvachev. Comparative figures were available for 23 cities in all. These showed extraordinarily good qualitative agreement between predictions and observations. Observed and predicted epidemic curves are exhibited for 10 cities in Rvachev (1971), and for 21 cities in Baroyan *et al.* (1970). Further confirmations over a fifteen-year period were reported by Baroyan *et al.* (1972).

It should be mentioned here that all the secondary outbreaks, both observed and predicted, occurred within a relatively short space of time. Most of the curves had peaks around the end of the first week in February, though in two cities the outbreaks occurred about two weeks later. It is the latter type of occurrence which, when accurately predicted, is especially convincing. Additional support for this type of modelling, in which there is a major migrational feature, would come from situations in which reasonably accurate predictions could be made with appreciably longer time-lags, of several months, say, such as may occur in the transmission of disease from one country to another.

The foregoing discussion presents the main features of this large-scale modelling of the spread of influenza, utilizing the structure of the transportation network. For further elaboration of the epidemiological and statistical minutiae the reader should consult the references cited, especially Rvachev (1968b), Baroyan *et al.* (1969, 1970, 1971, 1972), and Rvachev (1971). It is obvious that this whole approach is of considerable importance to the forecasting and possible control of serious epidemic diseases, both within countries and on a world-wide scale.

Further research is certainly required, especially on statistical problems of estimating the many unknown parameters, both epidemiological and transportational, and of testing more thoroughly the reliability and validity of the variety of models that might be needed for different diseases.

20
Immunization programs

20.1 Introduction

One of the major weapons against the spread of infectious disease is the use of some form of immunization which creates an artificial immunity amongst those who would otherwise be susceptible. This protection takes several forms. In discussing the modelling of tuberculosis in Section 16.2 we saw that an important control factor was the use of BCG vaccination. This did not prevent susceptibles becoming infected, but did reduce the probability of their becoming active cases if infected. Immunization against typhoid and tetanus was also mentioned in Section 16.3. In the case of cholera, improvements in sanitation were liable to be more effective than existing immunization procedures.

The development of multistate models, as in Chapter 16, allows one to forecast the possible consequences of a variety of public health interventions. But when immunization as such is carried out on a vast scale in the attempt to hold down a disease to a very low endemic level, or even eradicate it altogether, there comes a point when the costs of the intervention measures and the small but real risks inherent in these measures begin to outweigh the disadvantages of the disease. This is the case with smallpox in some countries.

As a matter of historical interest, a brief account is given in Section 20.2 of the 18th century controversy about the practice of inoculation, or variolation, against smallpox. It seems to have been effective, but the risks were by no means inappreciable. Section 20.3 introduces the 20th century problem of smallpox vaccination, and gives the general reasons why it has been considered appropriate to abandon this procedure as a routine measure in recent years in countries like the USA.

A detailed discussion of a vaccination model, based on the work of Becker (1972), is given in Section 20.4. This is primarily developed in the context of smallpox vaccination, with a numerical illustration in Section 20.5, but would be applicable to other diseases as well.

Some further developments are indicated in Section 20.6. These include certain refinements to Becker's model, and the more recent work done by Griffiths

(1973b) on the effects of measles vaccination using the recurrent epidemic models of Chapter 7.

20.2   Smallpox inoculation in the 18th century

The first recorded attempt to use a mathematical method for evaluating a public health policy appears to be that of Daniel Bernoulli (1760), who investigated the effectiveness of variolation (also referred to as "inoculation") against smallpox. This practice, which had been used in both China and India in ancient times, began to be adopted on an increasing scale in Europe in the first half of the 18th century. It consisted of inoculating a susceptible with material taken from a smallpox pustule in an active case, with a view to provoking a mild attack in the susceptible followed by recovery and permanent immunity. Such methods were of course superseded later by the more reliable technique of vaccination. The practice of variolation was not without risk. A variolated individual might die from the disease acquired, though rarely. He could also give rise to outbreaks of smallpox amongst the susceptibles with whom he was in contact. By 1760 there was considerable controversy as to the efficiency of the procedure and the potential dangers to inoculated individuals and to the community in general.

Bernoulli read his memoir to the Académie Royale des Sciences in Paris on 30th April 1760, though the actual publication did not appear until 1765. A vigorous attack was delivered by d'Alembert at a further session on 12 November 1760, and this was printed privately in his own *Opuscules Mathématiques* (d'Alembert, 1761) soon afterwards. Bernoulli's published paper contained a reply to d'Alembert's criticisms. On the whole, the latter's attacks would probably not be regarded as carrying much weight to-day, and indeed some of his arguments verge on the self-contradictory. Bradley (1971) has recently produced an English translation of the whole of Bernoulli's paper and d'Alembert's memoir referred to above, plus a part of the latter's voluminous notes and subsequent writings on the subject. See also Brambilla (1962, p. 103).

It is of some interest to consider in outline what Bernoulli actually wrote. He dealt not with the population dynamics of smallpox in the whole community, but discussed instead the fate of a cohort of newborn children. In modern notation the argument runs as follows. Suppose that at time t we have a total of $n(t)$ individuals surviving from the original cohort of $n(0) = n$, say. Let the number of susceptibles remaining at time t be $x(t)$. Evidently $x(0) = n(0)$, if all newborns can be considered susceptible. Now let us assume a deterministic model in which the rate per individual, at which susceptibles in the cohort acquire infection from the surrounding community, is β; the death-rate from causes other than smallpox is $\mu(t)$; and the case-fatality rate is ν. This means that we are using the fairly realistic concept of an age-specific death-rate.

It follows that the number of new infections in Δt is $\beta x \, \Delta t$; the number of susceptibles dying from causes other than smallpox is $\mu(t)x \, \Delta t$; and the number dying in the whole cohort from other causes is $\mu(t)n\,\Delta t$. We further interpret the case-fatality rate as meaning that the number of individuals dying of small-pox in Δt is $\nu\beta x\,\Delta t$, while those who survive and become immune are $(1 - \nu)\beta x\,\Delta t$. Given this slightly simplified model, we can immediately write down the deterministic equations

$$\frac{dx}{dt} = -\{\beta + \mu(t)\}x, \qquad (20.1)$$

$$\frac{dn}{dt} = -\nu\beta x - \mu(t)n, \qquad (20.2)$$

subject to the initial conditions

$$x(0) = n(0) = n. \qquad (20.3)$$

Next, let us write

$$f = x/n \qquad (20.4)$$

for the proportion of survivors at time t who are still susceptible to smallpox. Differentiating (20.4) with respect to t, and using (20.1) and (20.2), quickly leads to the equation in f given by

$$\frac{df}{dt} = \beta f(\nu f - 1), \qquad (20.5)$$

which incidentally does not involve $\mu(t)$, the initial condition being

$$f(0) = 1. \qquad (20.6)$$

The solution of (20.5) is the logistic curve

$$f(t) = \frac{1}{\nu + (1 - \nu)e^{\beta t}}. \qquad (20.7)$$

Using information available to him, Bernoulli chose the estimates $\nu = \beta = \frac{1}{8}$. He then used (20.7) to extend Halley's Life Table for Breslau (which was the best available at the time, and which was based on deaths from all causes) to estimate the numbers catching smallpox each year and the numbers dying from it, for comparison with those dying from other causes. A further table was then constructed to show what results would follow if nobody died of smallpox, i.e. if inoculation were completely effective with $\nu = 0$. This of course would be the ideal solution, but Bernoulli also calculated what would happen if the risk of dying from the inoculation were 1/200, which he regarded as an upper limit. The final conclusions can be summarized by saying that the life expectancy at birth, on Halley's Table, was 26 years 7 months. If inoculation were completely effective this figure would be increased to 29 years 9 months, while the suggested upper limit of the risk of dying from inoculation would reduce the latter expectation by only 1 month 20 days.

Bernoulli came out clearly on the side of inoculation on the grounds that the good done far outweighed any harm caused. Whatever the rights and wrongs of this controversy from a modern clinical or epidemiological standpoint, Bernoulli's principle, of using a mathematical method of inquiry to review the available data in order to evaluate alternative public health strategies, is as valid to-day as it was 200 years ago.

20.3   Smallpox vaccination in the 20th century

As is well known, the variolation technique of protection against smallpox was superseded by vaccination with cowpox virus (vaccinia), as demonstrated by Edward Jenner at the end of the 18th century. This procedure gradually became the major weapon in the fight against smallpox, though it took about 150 years before the continuing spread of the disease was effectively halted. The World Health Organization's global eradication program against smallpox, first called for in 1958, is now well on the way to eliminating the disease.

Now vaccination itself carries with it comparatively little risk of complications or death. At least, these risks are quite negligible when one is faced with an actual or threatened outbreak of smallpox. But when vaccination programs involve millions of people, and when the incidence of smallpox approaches a comparatively low level, there comes a point when public health authorities have a real problem in balancing the advantages and disadvantages of continuing vaccination as a routine policy. Thus in the USA in 1968 (Lane, Ruben, Neff and Millar, 1969) approximately 14 168 000 individuals were vaccinated of whom 572 suffered from confirmed complications, including 9 deaths. Nevertheless, not a single case of smallpox was imported into the USA in the 21-year period 1950-70. In addition, the total estimated cost to the USA in 1968 of vaccine production, physicians' services in vaccination, medical care for those with complications, processing of international vaccination certificates, etc., amounted to some $150 000 000 (World Health Organization, 1972). The general impression created is that the cost and other risks associated with smallpox vaccination far outweigh the advantages, at least in a country like the United States.

On the other hand, the smallpox outbreak that occurred in England in the winter of 1961-62 caused 24 deaths. It also necessitated the opening of 11 special smallpox hospitals and the distribution of 5½ million doses of vaccine, the total cost of all special measures being nearly $4 000 000 (World Health Organization, 1972). Thus the penalties of outbreaks when they do occur can be very considerable.

Nevertheless, epidemic outbreaks in well-developed areas tend to be rather circumscribed. Thus, although on average less than 50 percent of the population in Europe was vaccinated, there were only 391 cases in 28 different outbreaks over the period January 1961—September 1970 (World Health Organization, 1970). The average number of cases per outbreak was therefore about 14.

Moreover, the average number of deaths per outbreak was only 0·5 over the five years 1966-1970 (Center for Disease Control, 1971).

A careful review of all the statistical facts concerning the mortality and morbidity due to smallpox itself and to smallpox vaccination led the US Public Health Service in October 1971 to discontinue compulsory measures relating to routine vaccination. The Center for Disease Control (1971) indicated that "Based on European experience, it would require 15 importations per year to produce the same mortality currently associated with smallpox vaccinations in the United States", whereas in fact there had been no importations for twenty years, and clearly stated that in the USA at any rate, "Vigilant surveillance and outbreak control are the keys to maintain freedom from smallpox".

In this example the appropriate public health action could be deduced fairly easily from the existing morbidity statistics. It might, however, be argued that several people had died unnecessarily before such irrefutable statistical records were built up, and that appropriate action could have been taken sooner. This raises the whole question of whether a better understanding of the theory of vaccination programs and more accurate forecasting of the consequences of any given vaccination strategy would not enable an improved overall service to be provided to the community.

A more difficult case would seem to be that of the UK, where routine vaccination was also discontinued in 1971. Records showed some 100 deaths from smallpox vaccination compared with approximately 37 deaths from smallpox itself in the twenty-year period 1951-1970 (Dick, 1971). The optimal strategy is not immediately obvious, though it seems likely that discontinuance of routine vaccination plus continued vaccination of high-risk groups would probably be an improvement.

There are many technical difficulties in undertaking a full mathematical analysis, but an excellent start has been made by Becker (1972) whose work is introduced in the following section.

20.4 Vaccination models

We have already referred in Section 9.4 to Neyman and Scott's (1964) model for a spatially distributed epidemic process using a position-dependent branching process with discrete-time parameter. The assumption was made, not unreasonably when only small outbreaks were considered, that the stock of susceptibles was not appreciably diminished by the spread of infection. With this assumption, and subject to certain other conditions, it was shown that the immunization of a random proportion θ of the population would reduce the expected epidemic size to a value less than $(1 - \theta)/\theta$. As remarked by Neyman and Scott, this seems a rather optimistic conclusion. It implies, for example, that immunizing ten percent of the population leads to an average outbreak of less than nine cases!

What seems more probable in practice is that many serious diseases will initially spread quite rapidly, so far as the basic infectious process is concerned, until the existence of the outbreak is recognized. When the latter occurs, public health action increases the removal rate sufficiently for the birth-and-death process for infectives to be subject to certain extinction. This critical refinement has been incorporated in the investigation of Becker (1972), who dealt explicitly with the problem of vaccination programs for relatively rare diseases like smallpox.

Thus, using a notation slightly more in conformity with the earlier usage in this book, we may proceed as follows.

Suppose first that there is a probability α that on any given day one or more infectious individuals arrive in a community of size N. We shall assume α to be constant, although in practice we might well want to deal with the case where α was subject to seasonal fluctuations. Let the random variable R represent the number of days that pass before an outbreak occurs, measuring from some fixed point of time. Thus R has the geometric probability distribution given by

$$\Pr\{R = r\} = \alpha(1-\alpha)^{r-1}, \quad r = 0, 1, 2, ..., \tag{20.8}$$

the mean value being

$$\bar{R} = \alpha^{-1}. \tag{20.9}$$

Let us suppose that the vaccination strategy normally followed during the days before an outbreak is aimed at keeping the number of susceptibles down to a fixed level n. The chance of death following from any one vaccination is taken to be ϕ, which is assumed to be small and constant. In reality ϕ may well vary somewhat according to age, state of health, vaccination status, etc. Let the average number of vaccinations carried out per day when there are n susceptibles be $\theta(n)$. For a given number of vaccinations in R days, the number of deaths due to vaccination will have a binomial distribution. However, since ϕ is small and the number of vaccinations large, we can approximate by a Poisson distribution with parameter $R\phi\theta(n)$. Hence when R varies, we can use (20.9) to give the average number of deaths $V(n)$ due to vaccination in the period before an outbreak as

$$V(n) = \phi\theta(n)/\alpha. \tag{20.10}$$

In general we expect $\theta(n)$ to be a non-increasing function of n. A reasonable form for this function can be derived as follows. Let the mean survival rate per year for each individual be ξ, and let us further suppose that individuals need to be revaccinated every k years in order to remain immune. The average number of deaths per year in a large population of size N is $N(1-\xi)$, of whom $n(1-\xi)$ are susceptibles and $(N-n)(1-\xi)$ are vaccinated. These losses are made good by $N(1-\xi)$ new susceptibles, due to birth or immigration, so as to maintain a constant population size. Of the $(N-n)\xi$ surviving immunes there will be

$(N-n)\xi/k$ who require revaccination, and there are of course $n\xi$ surviving susceptibles. In order to maintain a constant level of n susceptibles in the community it follows that, approximately,

$$N(1-\xi) + n\xi + (N-n)\xi/k - 365\theta(n) = n,$$

whence

$$\theta(n) = \frac{N-n}{365}\left(1 - \xi + \frac{\xi}{k}\right). \tag{20.11}$$

We now consider the actual spread of the epidemic, carefully distinguishing the situation before and after discovery. We are, by definition, assuming the possibility of only small epidemics, as with smallpox in Europe in recent years. Thus before discovery we can conveniently represent the spread of infection as a simple birth process, and after discovery we can use a birth–death process. This assumes that the latent period is effectively zero (or at any rate very short), a restriction that can be relaxed in a more sophisticated model.

Let the contact-rate in the prediscovery phase be β, so that, if $Y(t)$ represents the number of infectives at time t, the number of new infectives in Δt is $\beta n\, Y(t)\, \Delta t$. Thus we have a birth process with birth-rate βn. By a standard result (e.g. Bailey, 1964a, Sec. 8.2), the probability of a single initial infective at time $t = 0$ giving rise to a group of j infectives (including the initial one) at time t is

$$p_j(t) = e^{-\beta nt}(1 - e^{-\beta nt})^{j-1}, \quad j \geqslant 1. \tag{20.12}$$

Now suppose that the time to discovery is a random variable independent of the number of circulating infectives $Y(t)$, having distribution function $F(t)$. Then it follows that the probability of there being j infectives at the time of discovery (including the discovered infective) is given by

$$P_j = \int_0^\infty e^{-\beta nt}(1 - e^{-\beta nt})^{j-1} dF(t). \tag{20.13}$$

This result applies, for example, to the case when there is a natural constant incubation period τ. For then we can assume that discovery occurs when the initial infective immigrant exhibits symptoms. Let the time to discovery be uniformly distributed over the interval $(0, \tau)$, i.e.

$$\begin{aligned} F(t) &= 0, & t &< 0, \\ &= t/\tau, & 0 &\leqslant t < \tau, \\ &= 1, & \tau &\leqslant t. \end{aligned} \right\} \tag{20.14}$$

Substituting (20.14) into (20.13) gives by direct integration

$$P_j = \frac{(1 - e^{-\beta n\tau})^j}{\beta n\tau j}, \quad j \geqslant 1. \tag{20.15}$$

The average number of infectives circulating at the time of discovery, including the discovered case, is readily found to be

$$E(j) = \frac{e^{\beta n \tau} - 1}{\beta n \tau}.$$ (20.16)

As soon as the first case is discovered and removed we suppose that general public health vigilance causes further cases to be identified in such a way that the total number of infectives can be described by a birth–death process with birth-rate βn and death-rate, i.e. removal-rate in our context, γ. In general, if the epidemic is to be brought under control, we shall have $\gamma > \beta n$, when extinction is certain. The initial number of infectives for this birth-death process is of course $j - 1$. By a standard result (e.g. Bailey, 1964a, Sec. 10.3) the average final cumulative population size for this process, i.e. the average total number of infectives occurring, including the $j - 1$ initial ones, is $\gamma(j - 1)/(\gamma - \beta n)$. If the case mortality-rate is ν, it follows using (20.16) that the average number of deaths $D(n)$ due to the disease is

$$D(n) = \nu \left\{ 1 + \frac{\gamma}{\gamma - \beta n} \left(\frac{e^{\beta n \tau} - 1}{\beta n \tau} - 1 \right) \right\}.$$ (20.17)

A reasonable strategy to follow is to choose a vaccination program which minimizes with respect to n the total cost in terms of death given by

$$C(n) = V(n) + D(n),$$ (20.18)

the components $V(n)$ and $D(n)$ being given by (20.10) and (20.17), respectively, and also using (20.11). It will be realized that the chance of an infective immigrant arriving on any given day is independent of the number of susceptibles. Thus the time-interval between outbreaks does not depend on n. On the other hand, the duration of an epidemic does depend on n. But since these durations are small compared with the intervals between outbreaks, it is a reasonable approximation to evaluate the effectiveness of the vaccination program in terms of the total number of deaths per outbreak.

Let the proportion of susceptibles in the population be $s = n/N$. Then, as shown by Becker, the minimum value of $C(n)$ is given by $s = s^*$ (or $n = n^*$), where

$$
\left.
\begin{aligned}
s^* &= 0, \quad \text{if } 365\alpha\beta\tau\nu \geqslant 2\phi(1 - \xi + \xi/k), \\
&= \min(x, 1), \quad \text{otherwise,}
\end{aligned}
\right\}
$$ (20.19)

where $x > 0$ satisfies

$$
\frac{\phi}{365\alpha\beta\gamma\nu} \left(1 - \frac{k-1}{k} \xi \right)(\beta Nx)^2(\gamma - \beta Nx)^2
$$
$$
+ \{(\beta Nx)^2 - (\gamma + 2\tau^{-1})\beta Nx + \gamma\tau^{-1}\}(e^{\beta Nx\tau} - 1) = \beta Nx(\gamma - 2\beta Nx).
$$ (20.20)

Instead of assuming the incubation period to be constant in the prediscovery phase, we might prefer to assume an exponential distribution resulting from a constant removal rate ω, say. In this case the infectives would follow a birth–death process, with birth-rate βn and death-rate ω, terminating as soon as the first death occurred. The usual random walk embedded in this process would have transition probabilities of $\beta n/(\beta n + \omega)$ and $\omega/(\beta n + \omega)$ for birth and death respectively. The probability P_j of there being exactly j infectives at the time of discovery is the probability that the random walk undergoes $j - 1$ birth transitions followed by a death transition, i.e.

$$P_j = \frac{\omega}{\beta n + \omega} \left(\frac{\beta n}{\beta n + \omega}\right)^{j-1}. \tag{20.21}$$

Since this is a geometric distribution, like (20.8), we can immediately write down the mean value as

$$E(j) = \frac{\beta n + \omega}{\omega}. \tag{20.22}$$

We have already seen that the average total number of infectives following the discovery of the outbreak is $\gamma(j - 1)/(\gamma - \beta n)$, including the $j - 1$ initial ones. Thus the average number of deaths due to the disease is

$$D(n) = \nu \left\{1 + \frac{\gamma}{\gamma - \beta n}\left(\frac{\beta n + \omega}{\omega} - 1\right)\right\}$$

$$= \nu \left\{1 + \frac{\gamma \beta n}{\omega(\gamma - \beta n)}\right\}. \tag{20.23}$$

Using this value of $D(n)$ in (20.18), we find that the minimum cost is given by

$$\left.\begin{array}{l} s^* = 0, \quad \text{if } 365\alpha\beta\nu \geqslant \omega\phi(1 - \xi + \xi/k), \\[2mm] = \min\left[\frac{\gamma}{\beta}\left\{1 - \left(\frac{365\alpha\beta\nu}{\omega\phi(1 - \xi + \xi/k)}\right)^{\frac{1}{2}}\right\}, 1\right], \quad \text{otherwise.} \end{array}\right\} \tag{20.24}$$

20.5 Numerical illustration

In order to use the theory of the previous section to determine the optimal policy in any specific instance, we need to know the values of the parameters α, β, γ, ν, ξ, τ, ϕ, ω, k and N. Since the diseases in question are considered to be rare, there are little data available for estimating the parameters in a completely satisfactory statistical manner. However, in practice we are more concerned with the broad implications for overall policy than with the technical detail required for a scientific epidemiological inquiry; and in any case the existence of a quantitative model allows us to carry out a sensitivity analysis on any parameters for which appreciable uncertainty might have material practical repercussions. It is therefore reasonable to use any *a priori* estimates of the relevant parameters that may be available in order to get started, with the proviso that revised estimates may be needed later.

Becker (1972) uses the following parameter values for smallpox in the USA based on figures drawn from the epidemiological literature (see Becker's paper for references):

$\alpha = 10^{-3}$. This implies a mean inter-arrival time of about three years. Since there have in fact been no US cases for 20 years, the value is probably too high. However, it seems safer to be pessimistic.

β. This contact-rate parameter is very community-dependent. No estimate was available, and its value has been left arbitrary in the present discussion.

$\gamma = 2$. Although the period of infectiousness may be about three weeks, normal public health practice of contact tracing, early diagnosis, etc. considerably reduces the effective value of γ. The figure of $\gamma = 2$ corresponds to a mean infectious period before removal of 0·5 days.

$\nu = 10^{-1}$. The case mortality rate is roughly 1 in 10.

$\xi = 0.9906$. Survival-rate based on US population figures for 1965.

$\tau = 5$. Assumes that the initial infective is infectious for five days before discovery (constant incubation period).

$\phi = 10^{-6}$. Approximate death-rate from primary vaccinations in 1968.

$\omega = 0.2$. Based on the mean duration of infectious period prior to discovery being five days (exponential incubation period).

$k = 4$. Assuming revaccination necessary after 3-5 years.

$N = 2 \times 10^8$. Approximate population size of US.

For these parameter values the optimal values of s, the proportion of susceptibles in the population, were calculated for the two different models in Section 20.4, using either (20.19) and (20.20) or (20.24). Table 20.1 shows these results for a range of values of $\beta N \equiv 2 \times 10^8 \beta$, since no actual estimate of β was available.

Obviously such figures can be used only as a qualitative guide. However, if using somewhat pessimistic estimates of the parameters we arrive at a value of s^* near to unity, then this will certainly suggest a policy where one vaccinates only those at high risk, e.g. military recruits, hospital and health workers, and visitors to and from areas where the disease is known to occur. It will be realized that βN is the average number of new cases that would arise per day from a single infective in a population of N susceptibles. To make even an approximate estimate of this quantity *a priori* would entail knowing, first, the approximate rate of physical contact, which might be deducible from sociological considerations, and secondly, the probability of disease transmission given the specified degree of contact, for which there might be some epidemiological evidence.

Table 20.1   *Optimal values of the proportion of susceptibles s* for two different models, given the parametric values shown in the text*

βN	Model with constant incubation period	Model with exponential incubation period
1·24	0·999	-
1·4	0·870	-
1·6	0·747	-
1·8	0·653	1·000
2·0	0·578	0·916
3·0	0·362	0·598
5·0	0·198	0·347
10·0	0·086	0·162
20·0	0·036	0·073
50·0	0·011	0·023

20.6   Further developments

Both of the models introduced into the previous section made the simplifying assumption that the latent period was of zero duration. Some indirect allowance for the existence of a non-zero latent period could be made by suitable choice of the removal rates ω and γ, though this would not be entirely satisfactory. Becker (1972) also considered a modified model based on Bartoszyński's (1967) representation of an epidemic as a discrete-time Galton–Watson process with variable latent and infectious periods. As pointed out in Section 8.1, this treatment confines attention to the one-dimensional process describing the population of infectives and neglects the changing number of susceptibles. However, in the present context, this simplification does not matter, so an opportunity is provided of making the discussion of Section 20.5 more realistic. For a full discussion of this application the reader should consult Becker (1972). There are of course some differences in detail from the results shown in Table 20.1, but the broad qualitative conclusions are very similar.

Another approach to studying the qualitative consequences of a vaccination program has been made by Griffiths (1973b) in relation to measles, using the models of Chapter 7 for recurrent epidemics. If x_0 and y_0 are the deterministic equilibrium values of the numbers of susceptibles and infectives, respectively, then

$$x_0 = \gamma/\beta, \quad y_0 = \mu/\gamma, \tag{20.25}$$

(as in (7.2)), where β, γ, and μ are the infection-rate, removal-rate, and birth-rate for new susceptibles, respectively.

For a stochastic model with the reintroduction of infectives, the approximate recurrence time to zero infectives was investigated in Section 7.62. Even with *no* new infectives being introduced it was pointed out that (7.79) gave the order of magnitude of the passage-time to zero. If $x_0 \gg y_0$, we can approximate (7.79) by

$$\bar{R}(x_0, y_0) \sim \frac{(2\pi x_0)^{\frac{1}{2}}}{\gamma y_0} \exp \left\{ \frac{(y_0 + x_0/y_0)^2}{2x_0} \right\}, \tag{20.26}$$

to give the expected time to fade-out of the infection.

Suppose now that a proportion $1 - \psi$ of children born each year are protected by measles vaccination. This means that the entry of new susceptibles is a proportion ψ of its previous value, that is, the effective birth-rate of new susceptibles becomes $\psi\mu$ instead of μ. Equation (20.25) in turn implies that the new deterministic equilibrium values of the numbers of susceptibles and infectives are x_0 and ψy_0, respectively. Substituting in (20.26) easily shows that

$$\bar{R}(x_0, \psi y_0) \equiv \bar{R}(x_0/\psi^2, y_0). \tag{20.27}$$

Thus the new critical community size is multiplied by a factor ψ^{-2}. If there is 50 percent immunization, the critical level of 250 000, previously suggested as approximately valid for measles in both the UK and the USA, will increase to 1 000 000. The phenomenon of fade-out evidently becomes more important after the introduction of immunization, and enhances the possibility of eradicating the disease.

It further follows from (7.45) and the subsequent remarks that, for small ϵ, the average inter-epidemic interval is, approximately,

$$\bar{t} \sim \left(\frac{\gamma}{\epsilon\beta\mu} \right)^{\frac{1}{2}}. \tag{20.28}$$

Now suppose that vaccination is nation-wide, so that when the infection fades from one community below the critical size, it is reintroduced from another community. If we can assume that the rate of entry is proportional to the outside endemic level, then the pre-vaccination entry rate ϵ will be replaced by $\psi\epsilon$ after vaccination. Thus, during a vaccination program both μ and ϵ in (20.28) will be replaced by $\psi\mu$ and $\psi\epsilon$, so that $\bar{t}$ is replaced by $\bar{t}/\psi$.

With a 50 percent vaccination-rate, the inter-epidemic interval will be doubled. Unless there is permanent fade-out, practically all susceptibles will eventually catch the disease. In a given period of time there will be half as many epidemics affecting half as many susceptibles as before. This means that the individual epidemics will be about the same size after the introduction of vaccination as before, although of course the susceptible population has been halved. A corollary of this phenomenon (Griffiths, 1971a, b; 1973b) is that the increase in period will tend to put up the average age of attack for those susceptibles who catch measles, with a resultant rise in the probability of side-effects and complications arising from the disease.

It is evident that there are many unsolved problems in this general area of immunization programs. Some of the theoretical work done so far has a very direct practical bearing on the choice of optimal intervention strategies. Further research could well combine mathematically interesting and challenging problems with the development of important new tools for public health action.

21
Public health control

21.1 General discussion

As we have already seen, Part 2 of this book develops the general theory of epidemics. It provides a broad quantitative background for more specific studies, but even at a theoretical level it provides some general insights of practical value: the various threshold theorems or the modelling of recurrent outbreaks, for example. (See Chapter 12 for detailed discussion.) However, it is in the present Part 3 that more specific epidemiological applications have been considered. The over-simplified models of Part 2 attempt to elucidate the general implications of major factors, such as spatial distributions of susceptibles and infectives, the existence of carriers, the consequences of migration, the complications of host-and-vector situations, etc. In Part 3 we have tried to get closer to individual diseases; to fit models to actual data where possible, as with measles, infectious hepatitis or malaria; or to investigate more realistically structured systems-type models, as with tuberculosis, typhoid, tetanus, or the geographical spread of influenza.

Such detailed epidemiological applications not only increase general scientific knowledge, but provide the kind of understanding that can be used to facilitate public health control. We are at present only at the beginning of this phase. Thus, the statistical methods of Chapters 14 and 15 allow us to develop and fit models involving parameters for the chance of adequate contact; the degree of variation in this chance within or between households; the length of latent, infectious and incubation periods, etc. The more extensive use of such techniques, both before and after the experimental use of public health interventions like immunization and vaccination, would provide information on how the natural history of the disease had been affected. This, in turn, could have valuable consequences for forecasting the probable effects of large-scale public health action affecting a whole region or country. It might turn out, for example, that immunization produced *inter alia* a small, but measurable, decrease in the length of the infectious period, or in the infection-rate itself. We could then calculate more accurately the implications of immunizing a given proportion of a large

371

population in a mass campaign, followed by an appropriate maintenance strategy.

Actually, the adoption of immunization procedures on a large scale introduces further complications, as we have seen in Chapter 20, since the procedures themselves often entail certain risks. In Section 20.3 we reviewed briefly some of the statistical data on the relative risks of death from smallpox compared with the dangers of dying from the vaccination or suffering from unpleasant side-effects. The problem of deciding on an optimal strategy is an important one, and relatively little quantitative work has yet been devoted to this aspect of public health decision-making.

Again, in Chapter 16, we have seen how multistate models can be developed to give guidance on the choice between alternative public health strategies. Some detail was given on the construction of a tuberculosis model, with indications of how this has been used to back up studies on the optimal allocation of resources, using linear programming techniques. Other diseases, such as typhoid, tetanus and cholera, have also been modelled in a similar way. So far, the calculations entailed have always been performed on artificially constructed models, using parameters estimated from various sources, or perhaps intelligently guessed. Such models therefore tend to be typical of certain kinds of situation, e.g. the spread of tetanus in a developing country, but can rarely be used to draw highly specific conclusions about any given community. For this purpose we need to estimate the parameters which relate to the community in question, and also to be reasonably sure that the model is sufficiently accurate and reliable.

These circumstances seem so far to have discouraged the widespread application of many undoubtedly useful multistate models. Of course, further efforts should be made to improve the detailed fitting of these models to local situations. However, many important problems of planning, policy analysis and strategy choice can be elucidated by means of quite straightforward computer simulations of general, rather than specific, disease models.

A hopeful development is the recent work described in Section 17.5 on the modelling of malaria, which has been conducted in the context of specific Nigerian villages. Parameters have been estimated, and modifications made in the structure of the original model so as to permit a closer fit between the model simulations and the empirical field data. This work, still in progress at the time of writing, relates to the effectiveness of control measures such as the use of larvicides and adulticides for eliminating mosquitoes, and various drugs for curing people. The ultimate importance for the public health control, or eradication, of malaria is self-evident. But exactly how the technical mathematical and epidemiological knowledge is to be used in order to promote effective public health action is a matter that requires further development.

Again, it frequently happens in developing countries that there is not just one, but several, widespread and possibly interacting diseases to be dealt with. This raises problems of practical importance that have as yet received scant attention. It seems probable that we need not only theoretical research, but also empirical field investigations of the major epidemiological and public health issues in this area.

We have so far in this section examined some of the more general aspects of public health control, with special reference to the implications of the detailed modelling already described in earlier chapters. For a short review of the potentialities in planning and evaluating control measures, with special emphasis on the simulation of control measures and the use of cost-effectiveness and cost-benefit analyses, see Cvjetanović (1972). A number of workers have, however, recently begun to look more closely at the possibility of applying the mathematical methods of standard control theory, including Taylor (1968); Jacquette (1970); Sanders (1971); Gupta and Rink (1971); Gupta (1972); Abakuks (1973); Gupta and Rink (1973); Hethcote and Waltman (1973); and Morton and Wickwire (1974). It would take us too far afield to discuss these developments in detail, especially as the extent to which highly sophisticated control theory is really relevant to the actual processes of health decision-making is a matter which requires much more investigation. Nevertheless, it is to be expected that further work in this direction will undoubtedly assist in our understanding of the way control measures should be implemented.

There is also the possibility of extending the principles of epidemic theory to other areas of the health field. A number of quantitative sociological studies have already been made on the diffusion of ideas, news and rumours (see Bartholomew, 1973, Chapter 10, for discussion and references). Some of this work has obvious public health applications. In addition, adaptations of epidemiological concepts and modelling have recently been used to investigate the spread of the addiction to drugs, notably heroin, by Hughes, Senay and Parker (1972) and Hughes and Crawford (1972). This seems to be an important field of application with much potential for further development.

21.2 Prospects for the future

This final section must inevitably be a rather personal view, partly of how existing trends are developing, and partly of what ought to be done if humanly possible.

The choice of material for this book has already exhibited the author's own predilections for (1) theoretical results which are relatively simple to understand, aesthetically appealing, and hopefully providing insight into basic epidemiological mechanisms; and (2) practical applications which minister directly to scientific epidemiological inquiry or have clear implications for public health intervention and control.

There appear to be two major trends in the development of the whole subject at the present time. The first is an ever-increasing flow of largely mathematical papers, the results of which have been pursued for their intrinsic mathematical interest, and can be applied to practical problems only occasionally when by chance the assumptions happen to fit some actual situation with sufficient realism. If this tendency is unchecked, we shall soon be faced with a vast abstract literature which contains little of fundamental mathematical importance and has virtually no practical relevance either. From a social point of view this would represent an unwarrantable waste of mathematical resources.

The second trend is in a more realistic direction and involves the careful modelling of specific diseases. Unfortunately it has rarely been possible, so far, to estimate all the critical parameters for any specific situation. Investigators then fall back on the analysis of typical models, applicable to developing countries, say, often having to resort to simulation studies backed up by computerized computations. While such studies can provide genuine insight into many of the factors affecting public health decision-making, one can never be sure that the general conclusions reached will apply in practice to any particular instance.

It is unnecessary, and would perhaps be invidious, to give here specific examples of these two trends. There are, moreover, a number of noteworthy exceptions. The reader can easily supply his own illustrations by a perusal of the foregoing discussions in Parts 2 and 3.

Another aspect to which more attention should be paid is the problem of training and education. If epidemiologists and public health authorities are to appreciate better what the right kind of epidemic modelling has to offer by way of support for practical planning and control, then there has to be an improved understanding of the whole approach. The possibilities for using simulation models and operational gaming have been discussed by Bogdanoff (1964), Lynn (1972), and Swain *et al.* (1972), but more effort is needed to incorporate such ideas into public health training programs.

The present book deals of course largely with the technical mathematical background to practical applications. But if the latter are to be pursued with vigour and imagination, much will have to be done to translate the implications of technical mathematics both into easily assimilable concepts couched in everyday language, and into usable technical instruments that can be incorporated into system dynamics approaches (see end of Chapter 4) to policy analyses and organizational studies involving multisectoral projections and forecasts. Such work has as yet hardly begun, though its potential contributions are urgently needed.

If the further development of the mathematical theory of epidemics is not to remain a purely academic curiosity, scientific insight into and understanding of the population dynamics of communicable disease spread must be effectively translated into public health action for intervention and control. "Die Philosophen" (and we might add, "Die Mathematiker") "haben die Welt nur verschieden interpretiert, es kommt aber darauf an, sie zu verändern", wrote Karl Marx in his eleventh Thesis on Feuerbach. It is significant, as can be seen from Chapter 2, that the origins of mathematical and statistical investigations into the spread of communicable diseases in the 17th and 18th centuries lay very much in primitive attempts to understand and control actual outbreaks. It is the belief of the present writer that the major mathematical efforts in the future should be directed towards those theoretical problems which, if solved, would contribute in a substantive way towards the eradication or control of the principal epidemic and endemic scourges of mankind. There are, of course, intellectual and aesthetic satisfactions in understanding the mechanisms and processes underlying the natural world; but, in the face of misery and suffering on a monumental scale, epidemic theory for its own take is a luxury mankind can ill afford. The world must not only be interpreted: it must be changed.

APPENDIX TABLES

The derivation and use of these tables is described in Section 6.81. They are employed in the maximum-likelihood estimation of the relative removal-rate from data on the total size of an intra-household epidemic. Score coefficients S_w are given for $n = 2, 3, 4$ and 5, over the range $\rho = 1 \cdot 0(0 \cdot 1)10 \cdot 0$. The tables were originally computed on EDSAC and are published here by kind permission of the Director of the University Mathematical Laboratory, Cambridge.

Table A.1 *Values of S_w for $n = 2$*

ρ	S_0	S_1	S_2	ρ	S_0	S_1	S_2
1.0	0.666667	0.666667	−0.666667	6.0	0.041667	−0.077381	−0.256868
1	0.586510	0.543220	−0.649962	1	0.040478	−0.077278	−0.253632
2	0.520833	0.445076	−0.633356	2	0.039339	−0.077148	−0.250475
3	0.466200	0.365866	−0.617040	3	0.038248	−0.076994	−0.247396
4	0.420168	0.301120	−0.601135	4	0.037202	−0.076818	−0.244390
5	0.380952	0.247619	−0.585714	5	0.036199	−0.076621	−0.241457
6	0.347222	0.202991	−0.570818	6	0.035236	−0.076407	−0.238592
7	0.317965	0.165460	−0.556466	7	0.034311	−0.076175	−0.235794
8	0.292398	0.133668	−0.542661	8	0.033422	−0.075929	−0.233060
9	0.269906	0.106566	−0.529399	9	0.032568	−0.075669	−0.230389
2.0	0.250000	0.083333	−0.516667	7.0	0.031746	−0.075397	−0.227778
1	0.232288	0.063317	−0.504448	1	0.030955	−0.075114	−0.225225
2	0.216450	0.045996	−0.492725	2	0.030193	−0.074820	−0.222728
3	0.202224	0.030946	−0.481476	3	0.029459	−0.074518	−0.220286
4	0.189394	0.017825	−0.470680	4	0.028752	−0.074208	−0.217896
5	0.177778	0.006349	−0.460317	5	0.028070	−0.073891	−0.215557
6	0.167224	−0.003716	−0.450366	6	0.027412	−0.073567	−0.213268
7	0.157604	−0.012566	−0.440806	7	0.026777	−0.073238	−0.211027
8	0.148810	−0.020363	−0.431619	8	0.026164	−0.072903	−0.208832
9	0.140746	−0.027247	−0.422784	9	0.025572	−0.072565	−0.206682
3.0	0.133333	−0.033333	−0.414286	8.0	0.025000	−0.072222	−0.204575
1	0.126502	−0.038722	−0.406106	1	0.024447	−0.071877	−0.202511
2	0.120192	−0.043498	−0.398228	2	0.023912	−0.071528	−0.200488
3	0.114351	−0.047735	−0.390638	3	0.023395	−0.071177	−0.198505
4	0.108932	−0.051495	−0.383320	4	0.022894	−0.070825	−0.196560
5	0.103896	−0.054834	−0.376263	5	0.022409	−0.070470	−0.194653
6	0.099206	−0.057798	−0.369452	6	0.021939	−0.070115	−0.192783
7	0.094832	−0.060430	−0.362875	7	0.021485	−0.069758	−0.190948
8	0.090744	−0.062765	−0.356522	8	0.021044	−0.069401	−0.189147
9	0.086919	−0.064834	−0.350382	9	0.020616	−0.069044	−0.187380
4.0	0.083333	−0.066667	−0.344444	9.0	0.020202	−0.068687	−0.185646
1	0.079968	−0.068286	−0.338700	1	0.019800	−0.068330	−0.183943
2	0.076805	−0.069715	−0.333140	2	0.019410	−0.067973	−0.182271
3	0.073828	−0.070972	−0.327755	3	0.019031	−0.067617	−0.180630
4	0.071023	−0.072075	−0.322539	4	0.018664	−0.067261	−0.179017
5	0.068376	−0.073038	−0.317483	5	0.018307	−0.066906	−0.177433
6	0.065876	−0.073875	−0.312580	6	0.017960	−0.066553	−0.175876
7	0.063512	−0.074599	−0.307823	7	0.017623	−0.066200	−0.174347
8	0.061275	−0.075220	−0.303207	8	0.017295	−0.065849	−0.172844
9	0.059154	−0.075747	−0.298725	9	0.016976	−0.065500	−0.171366
5.0	0.057143	−0.076190	−0.294372	10.0	0.016667	−0.065152	−0.169913
1	0.055233	−0.076557	−0.290142				
2	0.053419	−0.076854	−0.286031				
3	0.051693	−0.077088	−0.282033				
4	0.050050	−0.077265	−0.278144				
5	0.048485	−0.077389	−0.274359				
6	0.046992	−0.077466	−0.270675				
7	0.045568	−0.077500	−0.267087				
8	0.044209	−0.077495	−0.263593				
9	0.042909	−0.077454	−0.260187				

376

Table A.2 *Values of S_w for $n = 3$*

ρ	S_0	S_1	S_2	S_3
1.0	0.750000	1.083333	0.983333	-0.675926
1	0.665188	0.929118	0.794253	-0.674164
2	0.595238	0.803571	0.643639	-0.670228
3	0.536673	0.699843	0.521869	-0.664666
4	0.487013	0.613063	0.422177	-0.657895
5	0.444444	0.539683	0.339683	-0.650238
6	0.407609	0.477053	0.270788	-0.641944
7	0.375469	0.423164	0.212788	-0.633206
8	0.347222	0.376462	0.163619	-0.624173
9	0.322234	0.335729	0.121680	-0.614961
2.0	0.300000	0.300000	0.085714	-0.605660
1	0.280112	0.268498	0.054724	-0.596340
2	0.262238	0.240593	0.027908	-0.587055
3	0.246103	0.215770	0.004619	-0.577847
4	0.231481	0.193603	-0.015673	-0.568747
5	0.218182	0.173737	-0.033405	-0.559779
6	0.206044	0.155877	-0.048939	-0.550963
7	0.194932	0.139770	-0.062575	-0.542309
8	0.184729	0.125205	-0.074567	-0.533829
9	0.175336	0.112000	-0.085130	-0.525528
3.0	0.166667	0.100000	-0.094444	-0.517410
1	0.158646	0.089070	-0.102665	-0.509477
2	0.151210	0.079094	-0.109925	-0.501729
3	0.144300	0.069972	-0.116339	-0.494165
4	0.137868	0.061615	-0.122004	-0.486783
5	0.131868	0.053946	-0.127006	-0.479582
6	0.126263	0.046898	-0.131420	-0.472557
7	0.121017	0.040410	-0.135310	-0.465706
8	0.116099	0.034429	-0.138733	-0.459025
9	0.111483	0.028910	-0.141740	-0.452508
4.0	0.107143	0.023810	-0.144372	-0.446154
1	0.103057	0.019091	-0.146670	-0.439956
2	0.099206	0.014721	-0.148668	-0.433912
3	0.095572	0.010670	-0.150396	-0.428015
4	0.092138	0.006910	-0.151881	-0.422263
5	0.088889	0.003419	-0.153147	-0.416652
6	0.085812	0.000173	-0.154215	-0.411175
7	0.082896	-0.002846	-0.155105	-0.405831
8	0.080128	-0.005656	-0.155834	-0.400614
9	0.077499	-0.008274	-0.156417	-0.395522
5.0	0.075000	-0.010714	-0.156868	-0.390549
1	0.072622	-0.012990	-0.157200	-0.385692
2	0.070356	-0.015114	-0.157423	-0.380949
3	0.068197	-0.017096	-0.157548	-0.376314
4	0.066138	-0.018948	-0.157585	-0.371785

APPENDIX TABLES

Table A.2 *Values of S_w for $n = 3$ (contd.)*

ρ	s_0	s_1	s_2	s_3
5.5	0.064171	−0.020677	−0.157540	−0.367359
6	0.062292	−0.022294	−0.157423	−0.363033
7	0.060496	−0.023806	−0.157239	−0.358802
8	0.058777	−0.025219	−0.156995	−0.354665
9	0.057132	−0.026541	−0.156697	−0.350619
6.0	0.055556	−0.027778	−0.156349	−0.346661
1	0.054044	−0.028935	−0.155957	−0.342788
2	0.052595	−0.030017	−0.155524	−0.338997
3	0.051203	−0.031030	−0.155054	−0.335287
4	0.049867	−0.031978	−0.154551	−0.331654
5	0.048583	−0.032865	−0.154019	−0.328097
6	0.047348	−0.033695	−0.153459	−0.324613
7	0.046161	−0.034470	−0.152876	−0.321200
8	0.045018	−0.035196	−0.152271	−0.317857
9	0.043917	−0.035874	−0.151646	−0.314580
7.0	0.042857	−0.036508	−0.151004	−0.311369
1	0.041835	−0.037100	−0.150346	−0.308221
2	0.040850	−0.037653	−0.149675	−0.305134
3	0.039899	−0.038169	−0.148992	−0.302108
4	0.038981	−0.038650	−0.148298	−0.299139
5	0.038095	−0.039098	−0.147594	−0.296227
6	0.037239	−0.039515	−0.146883	−0.293370
7	0.036412	−0.039903	−0.146165	−0.290566
8	0.035613	−0.040264	−0.145441	−0.287815
9	0.034839	−0.040599	−0.144712	−0.285114
8.0	0.034091	−0.040909	−0.143979	−0.282463
1	0.033367	−0.041196	−0.143243	−0.279859
2	0.032666	−0.041462	−0.142505	−0.277303
3	0.031986	−0.041706	−0.141764	−0.274791
4	0.031328	−0.041932	−0.141023	−0.272325
5	0.030691	−0.042139	−0.140281	−0.269901
6	0.030072	−0.042328	−0.139539	−0.267520
7	0.029472	−0.042501	−0.138798	−0.265179
8	0.028891	−0.042658	−0.138057	−0.262879
9	0.028326	−0.042801	−0.137318	−0.260617
9.0	0.027778	−0.042929	−0.136580	−0.258394
1	0.027245	−0.043045	−0.135845	−0.256208
2	0.026728	−0.043147	−0.135111	−0.254058
3	0.026226	−0.043238	−0.134381	−0.251943
4	0.025738	−0.043318	−0.133653	−0.249863
5	0.025263	−0.043387	−0.132929	−0.247816
6	0.024802	−0.043446	−0.132208	−0.245803
7	0.024353	−0.043495	−0.131490	−0.243821
8	0.023916	−0.043535	−0.130776	−0.241871
9	0.023491	−0.043566	−0.130066	−0.239951
10.0	0.023077	−0.043590	−0.129360	−0.238062

Table A.3 *Values of S_w for $n = 4$*

ρ	S_0	S_1	S_2	S_3	S_4
1.0	0.800000	1.300000	1.585714	1.394340	-0.610675
1	0.713012	1.134299	1.353425	1.135261	-0.623275
2	0.641026	0.998169	1.164272	0.928096	-0.632361
3	0.580552	0.884666	1.007964	0.759946	-0.638533
4	0.529101	0.788841	0.877184	0.621729	-0.642297
5	0.484848	0.707071	0.766595	0.506887	-0.644079
6	0.446429	0.636646	0.672215	0.410576	-0.644231
7	0.412797	0.575500	0.591020	0.329150	-0.643047
8	0.383142	0.522031	0.520671	0.259822	-0.640770
9	0.356824	0.474977	0.459335	0.200425	-0.637600
2.0	0.333333	0.433333	0.405556	0.149257	-0.633705
1	0.312256	0.396290	0.358164	0.104962	-0.629224
2	0.293255	0.363185	0.316211	0.066453	-0.624270
3	0.276052	0.333477	0.278918	0.032844	-0.618941
4	0.260417	0.306713	0.245643	0.003413	-0.613316
5	0.246154	0.282517	0.215851	-0.022439	-0.607461
6	0.233100	0.260573	0.189093	-0.045207	-0.601432
7	0.221117	0.240610	0.164990	-0.065306	-0.595276
8	0.210084	0.222399	0.143221	-0.083085	-0.589032
9	0.199900	0.205745	0.123512	-0.098839	-0.582731
3.0	0.190476	0.190476	0.105628	-0.112820	-0.576401
1	0.181736	0.176447	0.089364	-0.125243	-0.570065
2	0.173611	0.163530	0.074546	-0.136293	-0.563741
3	0.166044	0.151614	0.061020	-0.146127	-0.557445
4	0.158983	0.140600	0.048654	-0.154884	-0.551190
5	0.152381	0.130403	0.037329	-0.162683	-0.544987
6	0.146199	0.120946	0.026944	-0.169630	-0.538844
7	0.140400	0.112163	0.017408	-0.175814	-0.532769
8	0.134953	0.103993	0.008640	-0.181316	-0.526768
9	0.129828	0.096383	0.000569	-0.186207	-0.520844
4.0	0.125000	0.089286	-0.006868	-0.190549	-0.515003
1	0.120446	0.082658	-0.013728	-0.194396	-0.509246
2	0.116144	0.076461	-0.020061	-0.197798	-0.503575
3	0.112076	0.070662	-0.025912	-0.200798	-0.497993
4	0.108225	0.065228	-0.031322	-0.203435	-0.492500
5	0.104575	0.060131	-0.036328	-0.205743	-0.487096
6	0.101112	0.055346	-0.040963	-0.207753	-0.481782
7	0.097823	0.050849	-0.045257	-0.209493	-0.476558
8	0.094697	0.046620	-0.049237	-0.210987	-0.471422
9	0.091722	0.042639	-0.052927	-0.212259	-0.466376
5.0	0.088889	0.038889	-0.056349	-0.213327	-0.461417
1	0.086188	0.035353	-0.059525	-0.214212	-0.456544
2	0.083612	0.032017	-0.062472	-0.214928	-0.451758
3	0.081152	0.028868	-0.065207	-0.215490	-0.447055
4	0.078802	0.025892	-0.067746	-0.215913	-0.442436

APPENDIX TABLES

Table A.3 *Values of S_w for $n = 4$ (contd.)*

ρ	s_0	s_1	s_2	s_3	s_4
5.5	0.076555	0.023079	-0.070103	-0.216209	-0.437899
6	0.074405	0.020418	-0.072291	-0.216388	-0.433442
7	0.072346	0.017899	-0.074321	-0.216461	-0.429064
8	0.070373	0.015514	-0.076206	-0.216437	-0.424764
9	0.068481	0.013254	-0.077954	-0.216324	-0.420540
6.0	0.066667	0.011111	-0.079575	-0.216131	-0.416390
1	0.064925	0.009079	-0.081078	-0.215863	-0.412314
2	0.063251	0.007150	-0.082471	-0.215528	-0.408309
3	0.061643	0.005319	-0.083760	-0.215132	-0.404374
4	0.060096	0.003580	-0.084953	-0.214680	-0.400508
5	0.058603	0.001923	-0.086056	-0.214176	-0.396709
6	0.057176	0.000357	-0.087075	-0.213625	-0.392976
7	0.055796	-0.001136	-0.088014	-0.213032	-0.389307
8	0.054466	-0.002557	-0.088880	-0.212400	-0.385701
9	0.053184	-0.003908	-0.089676	-0.211733	-0.382157
7.0	0.051948	-0.005195	-0.090408	-0.211034	-0.378673
1	0.050755	-0.006420	-0.091078	-0.210306	-0.375248
2	0.049603	-0.007586	-0.091692	-0.209552	-0.371831
3	0.048491	-0.008698	-0.092251	-0.208774	-0.368570
4	0.047416	-0.009757	-0.092760	-0.207975	-0.365314
5	0.046377	-0.010766	-0.093222	-0.207156	-0.362112
6	0.045372	-0.011728	-0.093639	-0.206320	-0.358963
7	0.044400	-0.012646	-0.094015	-0.205469	-0.355865
8	0.043459	-0.013521	-0.094351	-0.204604	-0.352818
9	0.042549	-0.014355	-0.094649	-0.203726	-0.349820
8.0	0.041667	-0.015152	-0.094913	-0.202838	-0.346870
1	0.040812	-0.015911	-0.095145	-0.201941	-0.343967
2	0.039984	-0.016636	-0.095345	-0.201035	-0.341110
3	0.039181	-0.017328	-0.095516	-0.200123	-0.338299
4	0.038402	-0.017989	-0.095659	-0.199204	-0.335531
5	0.037647	-0.018619	-0.095777	-0.198281	-0.332807
6	0.036914	-0.019221	-0.095870	-0.197353	-0.330125
7	0.036202	-0.019795	-0.095941	-0.196422	-0.327484
8	0.035511	-0.020344	-0.095990	-0.195489	-0.324883
9	0.034840	-0.020868	-0.096018	-0.194554	-0.322323
9.0	0.034188	-0.021368	-0.096027	-0.193617	-0.319800
1	0.033554	-0.021845	-0.096018	-0.192680	-0.317316
2	0.032938	-0.022301	-0.095992	-0.191744	-0.314869
3	0.032339	-0.022736	-0.095950	-0.190807	-0.312458
4	0.031756	-0.023151	-0.095893	-0.189872	-0.310083
5	0.031189	-0.023548	-0.095821	-0.188939	-0.307742
6	0.030637	-0.023926	-0.095736	-0.188007	-0.305436
7	0.030100	-0.024287	-0.095638	-0.187077	-0.303163
8	0.029577	-0.024632	-0.095528	-0.186150	-0.300922
9	0.029068	-0.024961	-0.095407	-0.185226	-0.298714
10.0	0.028571	-0.025275	-0.095275	-0.184306	-0.296537

Table A.4   *Values of S_w for $n = 5$*

ρ	S_0	S_1	S_2	S_3	S_4	S_5
1.0	0.833333	1.433333	1.905556	3.090741	1.866294	-0.516133
1	0.745156	1.262091	1.656865	2.701714	1.535278	-0.539043
2	0.672043	1.120761	1.452575	2.379645	1.269669	-0.558278
3	0.610501	1.002373	1.282263	2.109340	1.053300	-0.574217
4	0.558036	0.901951	1.138500	1.879847	0.874779	-0.587241
5	0.512821	0.815851	1.015851	1.683073	0.725872	-0.597715
6	0.473485	0.741342	0.910247	1.512906	0.600291	-0.605969
7	0.438982	0.676340	0.818585	1.364643	0.494048	-0.612300
8	0.408497	0.619225	0.738460	1.234609	0.403032	-0.616970
9	0.381388	0.568721	0.667977	1.119890	0.324710	-0.620209
2.0	0.357143	0.523810	0.605628	1.018149	0.256932	-0.622215
1	0.335345	0.483667	0.550194	0.927488	0.197985	-0.623163
2	0.315657	0.447621	0.500682	0.846351	0.146487	-0.623202
3	0.297796	0.415119	0.456277	0.773453	0.101317	-0.622461
4	0.281532	0.385698	0.416301	0.707722	0.061555	-0.621053
5	0.266667	0.358974	0.380186	0.648257	0.026442	-0.619075
6	0.253036	0.334622	0.347457	0.594298	-0.004656	-0.616609
7	0.240500	0.312363	0.317708	0.545196	-0.032269	-0.613728
8	0.228938	0.291963	0.290595	0.500399	-0.056843	-0.610495
9	0.218245	0.273218	0.265821	0.459429	-0.078758	-0.606964
3.0	0.208333	0.255952	0.243132	0.421876	-0.098336	-0.603183
1	0.199124	0.240014	0.222307	0.387380	-0.115855	-0.599191
2	0.190549	0.225271	0.203154	0.355632	-0.131552	-0.595025
3	0.182548	0.211606	0.185505	0.326357	-0.145632	-0.590714
4	0.175070	0.198917	0.169213	0.299317	-0.158275	-0.586287
5	0.168067	0.187115	0.154148	0.274299	-0.169636	-0.581766
6	0.161499	0.176119	0.140196	0.251118	-0.179850	-0.577172
7	0.155328	0.165858	0.127256	0.229605	-0.189036	-0.572522
8	0.149522	0.156269	0.115237	0.209615	-0.197300	-0.567831
9	0.144051	0.147296	0.104059	0.191015	-0.204733	-0.563113
4.0	0.138889	0.138889	0.093651	0.173687	-0.211417	-0.558380
1	0.134012	0.131001	0.083947	0.157526	-0.217424	-0.553642
2	0.129400	0.123592	0.074891	0.142436	-0.222820	-0.548907
3	0.125031	0.116626	0.066430	0.128331	-0.227661	-0.544183
4	0.120890	0.110067	0.058517	0.115134	-0.231998	-0.539477
5	0.116959	0.103887	0.051109	0.102776	-0.235879	-0.534794
6	0.113225	0.098058	0.044169	0.091191	-0.239343	-0.530140
7	0.109673	0.092554	0.037661	0.080323	-0.242427	-0.525518
8	0.106293	0.087353	0.031553	0.070119	-0.245166	-0.520933
9	0.103072	0.082434	0.025816	0.060531	-0.247589	-0.516387
5.0	0.100000	0.077778	0.020425	0.051515	-0.249723	-0.511882
1	0.097069	0.073367	0.015354	0.043031	-0.251594	-0.507422
2	0.094268	0.069185	0.010581	0.035042	-0.253222	-0.503008
3	0.091592	0.065217	0.006087	0.027516	-0.254628	-0.498641
4	0.089031	0.061451	0.001852	0.020420	-0.255832	-0.494323
5	0.086580	0.057872	-0.002140	0.013727	-0.256849	-0.490055
6	0.084232	0.054470	-0.005906	0.007410	-0.257694	-0.485837
7	0.081981	0.051234	-0.009460	0.001445	-0.258383	-0.481670
8	0.079821	0.048153	-0.012815	-0.004191	-0.258927	-0.477555
9	0.077748	0.045220	-0.015984	-0.009517	-0.259337	-0.473492

Table A.4   *Values of S_w for $n = 5$ (contd.)*

ρ	S_0	S_1	S_2	S_3	S_4	S_5
6.0	0.075758	0.042424	-0.018979	-0.014554	-0.259626	-0.469480
1	0.073844	0.039759	-0.021810	-0.019318	-0.259802	-0.465520
2	0.072005	0.037217	-0.024487	-0.023827	-0.259874	-0.461612
3	0.070235	0.034790	-0.027020	-0.028095	-0.259851	-0.457755
4	0.068531	0.032473	-0.029416	-0.032137	-0.259740	-0.453950
5	0.066890	0.030260	-0.031684	-0.035965	-0.259548	-0.450195
6	0.065308	0.028144	-0.033831	-0.039593	-0.259282	-0.446491
7	0.063784	0.026121	-0.035864	-0.043032	-0.258947	-0.442838
8	0.062313	0.024187	-0.037790	-0.046291	-0.258549	-0.439234
9	0.060894	0.022335	-0.039614	-0.049382	-0.258093	-0.435679
7.0	0.059524	0.020563	-0.041342	-0.052314	-0.257584	-0.432172
1	0.058200	0.018865	-0.042980	-0.055095	-0.257025	-0.428714
2	0.056922	0.017239	-0.044532	-0.057733	-0.256422	-0.425303
3	0.055685	0.015681	-0.046003	-0.060237	-0.255777	-0.421939
4	0.054490	0.014187	-0.047397	-0.062613	-0.255093	-0.418621
5	0.053333	0.012754	-0.048718	-0.064868	-0.254375	-0.415349
6	0.052214	0.011379	-0.049971	-0.067008	-0.253625	-0.412121
7	0.051130	0.010060	-0.051158	-0.069040	-0.252846	-0.408938
8	0.050080	0.008794	-0.052283	-0.070969	-0.252040	-0.405799
9	0.049063	0.007578	-0.053350	-0.072800	-0.251209	-0.402702
8.0	0.048077	0.006410	-0.054360	-0.074537	-0.250356	-0.399647
1	0.047121	0.005288	-0.055318	-0.076187	-0.249483	-0.396634
2	0.046194	0.004210	-0.056225	-0.077753	-0.248591	-0.393662
3	0.045294	0.003174	-0.057085	-0.079239	-0.247683	-0.390731
4	0.044421	0.002178	-0.057899	-0.080649	-0.246760	-0.387839
5	0.043573	0.001220	-0.058669	-0.081987	-0.245823	-0.384985
6	0.042750	0.000299	-0.059398	-0.083256	-0.244874	-0.382171
7	0.041950	-0.000588	-0.060088	-0.084460	-0.243914	-0.379393
8	0.041173	-0.001441	-0.060741	-0.085601	-0.242944	-0.376653
9	0.040417	-0.002262	-0.061358	-0.086683	-0.241966	-0.373950
9.0	0.039683	-0.003053	-0.061941	-0.087709	-0.240981	-0.371282
1	0.038968	-0.003814	-0.062492	-0.088681	-0.239989	-0.368649
2	0.038273	-0.004546	-0.063012	-0.089601	-0.238992	-0.366051
3	0.037597	-0.005252	-0.063503	-0.090472	-0.237990	-0.363487
4	0.036939	-0.005932	-0.063965	-0.091296	-0.236984	-0.360956
5	0.036298	-0.006587	-0.064401	-0.092076	-0.235974	-0.358459
6	0.035674	-0.007219	-0.064811	-0.092813	-0.234963	-0.355993
7	0.035066	-0.007827	-0.065197	-0.093509	-0.233949	-0.353559
8	0.034473	-0.008413	-0.065560	-0.094167	-0.232934	-0.351157
9	0.033896	-0.008979	-0.065900	-0.094787	-0.231919	-0.348785
10.0	0.033333	-0.009524	-0.066219	-0.095371	-0.230903	-0.346443

REFERENCES

An attempt has been made here to provide all relevant references that are mainly mathematical in character, though some are not explicitly mentioned in the text. With a rapidly expanding subject covering a wide field, there is inevitably a large group of borderline references about which there is doubt as to whether they should be included or not; in such cases arbitrary decisions have had to be made. Some works of a more clinical, epidemiological, or public health nature have also been added if they exemplify particular points in the text, or if they constitute comparatively non-technical introductions to the basic concepts involved in understanding the dynamics and background of the spread of infectious diseases.

Abakuks, A. (1973). An optimal isolation policy for an epidemic. *J. Appl. Prob.*, **10**, 247-62.

Abbey, Helen (1952). An examination of the Reed–Frost theory of epidemics. *Hum. Biol.*, **24**, 201-33.

Abe, O. (1973). A note on the methodology of Knox's tests of "time and space interaction". *Biometrics*, **29**, 66-77.

Abramowitz, M. and Stegun, I.A. (1964). *Handbook of Mathematical Functions*. U.S. Nat. Bur. Stand., Appl. Math. Ser., **55**.

Almond, Joyce (1954). A note on the χ^2 test applied to epidemic chains. *Biometrics*, **10**, 459-77.

Armitage, P. (1953). A note on the epidemiology of malaria. *Trop. Dis. Bull.*, **50**, 890-2.

Armitage, P., Meynell, G.G. and Williams, T. (1965). Birth–death and other models for microbial infection. *Nature*, **207**, 570-2.

Assaad, F.A. and Maxwell-Lyons, F. (1966). The use of catalytic models as tools for elucidating the clinical and epidemiological features of trachoma. *Bull. Wld Hlth Org.*, **34**, 341-55.

Atkinson, A.C. (1970). A method of discriminating between models. *J.R. Statist. Soc.*, Ser. B, **32**, 323-53.

Bailey, N.T.J. (1950). A simple stochastic epidemic. *Biometrika*, **37**, 193-202.

Bailey, N.T.J. (1951). A classification of methods of ascertainment and analysis in estimating the frequencies of recessives in man. *Ann. Eugen., Lond.*, **16**, 223-5.

Bailey, N.T.J. (1953a). The total size of a general stochastic epidemic. *Biometrika*, **40**, 177-85.

Bailey, N.T.J. (1953b). The use of chain-binomials with a variable chance of infection for the analysis of intra-household epidemics. *Biometrika*, **40**, 279-86.

Bailey, N.T.J. (1954a). A statistical method of estimating the periods of incubation and infection of an infectious disease. *Nature*, **174**, 139-40.

Bailey, N.T.J. (1954b). Maximum-likelihood estimation of the relative removal rate from the distribution of the total size of an intra-household epidemic. *J. Hyg., Camb.*, **52**, 400-2.

Bailey, N.T.J. (1955). Some problems in the statistical analysis of epidemic data. *J.R. Statist. Soc.*, Ser. B, **17**, 35-58.

Bailey, N.T.J. (1956a). On estimating the latent and infectious periods of measles. I. Families with two susceptibles only. *Biometrika*, **43**, 15-22.

Bailey, N.T.J. (1956b). On estimating the latent and infectious periods of measles. II. Families with three or more susceptibles. *Biometrika*, **43**, 322-31.

Bailey, N.T.J. (1956c). Significance tests for a variable chance of infection in chain-binomial theory. *Biometrika*, **43**, 322-6.

Bailey, N.T.J. (1957). *The Mathematical Theory of Epidemics* (1st edn). London: Griffin.

Bailey, N.T.J. (1963). The simple stochastic epidemic: a complete solution in terms of known functions. *Biometrika*, **50**, 235-40.

Bailey, N.T.J. (1964a). *The Elements of Stochastic Processes with Applications to the Natural Sciences*. New York: Wiley.

Bailey, N.T.J. (1964b). Some stochastic models for small epidemics in large populations. *Appl. Statist.*, **13**, 9-19.

Bailey, N.T.J. (1967a). The simulation of stochastic epidemics in two dimensions. *Proc. Fifth Berkeley Symp. Math. Statis. & Prob.*, **4**, 237-57. Berkeley and Los Angeles: Univ. California.

Bailey, N.T.J. (1967b). *The Mathematical Approach to Biology and Medicine.* London: Wiley.

Bailey, N.T.J. (1968). A perturbation approximation to the simple stochastic epidemic in a large population. *Biometrika,* **55,** 199-209.

Bailey, N.T.J. (1973a). The estimation of parameters from epidemic models. (Ch. 14 in *The Mathematical Theory of the Dynamics of Biological Populations,* ed. M.S. Bartlett and R.W. Hiorns, *q.v.*)

Bailey, N.T.J. (1973b). Modelos matemáticos para las enfermedades transmisibles. *Tribuna Medica-Revision* (14 December), 21-31.

Bailey, N.T.J. and Alff-Steinberger, C. (1970). Improvements in the estimation of latent and infectious periods of a contagious disease. *Biometrika,* **57,** 141-53.

Bailey, N.T.J. and Alff-Steinberger, C. (1972). The estimation of latent and infectious periods from a single epidemic outbreak. (Unpublished.)

Bailey, N.T.J. and Thomas, A.S. (1971). The estimation of parameters from population data on the general stochastic epidemic. *Theor. Pop. Biol.,* **2,** 253-70. (Summarized in *Adv. Appl. Prob.,* **3,** 211-14.)

Bain, A.D. (1963). The growth of demand for new commodities. *J.R. Statist. Soc.,* Ser. A, **126,** 285-99.

Barbour, A.D. (1972). The principle of the diffusion of arbitrary constants. *J. Appl. Prob.,* **9,** 519-41.

Barnard, G.A. (1953). Time intervals between accidents – a note on Maguire, Pearson and Wynn's paper. *Biometrika,* **40,** 212-13.

Baroyan, O.V., Basilevsky, U.V., Ermakov, V.V., Frank, K.D., Rvachev, L.A. and Shashkov, V.A. (1970). Computer modelling of influenza epidemics for large-scale systems of cities and territories. (Working paper for WHO Symposium on Quantitative Epidemiology, Moscow, 23-27 Nov. 1970. In English and Russian. Summarized in Baroyan *et al.,* 1971.)

Baroyan, O.V., Genchikov, L.A., Rvachev, L.A. and Shashkov, V.A. (1969). An attempt at large-scale influenza epidemic modelling by means of a computer. *Bull. Int. Epid. Assoc.,* **18,** 22-31.

Baroyan, O.V. and Rvachev, L.A. (1967). Deterministic epidemic models for a territory with a transport network. *Kibernetika,* **3,** 67-74. (In Russian.)

Baroyan, O.V. and Rvachev, L.A. (1968). Some epidemiological experiments carried out on an electronic computer. *Vestnik Akad. Med. Nauk,* **23** (5), 32-4. (In Russian.)

Baroyan, O.V., Rvachev, L.A., Basilevsky, U.V., Ermakov, V.V., Frank, K.D., Rvachev, M.A. and Shashkov, V.A. (1971). Computer modelling of influenza epidemics for the whole country (USSR). *Adv. Appl. Prob.,* **3,** 224-6.

Baroyan, O.V., Rvachev, L.A., Frank, K.D., Shashkov, V.A. and Basilevsky, U.V. (1973). Mathematical and computer modelling of influenza epidemics in the USSR. *Vestnik Akad. Med. Nauk,* **28** (5), 26-30. (In Russian.)

Baroyan, O.V. Zhdanov, V.M., Soloviev, V.D. Zakstelskaya, L.Ya., Rvachev, L.A., Urbakh, Yu, V., Ermakov, V.V. and Antonova, I.V. (1972). Prospects of machine modelling of influenza epidemics for the territory of the USSR. *Zh. Mikrobiol. Epidemiol. Immunobiol.,* **49** (5), 3-11. (In Russian.)

Bartholomay, A.F. (1964). The general catalytic queue process. In *Stochastic Models in Medicine and Biology* (ed. J. Gurland), 101-44. Madison: Univ. Wisconsin Press.

Bartholomew, D.J. (1955). Tests for departures from randomness in a sequence of events occurring in time and space. (Ph.D. Thesis: Univ. London.)

Bartholomew, D.J. (1973). *Stochastic Models for Social Processes* (2nd edn). Chichester: Wiley.

Bartlett, M.S. (1946). *Stochastic Processes.* (Notes of a course given at the Univ. of North Carolina, 1946.)

Bartlett, M.S. (1949). Some evolutionary stochastic processes. *J.R. Statist. Soc.*, Ser. B. **11**, 211-29.

Bartlett, M.S. (1952). The statistical significance of odd bits of information. *Biometrika*, **39**, 228-37.

Bartlett, M.S. (1953). Stochastic processes or the statistics of change. *Appl. Statist.*, **2**, 44-64.

Bartlett, M.S. (1954). Processus stochastiques ponctuels. *Ann. Inst. Poincaré*, **14** (Fasc. 1), 35-60.

Bartlett, M.S. (1955). *Stochastic Processes.* Cambridge Univ. Press.

Bartlett, M.S. (1956). Deterministic and stochastic models for recurrent epidemics. *Proc. Third Berkeley Symp. Math. Statist. & Prob.*, **4**, 81-109. Berkeley and Los Angeles: Univ. California Press.

Bartlett, M.S. (1957). Measles periodicity and community size. *J.R. Statist. Soc.*, Ser. A, **120**, 48-70.

Bartlett, M.S. (1960a). *Stochastic Population Models in Ecology and Epidemiology.* London: Methuen.

Bartlett, M.S. (1960b). Some stochastic models in ecology and epidemiology. In *Contributions to Probability and Statistics: Essays in Honor of Harold Hotelling* (ed. I. Olkin *et al.*,), 89-96. Stanford Univ. Press.

Bartlett, M.S. (1960c). The critical community size for measles in the United States. *J.R. Statist. Soc.*, Ser. A, **123**, 37-44.

Bartlett, M.S. (1961). Monte Carlo studies in ecology and epidemiology. *Proc. Fourth Berkeley Symp. Math. Statist. & Prob.*, **4**, 39-55. Berkeley and Los. Angeles: Univ. California Press.

Bartlett, M.S. (1964). The relevance of stochastic models for large-scale epidemiological phenomena. *Appl. Statist.*, **13**, 2-8.

Bartlett, M.S. (1966). Some notes on epidemiological theory. In *Research Papers in Statistics: Festschrift for J. Neyman* (ed. F.N. David), 25-36. New York: Wiley.

Bartlett, M.S. (1973). Equations and models of population change. (Ch. 1 in *The Mathematical Theory of the Dynamics of Biological Populations,* ed. M.S. Bartlett and R.W. Hiorns.)

Bartlett, M.S. and Hiorns, R.W. (Editors) (1973). *The Mathematical Theory of the Dynamics of Biological Populations.* London: Academic Press.

Barton, D.E. and David, F.N. (1966). The random intersection of two graphs. In *Research Papers in Statistics: Festschrift for J. Neyman* (ed. F.N. David), 445-59. New York: Wiley.

Barton, D.E., David, F.N., Fix, E., Merrington, M. and Mustacchi, P. (1967). Tests for space-time interaction and a power function. *Proc. Fifth Berkeley Symp. Math. Statist. & Prob.*, **4**, 217-27. Berkeley and Los Angeles: Univ. California Press.

Barton, D.E. David, F.N. and Merrington, M. (1965). A criterion for testing contagion in time and space. *Ann. Hum. Genet.*, **29**, 97-102.

Bartoszyński, R. (1967). Branching processes and the theory of epidemics. *Proc. Fifth Berkeley Symp. Math. Statist. & Prob.* **4**, 259-69. Berkeley and Los Angeles: Univ. California Press.

Bartoszyński, R. (1969). Branching processes and models of epidemics. *Dissertationes Mathematicae*, LXI. Warsaw.

Bartoszyński, R. (1972). On a certain model of an epidemic. *Applicationes Mathematicae*, **13**, 139-51.

Bartoszyński, R., Łoś, J. and Wycech-Łoś, M. (1965). Contributions to the theory of epidemics. In *Bernoulli–Bayes–Laplace* (ed. J. Neyman and L.M. LeCam), 1-8. Berlin: Springer.

Becker, N.G. (1968). The spread of an epidemic to fixed groups within the population. *Biometrics*, **24**, 1007-14.

Becker, N.G. (1970a). Mathematical models in epidemiology and related fields. (Ph.D. Thesis: Sheffield Univ.)

Becker, N.G. (1970b). A stochastic model for two interacting populations. *J. Appl. Prob.*, **7**, 544-64.

Becker, N.G. (1972). Vaccination programs for rare infectious diseases. *Biometrika*, **59**, 443-53.

Becker, N.G. (1973). Carrier-borne epidemics in a community consisting of different groups. *J. Appl. Prob.*, **10**, 491-501.

Benayoun, R. (1964a). Sur un modèle stochastique utilisé dans la théorie mathématique des épidémies. *C.R. Acad. Sci., Paris*, **258**, 5789-91.

Benayoun, R. (1964b). Contribution à la théorie mathématique des épidémies. (Thesis: Faculté des Sciences, Toulouse.)

Benayoun, R. and Monin, J.P. (1968). *Réflexions sur le phénomène de contagion, applications-modèles*. (Note de travail No. 85, SEMA, Paris.)

Bernoulli, D. (1760). Essai d'une nouvelle analyse de la mortalité causée par la petite vérole et des avantages de l'inoculation pour la prévenir. *Mém. Math. Phys. Acad. Roy. Sci., Paris*, 1-45.

Beye, H.K. and Gurian, J. (1960). The epidemiology and dynamics of *Wucheria bancrofti* and *Brugia malayi*. *Indian J. Malariol.*, **14**, 415-40.

Bharucha-Reid, A.T. (1956). On the stochastic theory of epidemics. *Proc. Third Berkeley Symp. Math. Statist. & Prob.*, **4**, 111-19. Berkeley and Los Angeles: Univ. California Press.

Bharucha-Reid, A.T. (1957). *An Introduction to the Stochastic Theory of Epidemics and some Related Statistical Problems*. Randolph Field, Texas: USAF School of Aviation Medicine.

Bharucha-Reid, A.T. (1958). Comparison of populations whose growth can be described by a branching stochastic process — with special reference to a problem in epidemiology. *Sankhyā*, **19**, 1-14.

Bharucha-Reid, A.T. (1960). *Elements of the Theory of Markov Processes and their Applications*. New York: McGraw-Hill.

Billard, Lynne (1973). Factorial moments and probabilities for the general stochastic epidemic. *J. Appl. Prob.*, **10**, 277-88.

Billingsley, P. (1961). *Statistical Inference for Markov Processes*. Univ. Chicago Press.

Black, F.L. (1966). Measles endemicity in insular populations: critical community size and its evolutionary implications. *J. Theor. Biol.*, **11**, 207-11.

Black, M.L. and Gay, J.D. (1965). Some kinetic properties of a deterministic epidemic confirmed by computer simulation. *Science*, **148**, 981-5.

Bogdanoff, E. (1964). Public health system training. *SDC Magazine* (Systems Development Corporation), **7**, 23-5.

Bolshev, L.N. and Kruopis, Yu. I. (1969). On the modelling of epidemic processes. *Lietuvos mathematikos rinkinys*, **9**, 243-53. (In Russian.)

Bradley, L. (1971). *Smallpox Inoculation: An Eighteenth Century Mathematical Controversy*. Adult Education Department: Univ. Nottingham.

Brambilla, F. (1960). Modelli deterministici e stocastici in epidemiologia. *Boll. Centro Ric. Operat. (Serie Metodol.)*, **4**, 3-28.

Brambilla, F. (1962). *Processi Stocastici in Economia e Sociologia* (pp. 102-13). Milano: Istituto Editoriale Cisalpino.

Brøgger, S. (1967). Systems analysis in tuberculosis control: a model. *Amer. Rev. Resp. Dis.*, **95**, 421-34.

Bross, I.D.J. (1958). How to use ridit analysis. *Biometrics*, **14**, 18-38.

Brownlea, A.A. (1972). Modelling the geographic epidemiology of infectious hepatitis. In *Medical Geography* (ed. N.D. McGlashan), 279-300. London: Methuen.

Brownlee, J. (1906). Statistical studies in immunity: the theory of an epidemic. *Proc. Roy. Soc. Edin.*, **26**, 484-521.

Brownlee, J. (1909). Certain considerations of the causation and course of epidemics. *Proc. Roy. Soc. Med. (Epid. Sec.)*, **2**, 243-58.

Brownlee, J. (1911). The mathematical theory of random migration and epidemic distribution. *Proc. Roy. Soc. Edin.*, **31**, 262-88.

Brownlee, J. (1914). Periodicity in infectious disease. *Proc. Roy. Phil. Soc. Glasgow*, **45**, 197-213.

Brownlee, J. (1915a). On the curve of the epidemic. *Brit. Med. J.*, **1**, 799-800.

Brownlee, J. (1915b). Historical note on Farr's theory of the epidemic. *Brit. Med. J.*, **2**, 250-2.

Brownlee, J. (1915c). Investigations into the periodicity of infectious diseases by the application of a method hitherto only used in physics. *Publ. Hlth, London,* **28,** 125-34.

Brownlee, J. (1916). On the curve of the epidemic. Supplementary note. *Brit. Med. J.,* **2,** 142-3.

Brownlee, J. (1918). Certain aspects of the theory of epidemiology in special relation to plague. *Proc. Roy. Soc. Med. (Sec. Epidem. and State Med.),* **11,** 85-132.

Bruce-Chwatt, L.J. (1969). Quantitative epidemiology of tropical diseases. *Trans. Roy. Soc. Trop. Med. Hyg.,* **63,** 131-43.

Budd, W. (1873). *Typhoid Fever: Its Nature, Mode of Spreading and Prevention.* London: Longmans (reprinted by Delta Omega Society, New York, 1931).

Bühler, W. (1966). A theorem concerning the extinction of epidemics. *Biom. Zeit.,* **8,** 10-14.

Bungeţianu, Gh. (1971). Mathematical models of tuberculosis. Vain expectations and fulfilled hopes. *Ftiziologia,* **20,** 573-82. (In Romanian.)

Bungeţianu, Gh. (1973). Mathematical modelling in tuberculosis. *Ftiziologia,* **22,** 561-84. (In Romanian.)

Burnet, F.M. and White, D.O. (1972). *The Natural History of Infectious Disease* (4th edn). Cambridge Univ. Press.

Cane, Violet (1966). On the size of an epidemic and the number of people hearing a rumour. *J.R. Statist. Soc.,* Ser. B, **28,** 487-90.

Center for Disease Control (1971). *Morbidity and Mortality,* **20,** 339-45.

Chassan, J.B. (1948). The autocorrelation approach to the analysis of the incidence of communicable diseases. *Human Biology,* **20,** 90-108.

Chassan, J.B. (1949). On a statistical approximation to the infection interval. *Biometrics,* **5,** 243-9.

Cheeseman, E.A. (1950). *Epidemics in Schools.* Medical Research Council Special Report, No. 271. London: H.M.S.O.

Chelsky, M. (1968). The propagating rate: a method of interpreting infectious disease incidence. (Ph.D. Thesis: School of Public Health, Univ. Michigan, Ann Arbor.)

Chelsky, M. (1969). A method of interpreting infectious disease incidence. *Amer. J. Publ. Hlth,* **59,** 1661-73.

Chelsky, M. and Angulo, J. (1973). Two models for estimation of some parameters of disease spread. *Math. Biosci.,* **18,** 119-31.

Chorba, R.W. and Sanders, J.L. (1971). Planning models for tuberculosis control programs. *Hlth Serv. Res.,* **6,** 144-64.

Cooke, K.L. (1967). Functional differential equations: some models and perturbation problems. In *Differential Equations and Dynamical Systems* (ed. J.K. Hale and J.P. LaSalle), 167-83. New York: Academic Press.

Cooke, K.L. and Yorke, J.A. (1973). Some equations modelling growth processes and gonorrhoea epidemics. *Math. Biosci.,* **16,** 75-101.

Cox, D.R. (1962). Further results on tests of separate familities of hypotheses. *J.R. Statist. Soc.,* Ser. B, **21,** 406-24.

Creighton, C. (1965). *A History of Epidemics in Britain,* 2 vol. (2nd edn). London: Cass.

Cristea, A., Copelovici, Y. and Cajal, N. (1973). Un modèle mathématique des cycles annuels et multiannuels de l'évolution des morbidités par certaines viroses. *Rev. Roum. Virol.,* **10,** 173-91.

Cruickshank, D.B. (1940). *Papworth Research Bulletin,* 36.

Cruickshank, D.B. (1947). Regional influences in cancer. *Brit. J. Cancer,* **1,** 109-28.

Cvjetanović, B. (1972). Use of mathematical models in the planning and evaluation of control measures against infectious diseases. *J. Egypt. Pub. Hlth Assoc.,* **47,** 121-8.

Cvjetanović, B., Grab, B. and Uemura, K. (1971). Epidemiological model of typhoid fever and its use in planning and evaluation of antityphoid immunization and sanitation programmes. *Bull. Wld Hlth Org.,* **45,** 53-75.

Cvjetanović, B., Grab, B., Uemura, K. and Bytchenko, B. (1972). Epidemiological model of tetanus and its use in the planning of immunization programmes. *Int. J. Epid.*, **1**, 125-37.

Cvjetanović, B., Uemura, K., Grab, B. and Sundaresan, T. (1973). Use of mathematical models in the evaluation of the effectiveness of preventive measures against some infectious diseases. *Proc. Sixth Int. Sci. Meeting, Int. Epid. Assoc.*, **2**, 913-33.

D'Alembert, J. (1761). *Opuscules Mathématiques*, **2**.

Daley, D.J (1967). Concerning the spread of news in a population of individuals who never forget. *Bull. Math. Biophys.*, **29**, 373-6.

Daley, D.J. and Kendall, D.G. (1964). Epidemics and rumours. *Nature*, **204**, 1118.

Daley, D.J. and Kendall, D.G. (1965). Stochastic rumours. *J. Inst. Math. Applns*, **1**, 42-55.

D'Ancona, U. (1954). *The Struggle for Existence*. Leiden: Brill.

Daniels, H.E. (1967). The distribution of the total size of an epidemic. *Proc. Fifth Berkeley Symp. Math. Statist. & Prob.*, **4**, 281-93. Berkeley and Los Angeles: Univ. California.

Daniels, H.E. (1971). A note on perturbation techniques for epidemics. *Adv. Appl. Prob.*, **3**, 214-18.

Daniels, H.E. (1972). An exact relation in the theory of carrier-borne epidemics. *Biometrika*, **59**, 211-13.

Daniels, H.E. (1974). The maximum size of a closed epidemic. *Adv. Appl. Prob.*, **6**, 607-21.

Davis, H.T. (1933, 1935). *Tables of Higher Mathematical Functions*, **1 & 2**. Indiana: Principia Press.

Denton, Gillian (1972). On Downton's carrier-borne epidemic. *Biometrika*, **59**, 455-61.

Dick, G. (1971). Routine smallpox vaccination. *Brit. Med. J.*, **3**, 163-6.

Dietz, K. (1966). On the model of Weiss for the spread of epidemics by carriers. *J. Appl. Prob.*, **3**, 375-82.

Dietz, K. (1967). Epidemics and rumours: a survey. *J.R. Statist. Soc.*, Ser. A, **130**, 505-28.

Dietz, K. (1969). Carrier-borne epidemics with immigration. II: immigration of susceptibles and birth of new carriers. (Unpublished.)

Dietz, K. (1970). Mathematical models for malaria in different ecological zones. (Seventh International Biometric Conference, Hannover, 16-21 August 1970.)

Dietz, K. (1971). Malaria models. *Adv. Appl. Prob.*, **3**, 208-10.

Dietz, K. and Downton, F. (1968). Carrier-borne epidemics with immigration. I: immigration of both susceptibles and carriers. *J. Appl. Prob.*, **5**, 31-42.

Dietz, K., Molineaux, L. and Thomas, A. (1974). A malaria model tested in the African Savannah. *Bull. Wld Hlth Org.*, **50**, 347-57.

Dionne, P.J. (1972). Epidemiology. *IEEE Trans. Biomed. Eng.*, **19**, 126-8.

Downton, F. (1967a). A note on the ultimate size of a general stochastic epidemic. *Biometrika*, **54**, 314-16.

Downton, F. (1967b). Epidemics with carriers: a note on a paper of Dietz. *J. Appl. Prob.*, **4**, 264-70.

Downton, F. (1968). The ultimate size of carrier-borne epidemics. *Biometrika*, **55**, 277-89.

Downton, F. (1972a). The area under the infectives trajectory of the general stochastic epidemic. *J. Appl. Prob.*, **9**, 414-17.

Downton, F. (1972b). A correction to "The area under the infectives trajectory of the general stochastic epidemic". *J. Appl. Prob.*, **9**, 873-6.

Duvillard, E.-E. (1806). *Analyse et tableaux de l'influence de la petite vérole sur la mortalité à chaque âge, et de celle qu'un préservatif tel que la vaccine peut avoir sur la population et la longévité*. Paris: Imprimerie Impériale.

Eden, M. (1961). A two-dimensional growth process. In *Proc. Fourth Berkeley Symp. Math. Statist. & Prob.*, **4**, 223-3). Berkeley and Los Angeles: Univ. California Press.

Ederer, F., Myers, M.H. and Mantel, N. (1964). A statistical problem in time and space: do leukemia cases come in clusters? *Biometrics*, **20**, 626-38.

Elveback, Lila (1971). Simulation of stochastic discrete-time epidemic models for two agents. *Adv. Appl. Prob.*, **3**, 226-8.

Elveback, Lila, Ackerman, E., Gatewood, L. and Fox, J.P. (1971). Stochastic two-agent epidemic simulation models for a community of families. *Amer. J. Epidem.*, **93**, 267-80.

Elveback, Lila, Ackerman, E., Young, G. and Fox, J.P. (1968). A stochastic model for competition between viral agents in the presence of interference. 1: Live virus vaccine in a randomly mixing population, model III. *Amer. J. Epidem.*, **87**, 373-84.

Elveback, Lila, Fox, J.P. and Varma, A. (1964). An extension of the Reed−Frost epidemic model for the study of competition between viral agents in the presence of inter-ference. *Amer. J. Hyg.*, **80**, 356-64.

Elveback, Lila, and Varma, A. (1965). Simulation of mathematical models for public health problems. *Public Hlth Rep.*, **80**, 1067-76.

Erdélyi, A. (ed.) (1953). *Higher Transcendental Functions*, 1 & 2. New York: McGraw-Hill.

Erdélyi, A. (ed.) (1954). *Tables of Integral Transforms*, 1. New York: McGraw-Hill.

Evans, G.H. (1875). Some arithmetical considerations of the progress of epidemics. *Trans. Epidem. Soc., London*, 1873-5, 551.

Ewy, W. (1971). A model and computer simulation system for epidemics of two competing agents in a structured population. (Ph.D. Thesis: Univ. Minnesota.)

Ewy, W., Ackerman, E., Gatewood, L.C., Elveback, L. and Fox J.P. (1972). A generalized stochastic model for simulation of epidemics in a heterogeneous population (model VI). *Comput. Biol. Med.*, **2**, 45-58.

Fanshel, S. (1972). A meaningful measure of health for epidemiology. *Int. J. Epid.*, **1**, 319-37.

Farr, W. (1840). Progress of epidemics. *Second Report of the Registrar General of England and Wales*, 91-8.

Feldstein, M.S., Piot, M.A. and Sundaresan, T.K. (1973). Resource allocation model for public health planning. *Bull. Wld Hlth Org.*, **48**, Supp., 3-108.

Feller, W. (1939). Die Grundlagen der Volterraschen Theorie des Kampfes ums Dasein in wahrscheinlichkeitstheoretischer Behandlung. *Acta Biotheoretica*, **5**, 11-40.

Feller, W. (1957). *An Introduction to Probability Theory and its Applications*, Vol. 1 (3rd edn, 1968). New York: Wiley.

Ferebee, Shirley (1967). An epidemiological model of tuberculosis in the United States. *NTA Bull.*, **53**, 4-7.

Firescu, D. and Tăutu, P. (1967). A stochastic model of focal epidemic. *Rev. Roum. Math. Pures Appl.*, **12**, 653-64.

Fisher, D.B. and Halstead, S.B. (1970). Observations related to pathogenesis of dengue haemorrhagic fever. V: Examination of age-specific sequential infection rates using a mathematical model. *Yale J. Biol. Med.*, **42**, 329-49.

Fisher, R.A. (1934). The effect of methods of ascertainment upon the estimation of frequencies. *Ann. Eugen., Lond.*, **6**, 13-25.

Foster, F.G. (1955). A note on Bailey's and Whittle's treatment of a general stochastic epidemic. *Biometrika*, **42**, 123-5.

Fox, J.P., Elveback, L., Scott, W., Gatewood, L. and Ackerman, E. (1971). Herd immunity: basic concept and relevance to public health immunization practice. *Amer. J. Epidem.*, **94**, 179-89.

Frisch, H.L. and Hammersley, J.M., (1963). Percolation processes and related topics. *J. Soc. Indust. Appl. Math.*, **11**, 894-918.

Gaffey, W.R. (1954). The probability of within-family contagion. (Thesis: Univ. California, Berkeley.)

Gani, J. (1965a). On a partial differential equation of epidemic theory, I. *Biometrika*, **52**, 617-22.

Gani, J. (1965b). On a partial differential equation of epidemic theory, II: The model with immigration. *Office of Naval Research Techn. Rep. RM-124*. Michigan State Univ.

Gani, J. (1966). On the stochastic epidemic with immigration. *Proc. Int. Cong. Math.* (Moscow).

Gani, J. (1967). On the general stochastic epidemic. *Proc: Fifth Berkeley Symp. Math. Statist. & Prob.*, **4**, 271-9. Berkeley and Los Angeles: Univ. California Press.

Gani, J. (1969). A chain binomial study of inoculation in epidemics. *Bull. I. S. I.*, **43** (2), 203-4.

Gani, J. (1971). Recent work in epidemiology at Sheffield. *Adv. Appl. Prob.*, **3**, 204-6.

Gani, J. (1973). Point processes in epidemiology. In *Stochastic Point Processes* (ed. P.A.W. Lewis), 756-73. New York: Wiley.

Gani, J. and Jerwood, D. (1971). Markov chain methods in chain binomial epidemic models. *Biometrics*, **27**, 591-604.

Gani, J. and Jerwood, D. (1972). The cost of a general stochastic epidemic. *J. Appl. Prob.* **9**, 257-69.

Garg, M.L., Thompson, D.J. and Gezon, H.M. (1967). Assessing the influence of treatment on the spread of staphylococci in newborn infants by simulation. *Amer. J. Epidem.*, **85**, 220-8.

Garrett-Jones, C. (1964). The human blood index of malaria vectors in relation to epidemiological assessment. *Bull. Wld Hlth Org.*, **30**, 241-61.

Garrett-Jones, C. and Shidrawi, G.R. (1969). Malaria vectorial capacity of a population of *Anopheles gambiae* — an exercise in epidemiological entomology. *Bull. Wld Hlth Org.* **40**, 531-45.

Gart, J.J. (1965). Some stochastic models relating time and dosage in response curves. *Biometrics*, **21**, 583-99.

Gart, J.J. (1968). The mathematical analysis of an epidemic with two kinds of susceptibles. *Biometrics*, **24**, 557-66.

Gart, J.J. (1971). Mathematical models in the interpretation of the interaction between infective agents. *Adv. Appl. Prob.*, **3**, 202-3.

Gart, J.J. (1972). The statistical analysis of chain-binomial epidemic models with several kinds of susceptibles. *Biometrics*, **28**, 921-30.

Gart, J.J. and Vries, J.L. de (1966). The mathematical analysis of concurrent epidemics of yaws and chickenpox. *J. Hyg., Camb.*, **64**, 431-9.

Gatewood, Laël, Ackerman, E., Ewy, W., Elveback, L. and Fox, J.P. (1971). Simulation of models of enteric virus epidemics. *Bio-Med. Comp.*, **2**, 201-13.

Goffman, W. (1965). An epidemic process in an open population. *Nature*, **205**, 831-2.

Goffman, W. (1966a). A mathematical model for describing the compatibility of infectious diseases. *J. Theor. Biol.*, **11**, 349-61.

Goffman, W. (1966b). Mathematical approach to the spread of scientific ideas — the history of mast cell research. *Nature*, **212**, 449-52.

Goffman, W. (1966c). Stability of epidemic processes. *Nature*, **210**, 786-7.

Goffman, W. and Newill, V.A. (1964). Generalization of epidemic theory. An application to the transmission of ideas. *Nature*, **204**, 225-8.

Goffman, W. and Newill, V.A. (1967). Communication and epidemic processes. *Proc. Roy. Soc.*, A, **298**, 316-34.

Goffman, W. and Warren, K.S. (1970). An application of the Kermack–McKendrick theory to the epidemiology of schistosomiasis. *Amer. J. Trop. Med. Hyg.*, **19**, 278-83.

Goodall, E.W. (1931). Incubation period of measles. *Brit. Med. J.*, **1**, 73-4.

Gordon, G., O'Callaghan, M. and Tallis, G.M. (1970). A deterministic model for the life cycle of a class of internal parasites of sheep. *Math. Biosci.*, **8**, 209-26.

Gould, K.L., Herrman, K.L. and Witte, J.J. (1971). The epidemiology of measles in the U.S. Trust Territory of the Pacific Islands. *Amer. J. Publ. Hlth*, **61**, 1602-14.

Grab, B. and Cvjetanović, B. (1971). Simple method for rough determination of the cost-benefit balance point of immunization programmes. *Bull. Wld Hlth Org.*, **45**, 536-41.

Grab, B. and Cvjetanović, B. (1975). Epidemiological model of cerebrospinal meningitis. (In preparation).

Greenwood, M. (1931). On the statistical measure of infectiousness. *J. Hyg., Camb.*, **31**, 336-51,

Greenwood, M. (1935). *Epidemics and Crowd Diseases*. London: Williams & Norgate.

Greenwood, M. (1946). The statistical study of infectious diseases. *J. R. Statist. Soc.*, Part II, **109**, 85-103.

Greenwood, M. (1949). The infectiousness of measles. *Biometrika,* **36**, 1-8.

Greenwood, M., Bradford Hill, A., Topley, W.W.C. and Wilson, J. (1936). *Experimental Epidemiology.* Medical Research Council Special Report, No. 209. London: H.M.S.O.

Griffiths, D.A. (1971a). Epidemic models. (Ph.D. Thesis: Univ. Oxford.)

Griffiths, D.A. (1971b). Measles in vaccinated communities. *Lancet,* **2**, 1423-4.

Griffiths, D.A. (1972a). A bivariate birth–death process which approximates to the spread of a disease involving a vector. *J. Appl. Prob.,* **9**, 65-75.

Griffiths, D.A. (1972b). A further note on the probability of disease transmission. *Biometrics,* **28**, 1133-9.

Griffiths, D.A. (1973a). Multivariate birth-and-death processes as approximations to epidemic processes. *J. Appl. Prob.,* **10**, 15-26.

Griffiths, D.A. (1973b). The effect of measles vaccination on the incidence of measles in the community. *J.R. Statistic. Soc.,* Ser. A, **136**, 441-9.

Griffiths, D.A. (1973c). Maximum likelihood estimation for the beta-binomial distribution and an application to the household distribution of the total number of cases of a disease. *Biometrics,* **29**, 637-48.

Grundy, F. and Reinke, W.A. (1973). *Health Practice Research.* Geneva: WHO.

Gupta, N.K. (1972). Modeling and optimum control of epidemics. (Ph.D. Thesis: Univ. Alberta.)

Gupta, N.K. and Rink, R.E. (1971). A model for communicable disease control. *Proc. 24th Ann. Conf. Eng. Med. Biol.,* Las Vegas.

Gupta, N.K. and Rink, R.E. (1973). Optimal control of epidemics. *Math. Biosci.,* **18**, 383-96.

Gurland, J. (ed.) (1964). *Stochastic Models in Medicine and Biology.* Madison: Univ. Wisconsin Press.

Haggett, P. (1972). Contagious processes in a planar graph: an epidemiological application. In *Medical Geography* (ed. N.D. McGlashan), 307-24. London: Methuen.

Hairston, N.G. (1962). Population ecology and epidemiological problems. In *CIBA Foundation Symposium on Bilharziasis* (ed. C.E.W. Wolstenholme and M. O'Connor), 36-62. London: Churchill.

Hairston, N.G. (1965a). On the mathematical analysis of schistosome populations. *Bull. Wld Hlth Org.,* **33**, 45-62.

Hairston, N.G. (1965b). An analysis of age-prevalence data by catalytic models. A contribution to the study of bilharziasis. *Bull. Wld Hlth Org.,* **33**, 163-75.

Hamer, W.H. (1906). Epidemic disease in England. *Lancet,* **1**, 733-9.

Hammersley, J.M. (1966). First-passage percolation. *J.R. Statist. Soc.,* Ser. B, **28**, 491-6.

Hammersley, J.M. and Welsh, D.J.A. (1965). First-passage percolation, subadditive processes, stochastic networks and generalized renewal theory. In *Bernoulli–Bayes–Laplace* (ed. J. Neyman and L.M. LeCam), 61-110. Berlin: Springer.

Hammond, B.J. and Tyrrell, D.A.J. (1971). A mathematical model of common-cold epidemics on Tristan da Cunha. *J. Hyg., Camb.,* **69**, 423-33.

Hare, Ronald (1954). *Pomp and Pestilence.* London: Gollancz.

Harris, T.E. (1963). *The Theory of Branching Processes.* Berlin: Springer.

Haskey, H.W. (1954). A general expression for the mean in a simple stochastic epidemic. *Biometrika,* **41**, 272-5.

Haskey, H.W. (1957). Stochastic cross-infection between two otherwise isolated groups. *Biometrika,* **44**, 193-204.

Heasman, M.A. and Reid, D.D. (1961). Theory and observation in family epidemics of the common cold. *Brit. J. Prev. Soc. Med.,* **15**, 12-16.

Hethcote, H.W. (1970). Note on determining the limiting susceptible population in an epidemic model. *Math. Biosci.,* **9**, 161-3.

Hethcote, H.W. (1973). Asymptotic behaviour in a deterministic epidemic model. *Bull. Math. Biol.,* **35**, 607-14.

Hethcote, H.W. and Waltman, P. (1973). Optimal vaccination schedules in a deterministic epidemic model. *Math. Biosci.*, **18**, 365-81.

Hill, B.M. (1963). The three-parameter lognormal distribution and Bayesian analysis of a point-source epidemic. *J. Amer. Statist. Assoc.*, **58**, 72-84.

Hill, R.T. and Severo, N.C. (1969). The simple stochastic epidemic for small populations with one or more initial infectives. *Biometrika*, **56**, 183-96.

Hope Simpson, R.E. (1948). The period of transmission in certain epidemic diseases. *Lancet*, **2**, 755-60.

Hope Simpson, R.E. (1952). Infectiousness of communicable diseases in the household. *Lancet*, **2**, 549-54.

Hope Simpson, R.E. and Sutherland, I. (1954). Does influenza spread within the household? *Lancet*, **1**, 721-6.

Hopf, E. (1952). Statistical hydromechanics and functional calculus. *J. Ration. Mech. Anal.*, **1**, 87-124.

Hoppensteadt, F. and Waltman, P. (1970). A problem in the theory of epidemics, I. *Math. Biosci.*, **9**, 71-91.

Hoppensteadt, F. and Waltman, P. (1971). A problem in the theory of epidemics, II. *Math. Biosci.*, **12**, 133-46.

Horiuchi, K. (ed.) (1962). *Contributions from the Department of Preventive Medicine and Public Health, Osaka City University Medical School,* **2** (Apr. 1959 – Mar. 1961). Osaka: Osaka City Univ. Med. School.

Horiuchi, K., Nishida, F., Ueshima, I., Yamamoto, K., Shibata, E., Masada, Y., Oki, Y. and Sugiyama, H. (1959). A study on the familiar aggregation of measles. *Jap. J. Pub. Hlth*, **6**, 276-8.

Horiuchi, K. and Sugiyama, H. (1957). On the importance of the Monte Carlo approach in the research of epidemiology. *Osaka City Med. J.*, **4**, 59-62.

Hughes, P.H. and Crawford, G.A. (1972). A contagious disease model for researching and intervening in heroin epidemics. *Arch. Gen. Psychiat.*, **27**, 149-55.

Hughes, P.H., Senay, E.C. and Parker, R. (1972). The medical management of a heroin epidemic. *Arch. Gen. Psychiat.*, **27**, 585-91.

Hugh-Jones, M.E. and Tinline, R.R. (1973). Studies on the 1967-68 Foot and Mouth disease epidemic. Incubation period and disease interval. (Unpublished.)

Iglehart, D.L. (1964). Multivariate competition processes. *Ann. Math. Statist.*, **35**, 350-61.

Indrayan, A., Srivastava, R.N. and Bagchi, S.R. (1970). Mathematical models in the assessment of infective force in filariasis. *Indian J. Med. Res.*, **58**, 1100-3.

Iosifescu, M. and Tăutu, P. (1968). *Procese Stohastice şi Applicaţii in Biologie şi Medicină.* Bucureşti. (In Romanian.)

Iosifescu, M. and Tăutu, P. (1973). *Stochastic Processes and Applications in Biology and Medicine*, II, New York: Springer.

Ipsen, J. (1959). Social distance in epidemiology – age of susceptible siblings as the determining factor in household infectivity of measles. *Hum. Biol.*, **31**, 162-79.

Ipsen, J. and Feigl, P. (1970). A biomathematical model for prevalence of *Trichomonas vaginalis*. *Amer. J. Epid.*, **91**, 175-84.

Irwin, J.O. (1954). A distribution arising in the study of infectious diseases. *Biometrika*, **41**, 266-8.

Irwin, J.O. (1963). The place of mathematics in medical and biological statistics. *J.R. Statist. Soc.*, Ser. A. **126**, 1-41.

Irwin, J.O. (1964). The contribution of G.U. Yule and A.G. McKendrick to stochastic process methods in biology and medicine. In *Stochastic Models in Medicine and Biology* (ed. J. Gurland), 147-63. Madison: Univ. Wisconsin Press.

Jaquette, D.L. (1970). A stochastic model for the optimal control of epidemics and pest populations. *Math. Biosci.*, **8**, 343-54.

Jerwood, D. (1970). A note on the cost of the simple epidemic. *J. Appl. Prob.*, **7**, 440-3.

Jerwood, D. (1971). Cost of epidemics. (Ph.D. Thesis: Sheffield Univ.)

Juchniewicz, M., Olakowski, T. and Mardoń, K. (1967). Prognostication of the epidemiological situation of tuberculosis based on an epidemiological model: preliminary report. *Gruźlica*, **35**, 961-7. (In Polish.)

Kampen, N.G. van (1973). Birth and death processes in large populations. *Biometrika*, **60**, 419-20.

Karlin, S. (1966). *A First Course in Stochastic Processes.* New York: Academic Press.

Kelker, D. (1973). A random walk epidemic simulation. *J. Amer. Statist. Assoc.*, **68**, 821-3.

Kemeny, J.G. and Snell, J.L. (1960). *Finite Markov Chains.* Princeton: Van Nostrand.

Kendall, D.G. (1948a). On the generalized "birth-and-death" process. *Ann. Math. Statist.*, **19**, 1-15.

Kendall, D.G. (1948b). On the role of variable generation time in the development of a stochastic birth process. *Biometrika*, **35**, 316-30.

Kendall, D.G. (1950). An artificial realization of a simple birth-and-death process. *J.R. Statist. Soc.*, Ser. B, **12**, 116-19.

Kendall, D.G. (1956). Deterministic and stochastic epidemics in closed populations. *Proc. Third Berkeley Symp. Math. Statist. & Prob.*, **4**, 149-65. Berkeley and Los Angeles: Univ. California Press.

Kendall, D.G. (1957). La propagation d'une épidémie ou d'un bruit dans une population limitée. *Publ. Inst. Statist. Univ. Paris*, **6**, 307-11.

Kendall, D.G. (1965). Mathematical models of the spread of infection. In *Mathematics and Computer Science in Biology and Medicine*, 213-25. London: H.M.S.O.

Kermack, W.O. and McKendrick, A.G. (1927-39). Contributions to the mathematical theory of epidemics. *Proc. Roy. Soc.*, A, **115**, 700-21. (Part I, 1927.) *Proc. Roy. Soc.*, A, **138**, 55-83. (Part II. 1932.) *Proc. Roy. Soc.*, A, **141**, 94-122. (Part III, 1933.) *J. Hyg., Camb.*, 37, 172-87. (Part IV, 1937.) *J. Hyg., Camb.*, **39**, 271-88. (Part V, 1939.)

Knox, E.G. (1959). Secular pattern of congenital oesophageal atresia. *Brit. J. Prev. Soc. Med.*, **13**, 222-6.

Knox, E.G. (1963a). Detection of low epidemicity: application to cleft lip and palate. *Brit. J. Prev. Soc. Med.*, **17**, 121-7.

Knox, E.G. (1963b). The family characteristics of children with clefts of lip and palate. *Acta Genet. (Basel)*, **13**, 299-315.

Knox, E.G. (1963c). Distribution of uncommon disorders. *Eugen. Rev.*, **55**, 29-32.

Knox, E.G. (1964a). Epidemiology of childhood leukaemia in Northumberland and Durham. *Brit. J. Prev. Soc. Med.*, **18**, 17-24.

Knox, E.G. (1964b). The detection of space–time interactions. *Appl. Statist.*, **13**, 25-9.

Knox, E.G. (1965). Recognition of outbreaks of acute leukaemia and congenital malformations. In *Mathematics and Computer Science in Biology and Medicine*, 227-33. London: H.M.S.O.

Krus, V.P. and Rvachev, L.A. (1971). The mathematical theory of epidemics: a study of the evolution of resistance in micro-organisms. *Adv. Appl. Prob.*, **3**, 206-8.

Kryscio, R.J. (1971). Computation and estimation procedures in multidimensional right-shift processes with application to epidemic theory. (Thesis: Dept. of Statistics, State Univ. New York, Buffalo.)

Kryscio, R.J. (1972a). The transition probabilities of the extended simple stochastic epidemic model and the Haskey model. *J. Appl. Prob.*, **9**, 471-85.

Kryscio, R.J. (1972b). On estimating the infection rate of the simple stochastic epidemic. *Biometrika*, **59**, 213-14.

Kryscio, R.J. (1974). On the extended simple stochastic epidemic model. *Biometrika*, **61**, 200-202.

Kryscio, R.J. and Severo, N.C. (1969). Some properties of an extended simple stochastic epidemic involving two additional parameters. *Math. Biosci.*, **5**, 1-8.

Landahl, H.D. (1953). On the spread of information with time and distance, *Bull. Math. Biophys.*, **15**, 367-81.

Landau, H.G. and Rapoport, A. (1953). Contribution to the mathematical theory of contagion and spread of information. I: Spread through a thoroughly mixed population. *Bull. Math. Biophys.,* **15,** 173-83.

Lane, J.M., Ruben, F.L., Neff, J.M. and Millar, J.D. (1969). Complications of smallpox vaccination, 1968. *New Eng. J. Med.,* **281,** 1201-8.

Lapage, G. (1963). *Animal Parasites in Man.* New York: Dover.

Larsen, R.J., Holmes, C.L. and Heath, C.W. (1973). A statistical test for measuring unimodal clustering: a description of the test and of its application to cases of acute leukaemia in metropolitan Atlanta, Georgia. *Biometrics,* **29,** 301-9.

Lechat, M.F. (1971). An epidemiometric approach for planning and evaluating leprosy control activities. *Int. J. Lepr.,* **39,** 603-7.

Lepine, P. (1971). Genèse et périodicité des grandes épidémies. *Médecine et Maladies Infectieuses,* **1** (9), 357-68.

Leyton, M.K. (1968). Stochastic models in populations of helminthic parasites in the definitive host. II: Sexual mating functions. *Math. Biosci.,* **3,** 413-19.

Lidwell, O.M. and Sommerville, T. (1951). Observations on the incidence and distribution of the common cold in a rural community during 1948 and 1949. *J. Hyg., Camb.,* **49,** 365-81.

Linhart, H. (1968). On some bilharzia infection and immunization models. *S. Afr. Statist. J.,* **2,** 61-6.

Linnert, L. (1954). A statistical report on measles notifications in Manchester, 1917-1951. (Unpublished Univ. Manchester Report.)

London, W.P. and Yorke, J.A. (1973). Recurrent outbreaks of measles, chickenpox and mumps. I: Seasonal variation in contact rates. *Amer. J. Epidem.,* **98,** 453-68. (See Yorke, J.A. and London, W.P.)

Lotka, A.J. (1923a). Martini's equations for the epidemiology of immunizing diseases. *Nature,* **111,** 633-4.

Lotka, A.J. (1923b). Contributions to the analysis of malaria epidemiology. *Amer. J. Hyg.,* **3** (Suppl. 1), 1-121.

Lotte, A. (1968). Intérêt des modèles et définition des paramètres entrant dans la constitution des modèles dans l'épidémiologie de la tuberculose. *Bull. INSERM,* **23,** 1093-8.

Lotte, A. and Uzan, J. (1973). Evolution of the rates of tuberculous infection in France and calculation of the annual risk by means of a mathematical model. *Int. J. Epid.,* **2,** 265-82.

Ludwig, D. (1973a). Stochastic approximation for the general epidemic. *J. Appl. Prob.,* **10,** 263-76.

Ludwig, D. (1973b). Mathematical models for the spread of epidemics. *Comput. Biol. Med.,* **3,** 137-9.

Ludwig, D. Final size distributions for epidemics. *Math. Biosci.,* (In preparation.)

Ludwig, D. Qualitative behavior of stochastic epidemics. *Math. Biosci.* (In preparation.)

Lvov, D.K., Bolshev, L.N., Rudik, A.P., Goldfarb, L.G. and Kruopis, Yu, I. (1968). An attempt at calculating the intensity of infection with tick-borne encephalitis. *Med. Parasit.,* **37,** 274-8. (In Russian.)

Lynn, W.R. (1972). *Epidemic Simulation for Students in Medicine.* New York: Cornell Univ. Medical College.

Lynn, W.R. and ReVelle, C.S. (1968). Workshop on model methodology for health planning, with particular reference to tuberculosis. *Amer. Rev. Resp. Dis.,* **98,** 687-91.

Macdonald, G. (1950a). The analysis of infection rates in diseases in which superinfection occurs. *Trop. Dis. Bull.,* **47,** 907-15.

Macdonald, G. (1950b). The analysis of malaria parasite rates in infants. *Trop. Dis. Bull.* **47,** 915-38.

Macdonald, G. (1952a). The analysis of the sporozoite rate. *Trop. Dis. Bull.,* **49,** 569-86.

Macdonald, G. (1952b). The analysis of equilibrium in malaria. *Trop. Dis. Bull.* **49,** 813-29.

Macdonald, G. (1953). The analysis of malaria epidemics. *Trop. Dis. Bull.* **50,** 871-89.

Macdonald, G. (1955). The measurement of malaria transmission. *Proc. Roy. Soc. Med.,* **48**, 295-301.

Macdonald, G. (1957). *The Epidemiology and Control of Malaria.* London: Oxford Univ. Press.

Macdonald, G. (1965a). The dynamics of helminth infections, with special reference to schistosomes. *Trans. Roy. Soc. Trop. Med. Hyg.,* **59**, 489-506.

Macdonald, G. (1965b). On the scientific basis of tropical hygiene. *Trans. Roy. Soc. Trop. Med. Hyg.,* **59**, 611-20.

Macdonald, G. (1965c). Eradication of malaria. *Pub. Hlth Rep.,* **80**, 870-80.

Macdonald, G. (1973). *Dynamics of Tropical Diseases.* London: Oxford Univ. Press.

Macdonald, G., Cuellar, C.B. and Foll, C.V. (1968). The dynamics of malaria. *Bull. Wld Hlth Org.,* **38**, 743-55.

Macdonald, G. and Göckel, C.W. (1964). The malaria parasite rate and interruption of transmission. *Bull. Wld Hlth Org.,* **31**, 365-77.

McFarlan, A.M. (1945). Time of occurrence of secondary familial cases of infective hepatitis. *Lancet,* **1**, 592.

McKendrick, A.G. (1926). Applications of mathematics to medical problems. *Proc. Edin. Math. Soc.,* **14**, 98-130.

McKendrick, A.G. (1940). The dynamics of crowd infections. *Edin. Med. J.,* New Series (IV), **47**, 117-36.

McNeil, D.R. (1972). On the simple stochastic epidemic. *Biometrika,* **59**, 494-7.

McNeil, D.R. and Schach, S. (1973). Central limit analogues for Markov population processes. *J.R. Statist. Soc.,* Ser. B, **35**, 1-15.

McPherson III, L.F. (1963). Urban yellow fever: an industrial dynamics study of epidemiology. (MIT: School of Industrial Management, Memo D-572.)

McQuarrie, D.A. (1967). Stochastic approach to chemical kinetics. *J. Appl. Prob.,* **4**, 413-78.

Maguire, B.A., Pearson, E.S. and Wynn, A.H.A. (1953). Further notes on the analysis of accident data. *Biometrika,* **40**, 213-16.

Mahler, H.T. and Piot, M.A. (1966a). Essais d'application de la recherche opérationnelle dans la lutte antituberculeuse. I: Formulation des problèmes, rassemblement des données, choix de modèles. *Bull. INSERM,* **21**, 855-81.

Mahler, H.T. and Piot, M.A. (1966b). Essais d'application de la recherche opérationnelle dans la lutte antituberculeuse. II: Programmation linéaire: problèmes conceptuels et d'application. *Bull. INSERM,* **21**, 1021-45.

Maia, J. de O.C. (1952). Some mathematical developments on the epidemic theory formulated by Reed and Frost. *Hum. Biol.,* **24**, 167-200.

Mansfield, E. and Hensley, C. (1960). The logistic process: tables of the stochastic epidemic curve and applications. *J.R. Statist. Soc.,* Ser. B, **22**, 332-7.

Mantel, N. (1967). The detection of disease clustering and a generalised regression approach. *Cancer Res.,* **27**, 209-20.

Marchand, H. (1956). Essai d'étude mathématique d'une forme d'épidémie. *Ann. Univ. Lyon,* A (3), **19**, 13-46.

Marcus, H.M. (1970). A stochastic model of the population dynamics of malaria parasites in the mammalian host. (Ph.D. Thesis: Johns Hopkins Univ.)

Martini, E. (1921). *Berechnungen und Beobachtungen zur Epidemiologie und Bekämpfung der Malaria.* Hamburg: Gente.

Masada, Y. (1960). An epidemiological study on the mode of prevalence of measles. *J. Osaka City Med. Center,* **9**, 909-27.

Mathen, K.K. and Chakraborty, P.N. (1950). A statistical study on multiple cases of disease in households. *Sankhyā,* **10**, 387-92.

Maxey, H.D. (1971). The no DDT problem, malaria – a model of the Ceylon malaria epidemic. (Techn. Rep., Center for Advanced Engineering Study, MIT, Cambridge, Mass.)

Meynell, G.G. and Maw, J. (1968). Evidence for a two-stage model of microbial infection. *J. Hyg., Camb.,* **66**, 273-80.

Meynell, G.G. and Meynell, E.W. (1958). The growth of micro-organisms *in vivo* with particular reference to the relation between dose and latent period. *J. Hyg., Camb.*, **56**, 323-46.

Meynell, G.G. and Williams, T. (1967). Estimating the date of infection from individual response time. *J. Hyg., Camb.*, **65**, 131-4.

Mode, C.J. (1971). *Multitype Branching Processes*. New York: American Elsevier.

Mollison, D. (1970). Spatial propagation of simple epidemics. (Ph. D. Thesis: Statistical Laboratory, Cambridge Univ.)

Mollison, D. (1972a). Possible velocities for a simple epidemic. *Adv. Appl. Prob.*, **4**, 233-57.

Mollison, D. (1972b). The rate of spatial propagation of simple epidemics. *Proc. Sixth Berkeley Symp. Math. Statist. & Prob.*, **3**, 579-614. Berkeley and Los Angeles: Univ. California Press.

Mollison, D. (1972c). Conjecture on the spread of infection in two dimensions disproved. *Nature*, **240**, 467-8.

Moor, P.P. de and Steffens, F.E. (1970). A computer simulated model of an arthropod-borne virus transmission cycle, with special reference to chikungunya virus. *Trans. Roy. Soc. Trop. Med. Hyg.*, **64**, 927-34.

Moran, P.A.P. (1947). The random division of an interval. Part I. *J.R. Statist. Soc. Suppl.*, **9**, 92-8.

Moran, P.A.P. (1948). The interpretation of statistical maps. *J.R. Statist. Soc.*, Ser. B, **10**, 243-51.

Moran, P.A.P. (1951a). Estimation methods for evolutive processes. *J.R. Statist., Soc.*, Ser. B, **13**, 141-6.

Moran, P.A.P. (1951b). The random division of an interval. Part II. *J.R. Statist. Soc.*, Ser. B, **13**, 147-50.

Moran, P.A.P. (1953). The estimation of the parameters of a birth and death process. *J.R. Statist. Soc.*, Ser. B, **15**, 241-5.

Morgan, R.W. (1964). A note on Dr Bailey's paper. *Appl. Statist.*, **13**, 20-4.

Morgan, R.W. (1965). The estimation of parameters from the spread of a disease by considering households of two. *Biometrika*, **52**, 271-4.

Morgan, R.W. and Welsh, D.J.A. (1965). A two-dimensional Poisson growth process. *J.R. Statist. Soc.*, Ser. B, **27**, 497-504.

Morton, R. and Wickwire, K.H. (1974). On the optimal control of a deterministic epidemic. *J. Appl. Prob.*, **6**, 622-35.

Moshkovskii, Sh.D. (1950). *Basic Laws of the Epidemiology of Malaria*. Moscow: AMN. (In Russian.)

Moshkovskii, Sh.D. (1967). A further contribution to the theory of malaria eradication. *Bull. Wld Hlth Org.*, **36**, 992-6.

Muench, H. (1959). *Catalytic Models in Epidemiology*. Harvard Univ. Press.

Muhomor, T.P. (1971). Local limit theorems for the size of a general epidemic. In *Random Processes and Related Questions*, **2**. (In Russian.)

Muhomor, T.P. and Nagaev, A.V. (1972). Limiting distribution for the duration time of an epidemic when the size is finite. In *Random Processes and Statistical Inference*, **2**, 84-8. Tashkent: FAN. (In Russian.)

Muhsam, H.V. (1970). Models for infectious diseases. In *Data Handling in Epidemiology* (ed. W.W. Holland). London: Oxford Univ. Press.

Mustacchi, P. (1965). Some intra-city variations in leukaemia incidence in San Francisco. *Cancer*, **18**, 362-8.

Mustacchi, P., David, F.N. and Fix, E. (1967). Three tests for space–time interaction: a comparative evaluation. *Proc. Fifth Berkeley Symp. Math. Statist. & Prob.*, **4**, 229-35. Berkeley and Los Angeles: Univ. California Press.

Nagaev, A.V. (1970). Asymptotic methods for problems in the mathematical theory of epidemics. (Working paper for WHO Symposium on Quantitative Epidemiology, Moscow, 23-27 November 1970. Summarized in Nagaev, 1971.)

Nagaev, A.V. (1971). Asymptotic methods for problems in the mathematical theory of epidemics. *Adv. Appl. Prob.*, **3**, 222-3.

Nagaev, A.V. and Startsev, A.V. (1968). A threshold theorem for an epidemic model. *Mat. Zametki*, **3**, 179-85. (In Russian.)

Nagaev, A.V. and Startsev, A.V. (1970). Asymptotic analysis of a stochastic epidemic model. *Theor. Verojat. Primen.*, **15**, 97-105. (In Russian.)

Nåsell, I. (1972). Mathematical models of some parasitic diseases involving an intermediate host. (Ph.D. Thesis: New York Univ.)

Nåsell, I. and Hirsch, W.M. (1971). Mathematical models of some parasitic diseases involving an intermediate host. (Report No. IMM393, Courant Institute of Mathematical Sciences, New York.)

Nåsell, I. and Hirsch, W.M. (1972). A mathematical model of some helminthic infections. *Comm. Pure Appl. Math.*, **25**, 459-77.

Nåsell, I. and Hirsch, W.M. (1973a). The transmission dynamics of schistosomiasis. *Comm. Pure Appl. Math.*, **26**, 395-453.

Nåsell, I. and Hirsch, W.M. (1973b). The transmission and control of schistosome infections (Working Proceedings of NATO Conference on "Mathematical Analysis of Decision Problems in Ecology", Istanbul, 9-13 July 1973.)

New York W.P.A. (1942). *Tables of Probability Functions, 2.*

Neyman, J. (1965). Certain chance mechanisms involving discrete distributions. *Sankhyā*, A, **27**, 249-58.

Neyman, J. and LeCam, L.M. (Editors) (1965). *Bernoulli—Bayes—Laplace.* Berlin: Springer.

Neyman, J. and Scott, E. (1964). A stochastic model of epidemics. In *Stochastic Models in Medicine and Biology.* (ed. J. Gurland), 45-85. Madison: Univ. Wisconsin Press.

Nishida, F. (1959). A method of forecasting the prevalence of measles – with applications to the forecasting in an isolated island. *J. Osaka City Med. Center*, **8**, 409-46.

O'Callaghan, M. and Fisher, N.I. (1974). A stochastic model for the development and immunological control of a class of parasites in sheep. *Math. Biosci.*, **19**, 287-97.

Ohlsen, Sally (1964). On estimating epidemic parameters from household data. *Biometrika*, **51**, 511-12.

Oki, Y. (1960). Studies on the incubation period of acute infectious diseases from the viewpoint of theoretical epidemiology. *J. Osaka City Med. Center*, **9**, 2341-68.

Owada, K., Sakamoto, K. and Tanaka, H. (1971). An epidemiological study on incubation period of influenza. *Jap. J. Hyg.*, **26**, 264-7. (In Japanese.)

Oyalese, Y.O. (1970). A stochastic model of epidemics involving an intermediate host (vector). (Ph.D. Thesis: Univ. California, Berkeley.)

Panchev, H. (1972). An attempt at modelling an elementary epidemiological process. *Med. Prob. (Plovdiv)*, **24** (3), 27-42. (In Bulgarian.)

Peller, S. (1967). *Quantitative Research in Human Biology and Medicine.* Bristol: John Wright.

Petersen, K. (1970). Die Bedeutung der seuchenhygienischen Dokumentation durch den Amtsarzt. *Das öffentliche Gesundheitswesen*, **32**, 86-95.

Pettigrew, H.M. (1971). On the mathematical theory of epidemics with two or more types of infectives. (Ph.D. Dissertation: George Washington Univ., Washington, D.C.)

Pettigrew, H.M. and Weiss, G.H. (1967). Epidemics with carriers: the large population approximation. *J. Appl. Prob.*, **4**, 257-63.

Pickles, W.N. (1939). *Epidemiology in Country Practice.* Bristol: John Wright.

Pike, M.C. and Smith, P.G. (1968). Disease clustering: a generalization of Knox's approach to the detection of space—time interactions. *Biometrics*, **24**, 541-54.

Pinkel, D. and Nefzger, D. (1959). Some epidemiological features of childhood leukaemia. *Cancer*, **12**, 351-8.

Puma, M. (1939). *Elementi per una teoria matematica del contagio.* Roma: Aeron.

Puri, P.S. (1966). On the homogeneous birth-and-death process and its integral. *Biometrika*, **53**, 61-71.

Puri, P.S. (1967). A class of stochastic models of response after infection in the absence of defense mechanism. *Proc. Fifth Berkeley Symp. Math. Statist. & Prob.*, **4**, 511-35. Berkeley and Los Angeles: Univ. California Press.

Pyke, R. (1965). Spacings. *J. R. Statist. Soc.*, Ser. B, **27**, 395-449.

Pyke, R. (1972). Spacings revisited. *Proc. Sixth Berkeley Symp. Math. Statist. & Prob.*, **1**, 417-27. Berkeley and Los Angeles: Univ. California Press.

Radcliffe, J. (1973). The initial geographical spread of host-vector and carrier-borne epidemics. *J. Appl. Prob.,* **10**, 703-17.

Radcliffe, J. (1974). The effective of the length of incubation period on the velocity of propagation of an epidemic wave. *Math. Biosci.,* **19**, 257-62.

Raman, S. and Chiang, C.L. (1973). On a solution of the migration process and the application to a problem in epidemiology. *J. Appl. Prob.,* **10**, 718-27.

Rao, C.R. (1952). *Advanced Statistical Methods in Biometric Research.* New York: Wiley.

Rapoport, A. (1953a). Spread of information through a population with socio-structural bias. I: Assumption of transitivity. *Bull. Math. Biophys.,* **15**, 523-33.

Rapoport, A. (1953b). Spread of information through a population with socio-structural bias. II: Various models with partial transitivity. *Bull. Math. Biophys.,* **15**, 535-46.

Rapoport, A. and Rebhun, L.J. (1952). On the mathematical theory of rumor spread. *Bull. Math. Biophys.,* **14**, 375-83.

Rashevsky, N. (1964). *Some Medical Aspects of Mathematical Biology.* Springfield, Illinois: Thomas.

Ratcliffe, L.H., Taylor, H.M., Whitlock, J.H. and Lynn, W.R. (1969). Systems analysis of a host–parasite interaction. *Parasitology,* **59**, 649-61.

Reuter, G.E.H. (1957). Denumerable Markov processes and the associated contraction semigroups on *l. Acta Math.,* **97**, 1-46.

Reuter, G.E.H. (1961). Competition processes. *Proc. Fourth Berkeley Symp. Math. Statist. & Prob.,* **2**, 421-30. Berkeley and Los Angeles: Univ. California Press.

ReVelle, C. (1967). The economic allocation of tuberculosis control activities in developing nations. (Ph.D. thesis: Cornell Univ.)

ReVelle, C., Feldmann, F. and Lynn, W. (1969). An optimization model of tuberculosis epidemiology. *Management Science,* **16**, B190-B211.

ReVelle, C., Lynn, W.R. and Feldmann, F. (1967). Mathematical models for the economic allocation of tuberculosis control activities in developing countries. *Amer. Rev. Resp. Dis.,* **96**, 893-909.

ReVelle, C. and Male, J. (1970). A mathematical model for determining case finding and treatment activities in tuberculosis control programs. *Amer. Rev. Resp. Dis.,* **102**, 403-11.

Ridler-Rowe, C.J. (1967). On a stochastic model of an epidemic. *J. Appl. Prob.,* **4**, 19-33.

Robson, D.S., Kahrs, R. and Baker, J. (1967). Bounds on the mean recurrence time of subclinical epidemics in dairy herds. *J. Theor. Biol.,* **17**, 47-56.

Ross, R. (1911). *The Prevention of Malaria* (2nd edn). London: Murray.

Ross, R. (1915). Some *a priori* pathometric equations. *Brit. Med. J.,* **1**, 546-7.

Ross, R. (1916). An application of the theory of probabilities to the study of *a priori* pathometry, I. *Proc. Roy. Soc.,* A, **92**, 204-30.

Ross, R. (1917). An application of the theory of probabilities to the study of *a priori* pathometry, II. *Proc. Roy. Soc.,* A, **93**, 212-25.

Ross, R. and Hudson, H.P. (1917). An application of the theory of probabilities to the study of *a priori* pathometry, III. *Proc. Roy. Soc.,* A, **93**, 225-40.

Rouillon, A. (1970). La place des modèles dans la prospective de la lutte contre la tuberculose. *Semaine des hôpitaux (Annales de pédiatrie),* **40**, 2473-80.

Rushton, S. and Mautner, A.J. (1955). The deterministic model of a simple epidemic for more than one community. *Biometrika,* **42**, 126-32.

Rusu, G. (1973a). A Markovian model in tuberculosis epidemiology. *Ftiziologia,* **22**, 585-92. (In Romanian.)

Rusu, G. (1973b). An operational research model in tuberculosis prevention. *Ftiziologia,* **22**, 593-8. (In Romanian.)

Rvachev, L.A. (1967). A model for the connection between processes in the organism and the structure of epidemics. *Kibernetika,* **3**, 75-8. (In Russian.)

Rvachev, L.A. (1968a). Modelling of the connection between epidemiological and infectious processes. *Vestnik Akad. Med. Nauk,* **23** (5), 34-7. (In Russian.)

Rvachev, L.A. (1968b). Computer modelling experiment on large scale epidemics. *Dokl. Akad. Nauk, SSSR,* **180** (2), 294-6. (In Russian.)

Rvachev, L.A. (1971). A computer experiment for predicting an influenza epidemic. *Dokl. Akad. Nauk, SSSR,* **198** (1), 68-70. (In Russian.)

Rvachev, L.A. (1972). Modelling medico-biological processes in a community in terms of the dynamics of continuous media. *Dokl. Akad. Nauk, SSSR*, **203** (3), 540-2. (In Russian.)

Saaty, T.L. (1961a). Some stochastic processes with absorbing barriers. *J.R. Statist. Soc.*, Ser. B, **23**, 319-34.

Saaty, T.L. (1961b). *Elements of Queueing Theory*. New York: McGraw-Hill.

Sakino, S. (1959). Epidemic model under the influence of damped oscillation. *Proc. Inst. Statist. Math.*, **6**, 117-24. (In Japanese.)

Sakino, S. (1962a). Historical development of epidemic models. *Proc. Inst. Statist. Math.*, **9**, 127-36. (In Japanese.)

Sakino, S. (1962b). On the analysis of epidemic model, II (theory and application). *Ann. Inst. Statist. Math.*, **13**, 147-63.

Sakino, S. (1962c). On the age distribution in epidemic, I. *Proc. Inst. Statist. Math.*, **10**, 33-9. (In Japanese.)

Sakino, S. (1963). On the age distribution of epidemic model and the prediction of poliomeylitis. *Proc. Inst. Statist. Math.*, **11**, 25-30. (In Japanese.)

Sakino, S. (1967). On the age distribution in epidemic, II. *Proc. Inst. Statist. Math.*, **15**, 126-33. (In Japanese.)

Sakino, S. (1968). On the solution of the epidemic equation. *Ann. Inst. Statist. Math.*, Suppl. V, 9-19.

Sakino, S. and Hayashi, C. (1959). On the analysis of epidemic model, I (theoretical approach). *Ann. Inst. Statist. Math.*, **10**, 261-75.

Sanders, J.L. (1971). Quantitative guidelines for communicable disease control programs. *Biometrics*, **27**, 883-93.

Sartwell, P.E. (1950). The distribution of incubation periods of infectious disease. *Amer. J. Hyg.*, **51**, 310-18.

Sartwell, P.E. (1966). The incubation period and the dynamics of infectious disease. *Amer. J. Epidem.*, **83**, 204-16.

Schrödter, H. and Ullrich, J. (1967). Eine mathematische-statistische Lösung des Problems der Prognose von Epidemien mit Hilfe meteorologischer Parameter, dargestellt am Beispiel der Kartoffelkrautfäule *(Phytophtora infestans)*. *Agr. Meteorol.*, **4**, 119-35.

Schwöbel, W., Geidel, H. and Lorenz, R.J. (1966). Ein Modell der Plaquebildung. *Zeit. Naturf.*, **21**, 953-9.

Seiden, E. (1957). On a mathematical model for a problem in epidemiology. *Bull. Amer. Math. Soc.*, **63**, 142-3.

Serfling, R.E. (1952). Historical review of epidemic theory. *Hum. Biol.*, **24**, 145-66.

Sevastyanov, B.A. (1951). Theory of branching stochastic processes. *Uspehi Mat. Nauk*, **6** (6), 47-99. (In Russian.)

Severo, N.C. (1967a). Two theorems on solutions of differential-difference equations and applications to epidemic theory. *J. Appl. Prob.*, **4**, 271-80.

Severo, N.C. (1967b). The probabilities of a carrier epidemic model with arbitrary initial distribution. (Res. Rep. No. 9, Dept. Math. Statist., State Univ. New York, Buffalo.)

Severo, N.C. (1969a). Generalizations of some stochastic epidemic models. *Math. Biosci.*, **4**, 395-402.

Severo, N.C. (1969b). The probabilities of some epidemic models. *Biometrika*, **56**, 197-201.

Severo, N.C. (1969c). A recursion theorem on solving differential-difference equations and applications to some stochastic processes. *J. Appl. Prob.*, **6**, 673-81.

Severo, N.C. (1969d). Right-shift processes. *Proc. Nat. Acad. Sci.*, **64**, 1162-4.

Severo, N.C. (1971). Multidimensional right-shift processes. *Adv. Appl. Prob.*, **3**, 200-1.

Sheene, P.R. and Feldman, H.A. (1969). Exposure model analysis of streptococcal acquisitions. *J. Infect. Dis.*, **119**, 172-81.

Shibata, E. (1960). Studies on an epidemic process of influenza among school children from a viewpoint of epidemic control. *J. Osaka City Med. Center*, **9**, 1339-50.

Silva, G.R. da (1969). A study on the epidemiological kinetics of the human infection by *Trypanosoma cruzi* through the application of a reversible catalytic model. *Rev. Saúde Públ.*, **3**, 23-9. (In Portuguese.)

Silver, K.A. (1968). A model for the incidence of venereal disease in a population of associated individuals. *IEEE Sys. Sci. Cyb. Conf.*, 202.

Siskind, V. (1965). A solution of the general stochastic epidemic. *Biometrika*, **52**, 613-16.

Smart, C.W. (1970). A computer model of wildlife rabies epizootics and an analysis of incidence patterns. (M.S. Thesis: Poly. Techn. Inst., Blacksburg, Virginia.)

Smith, Geddes (1943). *Plague on Us*. New York: Commonwealth Fund.

Snow, John (1855). *The Mode of Communication of Cholera* (2nd edn). London: Churchill.

Solomon, V.B. (1971). Some contributions to the mathematical theory of epidemics and related problems. (Thesis: Dept. of Statistics, Iowa State Univ.)

Soper, H.E. (1929). Interpretation of periodicity in disease-prevalence. *J.R. Statist. Soc.*, **92**, 34-73.

Spicer, C.C. (1967). Some empirical studies in epidemiology. *Proc. Fifth Berkeley Symp. Math. Statist. & Prob.*, **4**, 207-15. Berkeley and Los Angeles: Univ. California.

Spicer, C.C. and Lipton, S. (1958). Numerical studies on some contagious distributions. *J. Hyg., Camb.*, **56**, 516-22.

Startsev, A.N. (1970). The estimation of the regulating parameter in a stochastic epidemic model. *Izvestija Akd. Nauk Uzbek. SSR*, **14**, 53. (In Russian.)

Stocks, P. and Karn, M.N. (1928). A study of the epidemiology of measles. *Ann. Eugen., Lond.*, **3**, 361-98.

Störmer, H. (1964). Das Anwachsen des Verbrauchs von Wirtschaftsgütern als stochastischer Prozess. *Zeit. Angew. Math. Mech.*, **44**, 72-3.

Sugiyama, H. (1960). Some statistical contributions to the health sciences. *Osaka City Med. J.*, **6**, 141-58.

Sugiyama, H. (1961). Some statistical methodologies for epidemiological research of medical sciences. *Bull. Int. Statist. Inst.*, **38** (3), 137-51.

Sundaresan, T.K. and Assaad, F.A. (1973). The use of simple epidemiological models in the evaluation of disease control programmes: a case study of trachoma. *Bull. Wld Hlth Org.*, **48**, 709-14.

Sundaresan, T.K. Grab, B., Uemura, K. and Cvjetanović, B. (1974). Comparative epidemiological analysis of sanitation, immunization and chemoprophylaxis in the control of typhoid and cholera. *Amer. J. Publ. Hlth*, **64**, 910-12.

Swain, R.W., Lynn, W.R., Hodgson, T.A., Becker, N.G. and Johnson, K.G. (1972). Epidemic simulation for training in public health management. *IEEE Trans. Biomed. Eng.*, **19**, 120-5.

Tallis, G.M. (1970). Some stochastic extensions to a deterministic treatment of sheep parasite cycles. *Math. Biosci.*, **8**, 131-5.

Tallis, G.M. and Donald, A.D. (1970). Further models for the distribution on pasture of infective larvae of the strongyloid nematode parasites of sheep. *Math. Biosci.*, **7**, 179-90.

Tallis, G.M. and Leyton, M.K. (1966). A stochastic approach to the study of parasite populations. *J. Theor. Biol.*, **13**, 251-60.

Tallis, G.M. and Leyton, M.K. (1969). Stochastic models of populations of helminth parasites in the definitive host: I. *Math. Biosci.*, **4**, 39-48.

Taylor, H.M. (1968). Some models in epidemic control. *Math. Biosci.*, **3**, 383-98.

Taylor, I. and Knowelden, J. (1964). *Principles of Epidemiology* (2nd edn). London: Churchill.

Taylor, W.F. (1956). Problems in contagion. *Proc. Third Berkeley Symp. Math. Statist. & Prob.*, **4**, 167-79. Berkeley and Los Angeles: Univ. California Press.

Taylor, W.F. (1958). Some Monte Carlo methods applied to an epidemic of acute respiratory disease. *Hum. Biol.*, **30**, 185-200.

Tonascia, J.A. (1971). Contributions to the theory of chain-binomial epidemics. (Dept. of Biostatistics, Johns Hopkins Univ.)

Turing, A.M. (1952). The chemical basis of morphogenesis. *Phil. Trans.*, B, **237**, 37-72.

Voors, A.W. and Stewart, G.T. (1968). Biomathematical analysis of mycoplasmal infection in marine recruits. *Amer. Rev. Resp. Dis.*, **97**, 515-23.

Waaler, H.T. (1968a). Cost-benefit analysis of BCG-vaccination under various epidemio-
logical situations. *Bull. Int. Un. Tuber.*, **41**, 42-52.
Waaler, H.T. (1968b). A dynamic model for the epidemiology of tuberculosis. *Amer. Rev.
Resp. Dis.*, **98**, 591-600.
Waaler, H.T., Geser, A. and Andersen, S. (1962). The use of mathematical models in the
study of the epidemiology of tuberculosis. *Amer. J. Publ. Hlth*, **52**, 1002-13.
Waaler, H.T. and Piot, M.A. (1969). The use of an epidemiological model for estimating
the effectiveness of tuberculosis control measures: sensitivity of the effectiveness
of tuberculosis control measures to the coverage of the population. *Bull. Wld Hlth
Org.*, **41**, 75-93.
Waaler, H.T. and Piot, M.A. (1970). Use of an epidemiological model for estimating the
effectiveness of tuberculosis control measures: sensitivity of the effectiveness of
tuberculosis control measures to the social time of preference. *Bull. Wld Hlth Org.*,
43, 1-16.
Wada, Y. (1972a). Theoretical model for Japanese encephalitis epidemic. *Trop. Med.*, **14**,
41-54. (In Japanese.)
Wada, Y. (1972b). Theoretical considerations on the effects of pig immunization as
preventive measures for Japanese encephalitis. *Trop. Med.*, **14**, 141-63. (In Japanese.)
Waltman, P. *Deterministic Threshold Models in the Theory of Epidemics*. Springer. (In
preparation.)
Watson, G.N. (1923), Martini's equations for the epidemiology of immunizing diseases.
Nature, **111**, 808.
Watson, R.K. (1972). On an epidemic in a stratified population. *J. Appl. Prob.*, **9**, 659-66.
Waugh, W.A. O'N. (1958). Conditioned Markov processes. *Biometrika*, **45**, 241-9.
Weiss, G.H. (1965). On the spread of epidemics by carriers. *Biometrics*, **21**, 481-90.
Weiss, G.H. (1970). A perturbation technique for the stochastic theory of epidemics.
(Working paper for WHO Symposium on Quantitative Epidemiology, Moscow,
23-27 November 1970. Summarized in Weiss, 1971.)
Weiss, G.H. (1971). On a perturbation method for the theory of epidemics. *Adv. Appl.
Prob.*, **3**, 218-20.
Weiss, G.H. and Dishon, M. (1971a). Asymptotic behavior of a generalization of Bailey's
simple epidemic. *Adv. Appl. Prob.*, **3**, 220-1.
Weiss, G.H. and Dishon, M. (1971b). On the asymptotic behavior of the stochastic and
deterministic models of an epidemic. *Math. Biosci.*, **11**, 261-6.
Whittle, P. (1952). Certain nonlinear models of population and epidemic theory. *Skand.
Aktuar.*, **14**, 211-22.
Whittle, P. (1955). The outcome of a stochastic epidemic – a note on Bailey's paper.
Biometrika, **42**, 116-22.
Whittle, P. (1956). The estimation of age-specific infection rates from a curve of relative
infection. *Biometrics*, **12**, 154-62.
Wiesenfield, S.L. (1967). Sickle-cell trait in human biological and cultural evolution. Devel-
opment of agriculture causing increased malaria is bound to gene-pool changes causing
malaria reduction. *Science*, **157**, 1134-40.
Wilkins, J.E. (1945). The differential difference equation for epidemics. *Bull. Math. Biophys.*,
7, 149-50.
Williams, T. (1965a). The simple stochastic epidemic curve for large populations of suscep-
tibles. *Biometrika*, **52**, 571-9.
Williams, T. (1965b). The distribution of response times in a birth–death process. *Biometrika*,
52, 581-5.
Williams, T. (1965c). The basic birth-death model for microbial infections. *J. R. Statist.
Soc.*, Ser. B, **27**, 338-60.
Williams, T. (1970). An algebraic proof of the threshold theorem for the general stochastic
epidemic. (Working paper for WHO Symposium on Quantitative Epidemiology,
Moscow, 23-27 November 1970. Summarized in Williams, 1971.)
Williams, T. (1971). An algebraic proof of the threshold theorem for the general stochastic
epidemic. *Adv. Appl. Prob.*, **3**, 223.
Williams, T. and Bjerknes, R. (1971). Hyperplasia: the spread of abnormal cells through
a plane lattice. *Adv. Appl. Prob.*, **3**, 210-11.

Williams, T. and Bjerknes, R. (1972). Stochastic model for abnormal clone spread through epithelial basal layer. *Nature*, **236**, 19-21.

Williams, T. and Meynell, G.G. (1967). Time-dependence and count-dependence in microbial infection. *Nature*, **214**, 473-5.

Wilson, E.B. (1945). Some points in epidemiological theory. *Amer. Scientist*, **33**, 246-52.

Wilson, E.B. (1947). The spread of measles in the family. *Proc. Nat. Acad. Sci., Wash.*, **33**, 68-72.

Wilson, E.B., Bennett, C., Allen, M. and Worcester, J. (1939). Measles and scarlet fever in Providence, R.I., 1929-34 with respect to age and size of family. *Proc. Amer. Phil. Soc.*, **80**, 357-476.

Wilson, E.B. and Burke, M.H. (1942). The epidemic curve. *Proc. Nat. Acad. Sci., Wash.*, **28**, 361-7.

Wilson, E.B. and Burke, M.H. (1943). The epidemic curve, II. *Proc. Nat. Acad. Sci., Wash.*, **29**, 43-8.

Wilson, E.B. and Worcester, J. (1941a). Contact with measles. *Proc. Nat. Acad. Sci., Wash.*, **27**, 7-13.

Wilson, E.B. and Worcester, J. (1941b). Progressive immunizations. *Proc. Nat. Acad. Sci., Wash.*, **27**, 129-35.

Wilson, E.B. and Worcester, J. (1944a). A second approximation to Soper's epidemic curve. *Proc. Nat. Acad. Sci., Wash.*, **30**, 37-44.

Wilson, E.B. and Worcester, J. (1944b). The epidemic curve with no accession of susceptibles. *Proc. Nat. Acad. Sci., Wash.*, **30**, 264-9.

Wilson, E.B. and Worcester, J. (1945a). The law of mass action in epidemiology, I. *Proc. Nat. Acad. Sci., Wash.*, **31**, 24-34.

Wilson, E.B. and Worcester, J. (1945b). The law of mass action in epidemiology, II. *Proc. Nat. Acad. Sci., Wash.*, **31**, 109-16.

Wilson, E.B. and Worcester, J. (1945c). The variation of infectivity, I. *Proc. Nat. Acad. Sci., Wash.*, **31**, 142-7.

Wilson, E.B. and Worcester, J. (1945d). The variation of infectivity, II. *Proc. Nat. Acad. Sci., Wash.*, **31**, 203-8.

Wilson, E.B. and Worcester, J. (1945e). Damping of epidemic waves. *Proc. Nat. Acad. Sci., Wash.*, **31**, 294-8.

Wilson, E.B. and Worcester, J. (1945f). The spread of an epidemic. *Proc. Nat. Acad. Sci., Wash.*, **31**, 327-32.

Wilson, L.O. (1972). An epidemic model involving a threshold. *Math. Biosci.*, **15**, 109-21.

Winslow, C.E.A. (1943). *The Conquest of Epidemic Disease*. Princeton Univ. Press.

World Health Organization (1970). *Wkly Epid. Rec.*, **45**, 453-8.

World Health Organization (1972). *World Health*, Oct. 1972, 26-7.

Yamamoto, K. (1959). A theoretical epidemiological study on the mode of infection of influenza in the household. *J. Osaka City Med. Center*, **9**, 2179-90.

Yamamoto, K., Oki, Y., Masada, Y. and Shibata, E. (1960). A study on the mechanisms of the spreading of influenza in a large city. *Jap. J. Pub. Hlth*, **7**, 12-15.

Yang, Grace (1966). Contagion in stochastic models for epidemics. (Thesis: University of California, Berkeley.)

Yang, Grace (1968). Contagion in stochastic models for epidemics. *Ann. Math. Statist.*, **39**, 1863-89.

Yang, Grace (1972a). Empirical study of a non-Markovian epidemic model. *Math. Biosci.*, **14**, 65-84.

Yang, Grace (1972b). On the probability distributions of some stochastic epidemic models. *Theor. Pop. Biol.*, **3**, 448-59.

Yang, Grace and Chiang, C.L. (1972). A time-dependent simple stochastic epidemic. *Proc. Sixth Berkeley Symp. Math. Statist. & Prob.*, **6**, 147-58. Berkeley and Los Angeles. Univ. California Press.

Yorke, J.A. and London, W.P. (1973). Recurrent outbreaks of measles, chickenpox and mumps. II: Systematic differences in contact rates and stochastic effects. *Amer. J. Epidem.* **98**, 469-82.

ADDITIONAL REFERENCES ADDED IN PROOF

ABAKUKS, A. (1972). Some optimal isolation and immunization policies for epidemics. (D. Phil. Thesis, University of Sussex.)

ABAKUKS, A. (1974). Optimal immunization policies for epidemics. *Adv. Appl. Prob.*, **6**, 494−511.

ABAKUKS, A. (1974). A note on supercritical carrier-borne epidemics. *Biometrika*, **61**, 271−5.

BAILEY, N.T.J. (1975). Current trends in the modelling of infectious disease. *Proc. 8th Biometric Conf.*, Constanţa, 25−30 August, 1974. (To appear.)

BECKER, N. (1974). On parametric estimation for mortal branching processes. *Biometrika*, **61**, 393−9.

BILLARD, Lynne (1974). The recurrent epidemic. *J. Appl. Prob.*, **11**, 568−71.

DANIELS, H.E. (1974). An approximation technique for a curved boundary problem. *Adv. Appl. Prob.*, **6**, 194−6.

DAYANANDA, P.W.A. (1974). An approximate chain-binomial model for simple epidemics. *Biometrics*, **30**, 705−8.

DUTERTRE, J. and ALARY, J.-C. (1973). Essai d'élaboration d'un modèle épidémiométrique pour la méningite. *Méd. Trop.*, **33**, 105−15.

GRIFFITHS, D.A. (1974). A catalytic model of infection for measles. *Appl. Statist.*, **23**, 330−9.

HOPPENSTEADT, F.C. (1974). An age dependent epidemic model. *J. Franklin Inst.*, **297**, 325−33.

JERWOOD, D. (1974). The cost of a carrier-borne epidemic. *J. Appl. Prob.*, **11**, 642−51.

KANAMITSU, M. (1971). Epidemiologic methodology. *Saishin Igaku*, **26**, 1836−42. (In Japanese.)

NÁJERA, J.A. (1974). A critical review of the field application of a mathematical model of malaria eradication. *Bull. Wld Hlth Org.*, **50**, 449−57.

NASELL, I. (1975). A mathematical model of schistosomiasis with snail latency. (Report to Swedish−Czechoslovak Symposium on Applied Mathematics, Prague, 17−21 March 1975.)

PIKE, M.C. and SMITH, P.G. (1974). A case-control approach to examine diseases for evidence of contagion, including diseases with long latent periods. *Biometrics*, **30**, 263−79.

RADCLIFFE, J. (1974). A note on the recurrence of yellow fever epidemics in urban populations. *J. Appl. Prob.*, **11**, 170−3.

RADCLIFFE, J. (1974). The periodicity of malaria. *J. Appl. Prob.*, **11**, 562−7.

SPLAINE, M., LINTOTT, A.P. and ANGULO, J.J. (1974). On the use of contour maps in the analysis of spread of communicable disease. *J. Hyg. Camb.*, **73**, 15−26.

STIRZAKER, D. (1974). A singular perturbation analysis for models of schistosomiasis. *Math. Biosci.*, **21**, 183−205.

WALTER, S.D. (1974). On the detection of household aggregation of disease. *Biometrics*, **30**, 525−38.

WALTMAN, P. (1972). A deterministic model of the spread of an infection. (In *Delay and Functional Differential Equations*, ed. K. Schmitt, New York: Academic Press.)

WALTMAN, P. (1974). A threshold criterion for the spread of an infection in a two population model. *Math. Biosci.*, **21**, 119−25.

WOODS, A.J. (1974). Epidemic models in non-homogeneous populations. *Adv. Appl. Prob.*, **6**, 239.

INDEX OF AUTHORS

405

INDEX OF SUBJECTS

distribution of time-intervals, 233
household distribution of cases, 228
introduction, 225
space–time interactions, 17, 226, 227, 235, 238
standard epidemiological approach, 226
Infective hepatitis: *see* Infectious hepatitis
Influenza, 3, 4, 7, 18, 133, 268–70, 293
spread of, in USSR, 18, 350, 353
Intensity of epidemic, 86
Interference models, 7, 18, 332
chickenpox and yaws, 17, 18, 332
deterministic model, 333
enterovirus interference, 18, 348
generalized chain-binomial, 336
introduction, 332
poliomyelitis control, 18, 349
polio virus vaccine, 348
polio viruses, 7
simulation studies, 18, 345
sociological structure, allowance for, 348

Latent and infectious periods, measurement of, 271
computerized applications, 293
households of two, 275
measles data, 273, 279, 295
misclassification of chains, 282
missing data, 280
parameters, estimation of, 276
variations in
chance of infection, 281
infectious period, 282
latent period, 274
households of three, 283
infectious hepatitis, 296
influenza, 293
measles data, 284, 292, 295
parameters, estimation of, 287
variations in chance of infection, 290
introduction, 271
larger groups, extension to, 298
preliminary analysis of data, 273
simulation, use of, 299
Latent period, 7, 12, 14, 17, 21, 22, 81, 227, 239, 240, 271 *et seq.*
extended models, 271 *et seq.*
related to underlying pathogenic process, 273
Leprosy, 4, 311
Leukaemia, childhood, 227, 235, 237
London Bills of Mortality, 5, 9

Malaria, 3, 7, 11, 17, 23, 84, 207, 214
control and eradication of, 322

deterministic model of, 314
epidemiology of, 313
extended model of, 317
parameters, estimation of, 328
recent developments in modelling of, 18, 322
restrictions on homogeneous mixing, 210
superinfection, 317
Maps, statistical, 227
Maximum-likelihood estimation, 7
use of computerized optimization techniques for, 7, 25, 26, 124, 293
Measles, 7, 12, 14, 15, 23, 25, 133, 134, 143, 147, 154, 155, 174, 218, 239, 249 *et seq.*, 271 *et seq.*
vaccination, 368
Mechanical model of epidemic, 13
Methodological aspects, 24
Monte Carlo experiments: *see* Simulation studies
Multicompartment models: *see* Multistate models
Multidisease models, 26
importance for public health, 372
Multistate models, 7, 17, 301
applications to
cholera, 7, 17, 310, 311
leprosy, 311
tetanus, 7, 17, 310
tuberculosis, 7, 17, 302 *et seq.*
typhoid, 7, 17, 310, 311
control variables, 307
introduction, 301
optimization model, 308
Mumps, 239, 270, 271

Non-homogeneous mixing, 32, 75
Notifications of disease, asymmetry in, 88

Oesophageal atresia, 227
Onchocerciasis, 4, 331
Operational gaming, 374
Optimal resource allocation: *see* Resource allocation, optimal
Optimization program, computerized: *see* Computerized optimization program
Orientation, 1

Pandemic disease, 3, 176
Parasitic diseases, 3, 7, 17, 20, 23, 312
filariasis, 4, 331
malaria, 3, 7, 17, 23, 84, 207, 214, 312; *see also* Malaria
basic deterministic model of, 314
epidemiology of, 313
extended model of, 317
recent developments in modelling of, 18, 322